THE
BOOK
OF
LOOKS

SPECIAL THANKS TO:
PHOEBE PHILLIPS
CLAUDIA REILLY

ESPECIALLY TO STANLI
AND DIETER FOR MORAL SUPPORT

CONTRIBUTING WRITER: CHARLOTTE PARRY-CROOKE
EDITOR: HETTY EINZIG
SUB EDITOR: GABRIELLE TOWNSEND
MAKE-UP CONSULTANT: MARY ELLEN LAMB
PRODUCTION: RICHARD HAYES AT IMAGO PUBLISHING
PASTE UP: CLARE FINLAISON

THIS BOOK IS DEDICATED TO CLOTHES LOVERS EVERYWHERE

This edition First published
in Great Britain in 1984
by Michael Joseph Ltd.
44 Bedford Square
London WC1
1984

COPYRIGHT © 1983 BY JOHNSON EDITIONS LIMITED
LONDON, ENGLAND

ISBN 0 7181 2453 7

1 2 3 4 5 6 7 8 9

PRINTED AND BOUND IN SINGAPORE BY IMAGO PUBLISHING LTD

THE
BOOK
OF
LOOKS

by Lorraine Johnson
illustratated by Neil Greer

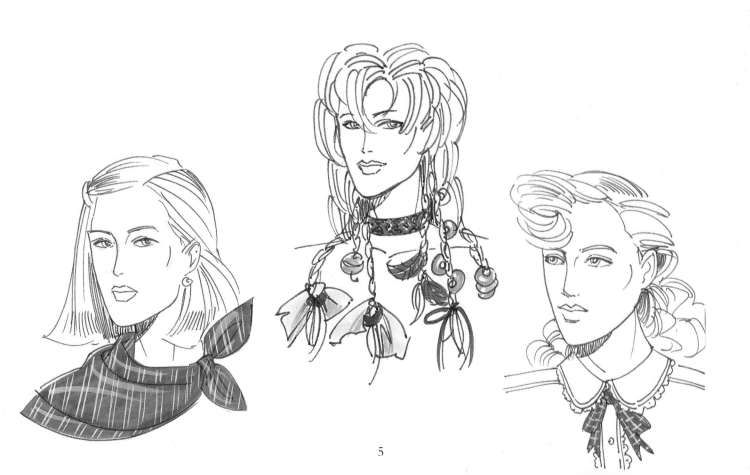

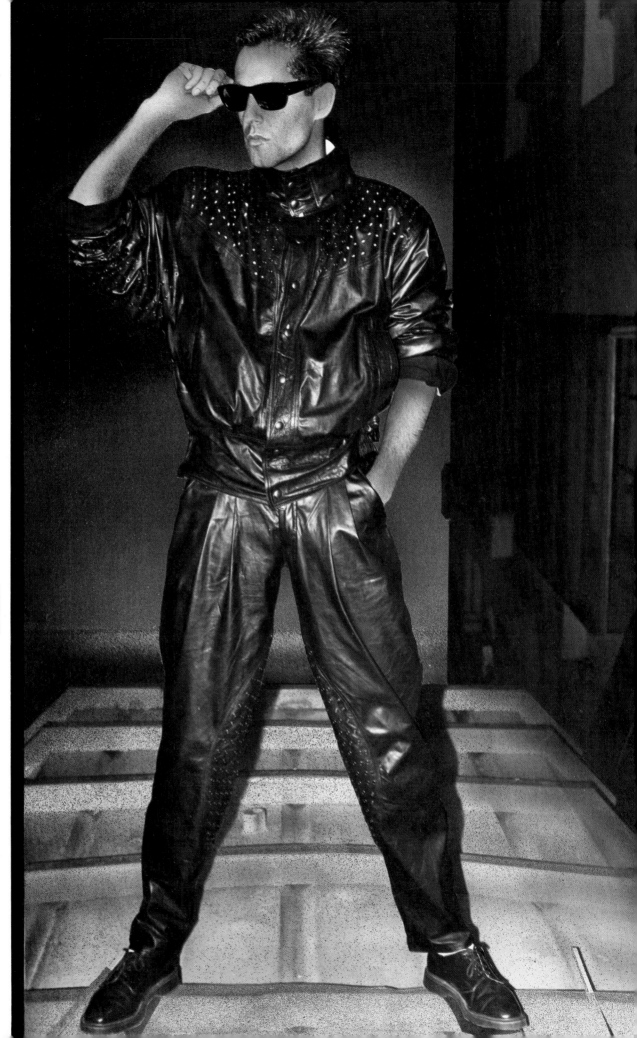

JACQUELINE HANCHER

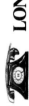

LONDON 388 5877

CONTENTS

INTRODUCTION

WHAT IS HAPPENING TO FASHION?

Fashion, as a part of history, repeats itself. Areas of the body emphasized one year are hidden and forgotten the next. Ethnically influenced styles come and go as the fortunes of each nation change, while the clothes you once thought looked dowdy or eccentric on your ancestors you may one day covet. Moreover, it is now impossible to avoid being influenced by the editorial and visual ploys of today's media: magazines intentionally set out to coax us into duplicating a particular look, which it seems can only be achieved by purchasing a completely new set of clothes. These factors, together with the contemporary relaxation of formal dress codes, have given rise to a plurality within fashion never known before and as a result the task of dressing today is more complicated than ever. The possibilities and interpretations seem endless.

The Book of Looks is therefore an attempt to create order out of chaos, by making you appreciate the versatility of the multitude of garments now available and adapt them to various styles of dress. It is a guidebook through a wardrobe, a self-help manual, a way of sorting dress components into categories, providing illustrations of the looks you might want to achieve. It also incorporates light-hearted references from literature, film and history, so that in the midst of any fashion revival, you can identify and study the garments, fabrics, accessories, hair and face treatments appropriate to any given look.

However, this freedom of choice does not mean that there are no rules, as some fashion journalists seem to suggest – you cannot really wear anything you like and still be à la mode. But you can adapt any look you like, whether from the past, present or future, and still be stylish, provided that you get the proportions right, in line with current idioms. Of course, when most of us are faced with this overwhelming choice and relative freedom, paralysing indecision is usually our response.

Like it or not, the length of skirts, the shape of shoes, the height of heels, the fullness or tightness of trousers, the entire proportions of clothes change every five years or so. To be in fashion, you must grow with the times, incorporating some new or revived styles as you go.

Admittedly, by categorizing the assorted ways of dressing into separate looks, we've had to establish dividing lines, in order to prevent repetition. There are, of course, innumerable variations to choose from. The forty-five looks which appear on the following pages are merely a distillation of the best from the past, present and future. For the purposes of defining each look, we have established a fairly tight set of rules, but do not assume they are rigid – who says, for instance, that you cannot wear a frilly white shirt from THE PIRATE with the jeans of THE COWGIRL? Of course you can, but only after studying the ingredients of the original look can you begin to be creative, to work out alternatives and evolve your own distinctive style of dressing.

It stands to reason that appearance is critical and that each of us needs to get our appearance right on our own terms. The occasion, your mood and the range of your wardrobe are all essential contributors to this final appearance, and the clothes which you select are immediate signals to those you encounter, indicating various aspects of your character. Before you begin to choose your style(s) ask yourself what you want your clothes to say. You may not be able to change many of your physical features, but you can capture the elusive quality called 'style'.

Some people seem to be born with an innate sense of style, knowing what looks good on them and when it is appropriate. Others readily admit that they have arrived at a sense of self and of fashion, after years of trial and error. However, one thing is certain: you'll find that as you take more care of your appearance, your confidence will rise; and out of this will emerge a very particular style which is uniquely yours.

Choose your drink to match your look

Whatever your look, there is no drink with more style than Malibu. On its own over ice, the chilled coconut taste comes through, reminding you of summer and sun-drenched islands.

Malibu is a friendly, fashionable mixer, too. If you take your new look out to a cocktail bar, there are a lot of ways to mix with Malibu. Bars, clubs and pubs have a choice as well, depending on your style. At home Malibu forms the foundation for a fashion that's all its own. If you would like to know more, send off for our offer and make Malibu part of *your* style.

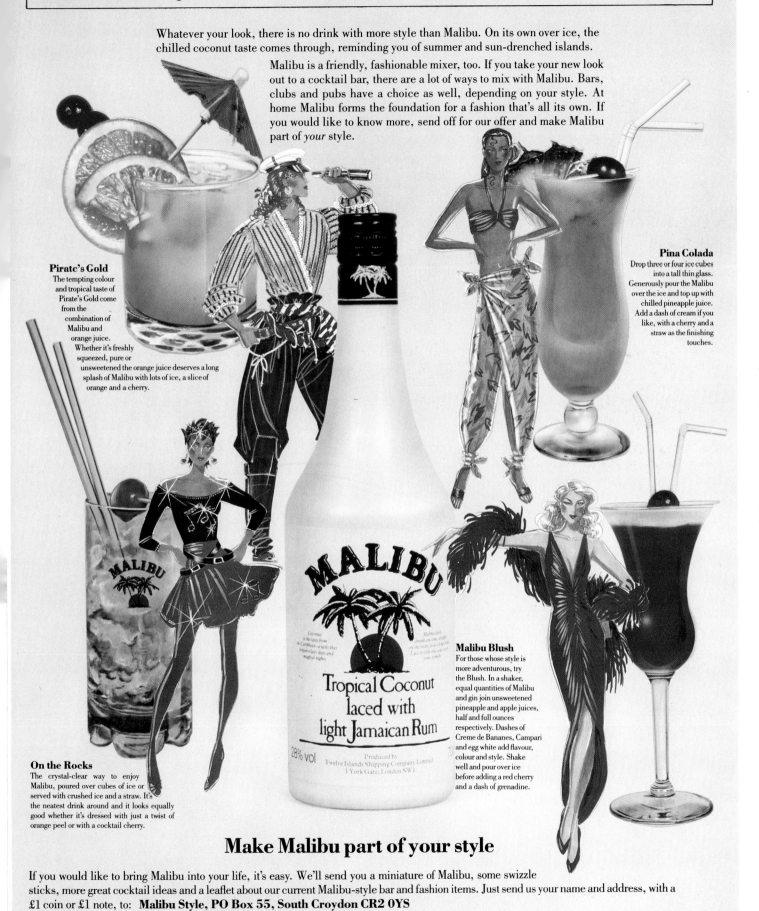

Pirate's Gold
The tempting colour and tropical taste of Pirate's Gold come from the combination of Malibu and orange juice. Whether it's freshly squeezed, pure or unsweetened the orange juice deserves a long splash of Malibu with lots of ice, a slice of orange and a cherry.

Pina Colada
Drop three or four ice cubes into a tall thin glass. Generously pour the Malibu over the ice and top up with chilled pineapple juice. Add a dash of cream if you like, with a cherry and a straw as the finishing touches.

On the Rocks
The crystal-clear way to enjoy Malibu, poured over cubes of ice or served with crushed ice and a straw. It's the neatest drink around and it looks equally good whether it's dressed with just a twist of orange peel or with a cocktail cherry.

Malibu Blush
For those whose style is more adventurous, try the Blush. In a shaker, equal quantities of Malibu and gin join unsweetened pineapple and apple juices, half and full ounces respectively. Dashes of Creme de Bananes, Campari and egg white add flavour, colour and style. Shake well and pour over ice before adding a red cherry and a dash of grenadine.

Make Malibu part of your style

If you would like to bring Malibu into your life, it's easy. We'll send you a miniature of Malibu, some swizzle sticks, more great cocktail ideas and a leaflet about our current Malibu-style bar and fashion items. Just send us your name and address, with a £1 coin or £1 note, to: **Malibu Style, PO Box 55, South Croydon CR2 0YS**

We'll RSVP by return but can only accept one application per person.

Applications are restricted to UK residents aged 18 or over and must reach the address above by 31 March 1985.

IDV (UK) Ltd, Registered in England, No. 1009388.

HOW TO FIND YOUR LOOK

In order to work out how you want to look, you will temporarily need to abandon your preconceptions about yourself and your clothes. Put aside your hang-ups about the colours you can wear, the length of your skirts, the cut of your trousers, the style of your shoes, the shade of your hair, and the palette of your make-up. Imagine that you have a clean slate, so to speak – what would you want to look like?

Although most of us aren't perfectly beautiful, we all possess special features. It is these you should be proud of and emphasize. Belts can cinch tiny waists, eye make-up can accent beautiful eyes, heels can add height, colour can add sparkle. And then, there are certain aspects of our appearance over which all of us have control: diet and exercise, in particular, contribute more to good looks than all the clothes you could hope for.

No one is perfect. You are probably over-critical of your faults and shortcomings because you constantly measure yourself against impossible standards, such as photographic illusions achieved by studio lighting, soft focus lenses, retouched negatives and many other tricks of the fashion photography trade. These photographs should inspire, not frustrate.

In trying to identify what pleases you, you will need to experiment. People who already have a highly developed sense of their own style manage to put a personal imprint on everything and you can learn to do the same.

HOW MANY CLOTHES DO YOU NEED?

No one will feel comfortable wearing all the looks in this book but some of them will appeal instantly and those are the ones you should explore first. As your clothing horizons expand, you will inevitably arrive at the dilemma clothes addicts know well – need versus greed. For the addict, there is no solution, but the rest of us can take action.

First of all, go to your wardrobe and remove everything that you haven't worn in the last year. Try to work out why it is that you no longer wear it. Pack it away – it will probably come back into style. Or perhaps you don't have anything to wear with it? As a rough guideline, each item in your wardrobe should go with at least two other things; if it doesn't and you like it, make a list of the things you could buy to go with it, then see if these in turn would go with clothes you already have.

Then experiment with styles by trying on your friends' clothes and by considering outfits you normally wouldn't the next time you are shopping. This is not to say that you should try on clothes which you would *never* wear. Rather, just go a little further beyond your normal range of clothing to see if you can add a new component to your wardrobe. For example, have you ever worn a boiler suit? Or a mini skirt? Or toreador trousers? Why not? Having assessed your figure type properly, go ahead and try them – preconceptions about the clothing which suits us are often the root of our dissatisfaction with our appearance.

However, before purchasing new clothes let us repeat what you've read in dozens of other fashion books: always buy the best quality you can afford, bearing in mind the number of times you will be wearing a specific garment. This does not mean that we are advising a wardrobe full of designer fashion; simply suggesting you buy clothes that have been well made in good quality fabrics.

Additionally, you should take advantage of sales to buy better quality clothes and accessories than you can normally afford. But don't develop sale mania and be tempted to purchase bargains which turn out to be money wasters rather than money savers.

HOW CAN WE KEEP FASHION IN ITS PLACE?

Once you have experimented successfully with a few new looks, your self-confidence will grow and you will be encouraged to take even more adventurous strides.

Admittedly, the world of fashion smacks of persuasion, exploitation and built-in obsolescence. Yet nobody – greedy manufacturer or sensation-seeking designer – can dictate the way we look. We may be influenced by fashion trends, but *The Book of Looks* suggests ways in which we can evolve an individual style. Today, more than ever before, fashion is an interaction with society at large. New trends evolve from trends that went before; sometimes they don't achieve popularity until their third or fourth season, and by that time other innovations are edging their way in. By studying the forty-five looks illustrated here you will also be able to recognize the various cultural influences at play in the fashion world and use them to develop your new style. Fashion is change, fashion is fun and fashion is individual. *The Book of Looks* is a book of possibilities. Explore and have fun.

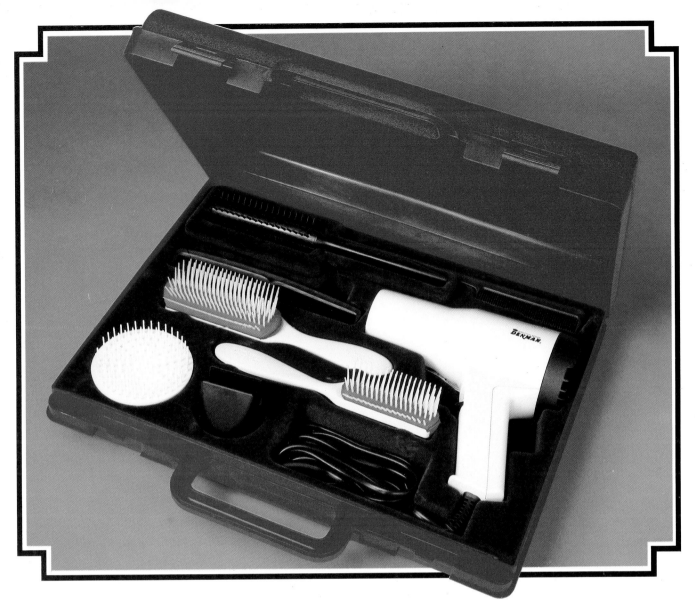

Introducing the F126
Complete Styling Kit by DENMAN®

D6 Shampoo/Massage
To stimulate the scalp, loosen dead skin and ensure shampoo and conditioner reach the hair roots.

D18 Cutting Comb
A general cutting/styling comb for sectioning and parting.

F126 Dryer
A powerful 1200 watt dryer forcing moisture from the hair using maximum temperatures, 4 heat/speed settings.

D3 Standard Brush (7 row)
The basic blow-dry tool for any KIT, controls hair perfectly and no static build up. For lifting and shaping.

D143 Mini Brush (5 row)
For shorter hair, works to control dificult sections, and for loose curls.

D37 Radial
To finish a style, tighter curls, fringes and sides.

D19 Tail Comb
For teasing hair into a final position.

A complete set of tools for all general styling in a compact case.

Made in the United Kingdom. DENROY INTERNATIONAL LTD.
Denroy House, 85, Brighton Road, Surbiton, Surrey. Tel: 01-399-4151. Telex 21786.

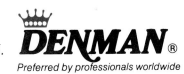

Preferred by professionals worldwide

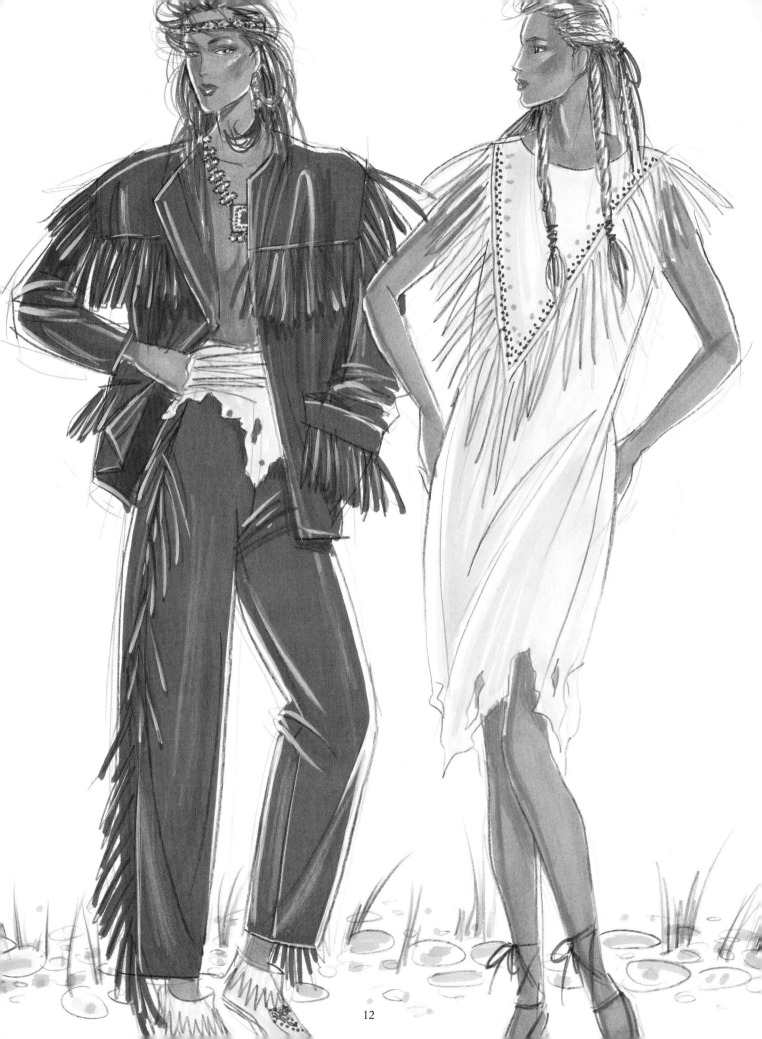

THE AMERICAN INDIAN

BACKGROUND

Before their numbers were decimated by white men, the North American Indians were the true noble savages; what we know of their culture commands the greatest respect. Various tribes inhabited virtually every area of North America, and though their way of life differed greatly from region to region, they all shared a close relationship with nature and the land. Predictably, lifestyle and habitat determined the crafts they practised and excelled in: weaving and silverworking developed among sedentary and agricultural tribes while hunters and nomads were skilled in carving, leather and textile ornamentation.

However, recognition of their rich tradition outside their culture did not occur until the early twentieth century, when the geometric designs of the Navaho, Zuni and Hopi tribes were adapted for Art Deco ornamentation. It is important to bear in mind that not all Indians dressed in the skins of the animals they hunted for food; the south-western tribes such as the Pueblo of New Mexico had very sophisticated weaving techniques and wore gorgeously coloured textiles as well as leather. Unfortunately, most of what we now know about them derives from Hollywood: we tend to think only of the Indians who lived on the Great Plains and made war on white men.

THE LOOK

The fashion look based on this image has been further diluted in recent years by mixing it with the plaids and denims of the cowboy (see THE COWGIRL). The two looks are compatible, but for our purposes, we will stick to the pure Indian. This look is ideal for casual outdoor

Below: Accessory items essential to **The American Indian**'s wardrobe have survived into the twentieth century and remain fashionable today. Moccasins, whether soled or not, fringed or beaded, look great with this look; bare, laced sandals look right with short chamois skirts; beadwork and feathers, even silver and turquoise, on belts, bags and jewellery can be as profuse as you like.

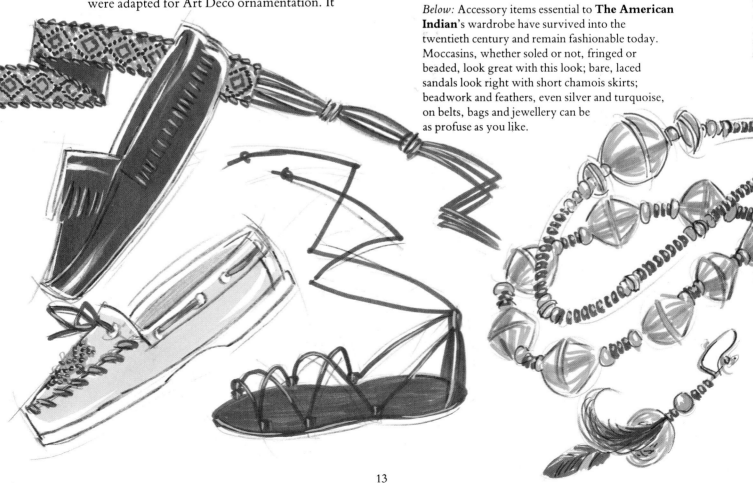

13

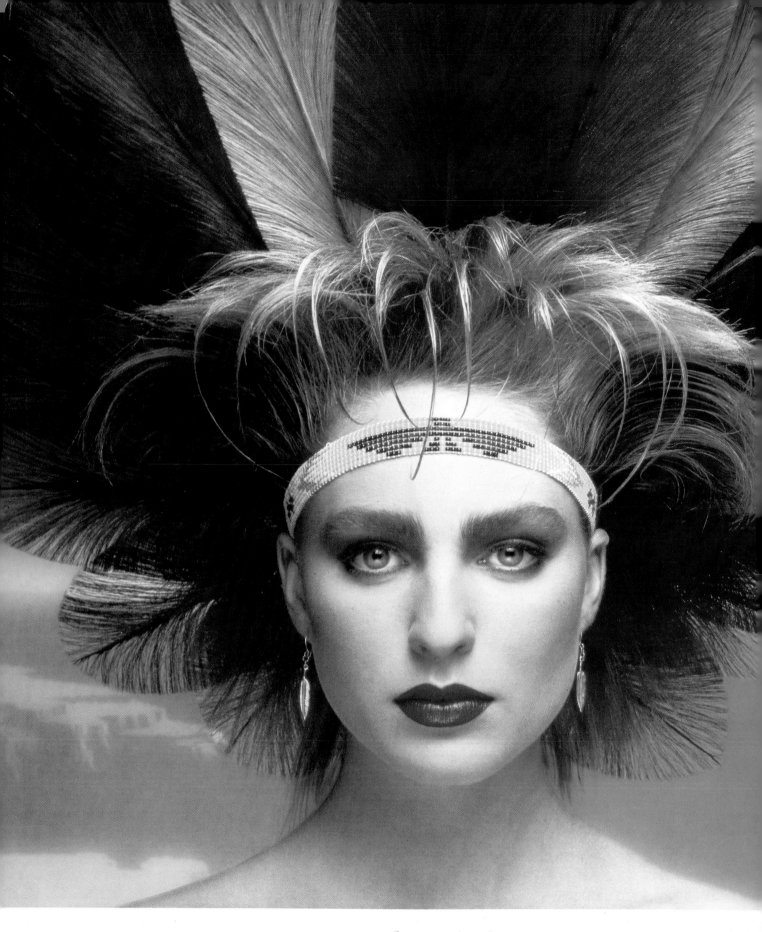

Harmony can colour hair in 14 diff

Shampoo Harmony in. Leave for ten to twenty minutes. Rinse. Harmony has at least four colours to suit your ow

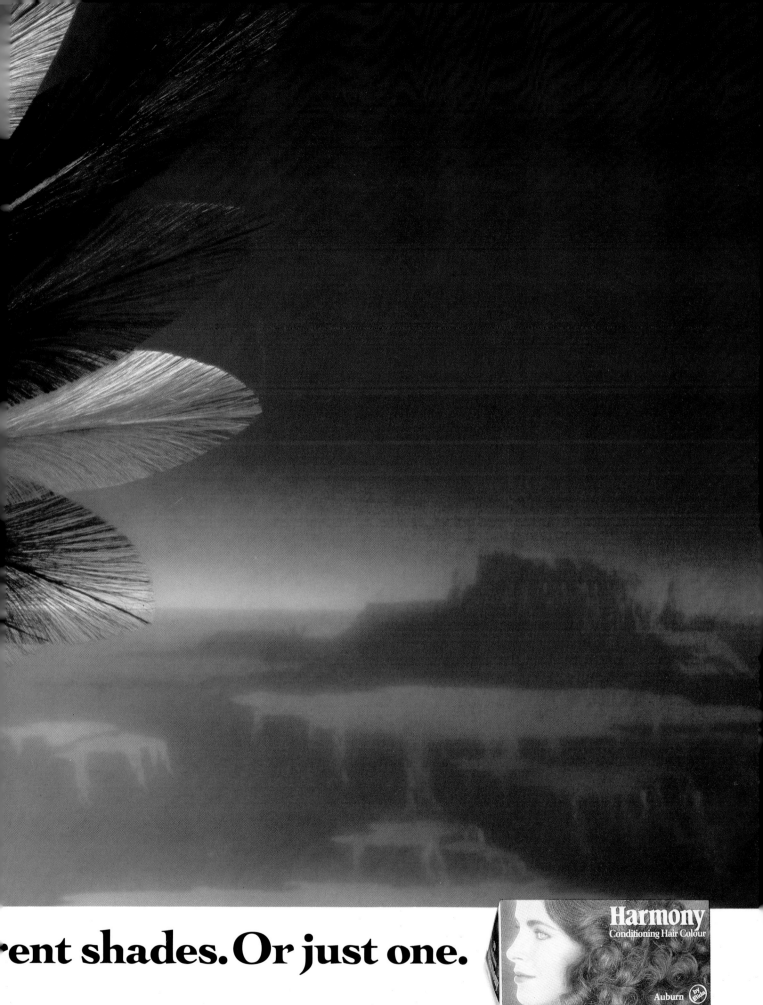

rent shades. Or just one.

Harmony
Conditioning Hair Colour

Auburn   by Elida

at'll condition and colour through six washes. And all the evenings in between.

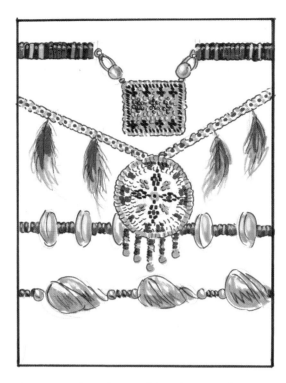

Left: A few ideas from traditional beadwork designs to provide inspiration for your own jewellery making: thread beads of any size and shape; twist on feathers of any hue; drill holes in shells and stone.

ACCESSORIES

Footwear should be soft – either ankle-length suede boots or traditional leather moccasins or booties. Ideally, these have fringed or beaded detailing. Colours for footwear can be bright, although desert shades of beige or tan are more in keeping. For hot summer days, flat sandals which laces up to the knee will work too, especially if worn with a short skirt, or if the legs of trousers can be wrapped round with the laces. For ornament, wear beaded belts, necklaces, earrings, wristbands and headbands.

Beadwork began in the eastern United States about 1675, with the Iroquois and the Algonquin tribes as the great beadwork traders. The precise purpose of beaded items remains lost in legend, but strings of abalone, clam and oyster beads seemed to have been involved in matrimonial ceremonies. Other semi-precious stones such as quartz, slate, soapstone, were also used, as were dried berries, fruit pits, bone and horn from animals. Even the colours of the beads were symbolic: white for peace and good health, purple for sorrow and red for war.

On the whole, these beautiful beaded accessories are cheap today, and add the much needed dash of colour to the muted tones of the clothing. Traditional accessories in silver and turquoise (recently popularized by the designer Ralph Lauren) can also be found, but they are usually prohibitively expensive, unless you plan to wear this look often. In your search for Indian accents, also look for jewellery made from feathers. Although the pieces may not be very durable, feathery ornaments look wild and wonderful, whether naturally-coloured or brightly-hued. Of course, you can easily add your own feathers to your Indian outfit – tuck them into headbands, belts, hair. Find them in the wild, or buy them from craft shops or milliner's supply houses.

For the perfect carry-all, choose a soft drawstring-style bag in suede, fabric or leather (see **Ideas**).

dressing. The colours of the Plains, such as pale tan, russet, honey beige, warm brown and gold, predominate, with turquoise, red and orange as accents in the form of ethnic jewellery.

Fringing is the predominant characteristic, whether on clothing or accessories, of suede, leather, wool, felt or cotton. In fact, a single article such as a fringed suede skirt, jacket, shirt or pants will impart the look instantly. However, if you like the look, and can't afford to invest in these more expensive pieces, try a fringed wool sweater, a fringed felt skirt or fringed wool trousers. Combine them with plain T-shirts or tailored cotton flannel shirts – although not authentic, they balance the fringed articles nicely. For example, should you have a fringed sweater or jacket, team it with straight-legged trousers and a top as described above, keeping to the suggested colour scheme. Alternatively, if you adore the idea of dressing exactly like THE AMERICAN INDIAN, you could invest in a suede or chamois straight-lined dress, with fringed hemline, sleeves and yoke front. Complete the look with beaded moccasins or low boots, (see below) and wear it in all but the hottest weather. For outer wear, a plain or Navajo-patterned blanket can be worn as a shawl over more prosaic clothing, perhaps held in place by a wide beadwork or leather belt. (See THE GYPSY for ideas on draping a large shawl in several different ways.)

FACE AND HAIR

Long hair is most characteristic of this look and should ideally be plaited in two with a headband around the forehead. If your hair is short, braid a lock or two and tie with colourful string or thread. If your hair is long enough, opt for two or more plaits, fastened at the ends with leather or suede shoelaces, then stuck with a couple of feathers.

Alternatively, a strand of small beads can be woven into your hair as you plait it. Single beads with large holes can be threaded on to strands of hair itself, while you are plaiting it. If your hair is short, or plaits are unsuitable, wear your hair wavy and free, tossed by the wind of the Plains, with just a beaded headband or leather strip across your forehead to keep it out of your eyes.

Choose make-up to give you a bronzed outdoor look. Apply a tinted moisturizer all over the face unless you have a naturally ruddy complexion or slight tan. To give yourself the characteristic high cheekbones of THE AMERICAN INDIAN, apply a dark taupe blusher under your cheekbone, then apply an ivory highlighter on top of the cheekbone, extending this up to the hairline. Complete the illusion with an orangeish-bronze blusher applied between the taupe and ivory strokes. Blend well, and finish the look with a slick of gold or apricot lipstick. If you're not shy of stares, draw a red zigzag (with lipbrush and lipstick) across one cheek.

IDEAS

● Jewellery is made from the things you'd find in the wild – feathers, string, grasses, stones, bones. The sketches below show several possibilities.

● For a quick effect, sew fringed braid to the outside seam of jeans – you'll find it in cotton, wool yarn, real and fake suede.

● For more instant jewellery, glue rather than sew small inexpensive beads, in traditional designs, to strips of leather, suede or felt to make wristbands, headbands, neckbands. (Wrap up your belongings by tying opposite corners of a square chamois leather together.)

● The lines of Indian clothing are simple, straight and untailored. Competent seamstresses might consider fashioning a skirt or dress by joining together inexpensive chamois from specialist suppliers. For appropriate decoration, use bone or horn buttons or thongs for joining at the waistband: wear the hem naturally uneven or fringe it by evenly cutting an inch or two up into the chamois. Finish your work by stringing large beads on to some strands of the fringe, knotting underneath the bead to keep it in place.

Below: Ways with beads and hair for the ultimate **American Indian** look: from the left, a beaded choker worn with four plaits, ornamented with feathers and beads as they were plaited; a beaded headband and single plait ornamented as above; a necklace worn with hair off the face, but plaited into several thin strands at the back; shorter hair with fake plaits added to give an impression similar to the first idea.

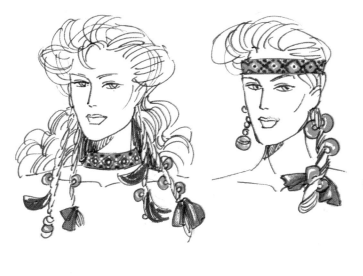

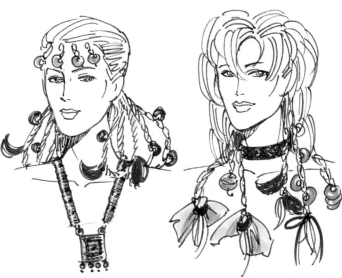

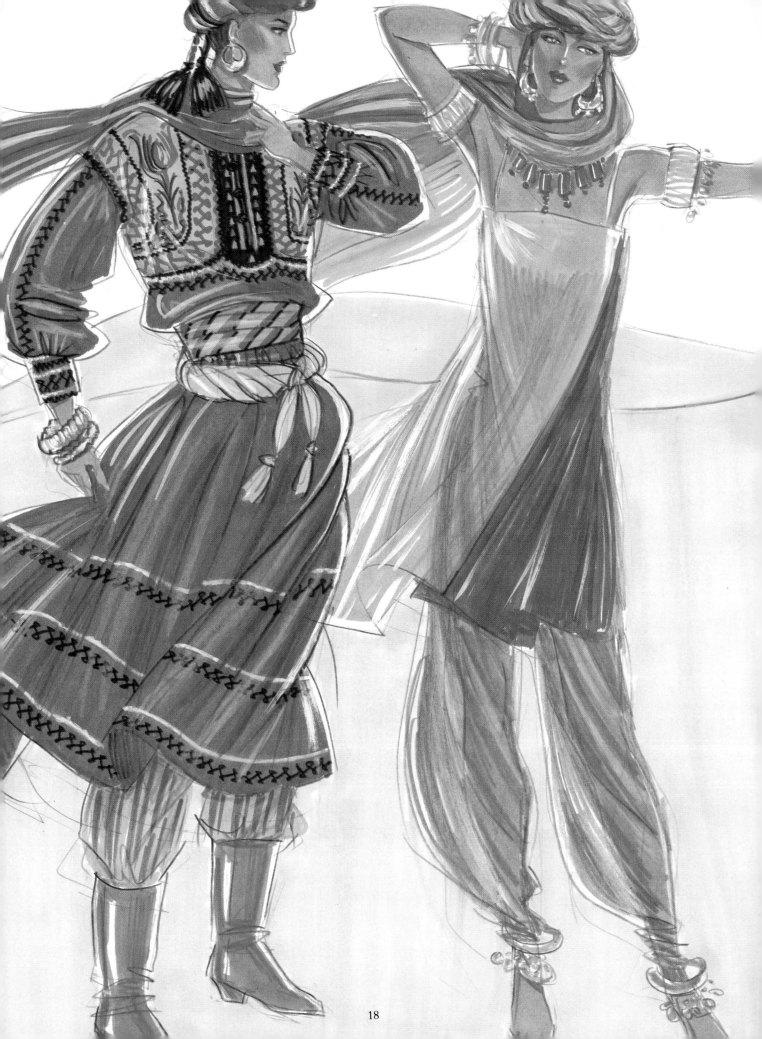

THE ARABIAN

BACKGROUND

The mystery of the Middle East has long fired the imaginations of travellers and explorers. Until this century only the most intrepid and fearless ventured into the unknown territories of the Arabian peninsula and neighbouring Islamic countries. In the nineteenth century tales came back via the pens of such legendary explorers as Charles Doughty and Sir Richard Burton of the lives and customs of the Arabian peoples and of their Islamic cultural traditions. Letters told of magnificent isolated cities, Baghdad, Sana'a and Esfahān, of vast undulating sand-duned deserts populated only by the fiercely proud nomadic Bedouin tribes, of camel caravans laden with exotic goods pausing for rest and replenishment at the scarce oasis pools. *A Thousand and One Nights* told of caliphs, sheiks and sultans, harems, odalisques and eunuchs, and travellers' journals described mirages, mosques and muezzins' calls from minaret tops to the faithful; of the impenetrable holy cities such as Mecca, barred to women and foreigners.

The air of mystery surrounding Arabia lingered into the early decades of this century.

Below: Jingle and jangle as you go, bedecked in gold or silver and semi-precious stones. You'll have 'jewels' on your ears, around your neck, on your shoes, on your fingers, and at your waist.

Most Westerners' knowledge of the area was still restricted to information supplied in the writings of flamboyant characters such as T.E. Lawrence in *The Seven Pillars of Wisdom* (later enacted by Peter O'Toole in the film *Lawrence of Arabia*), and in the accounts of early twentieth-century travellers such as H.St John Philby and two redoubtable ladies, Gertrude Bell and Freya Stark.

Since the revitalization of the Arabian civilization by Mohammed in the early seventh century A.D. and the adoption of the Moslem faith, religion has defined and ordained the behaviour of these women; only oil supremacy and the subsequent opening-up of the Middle East in the Sixties and Seventies have brought about an alteration in

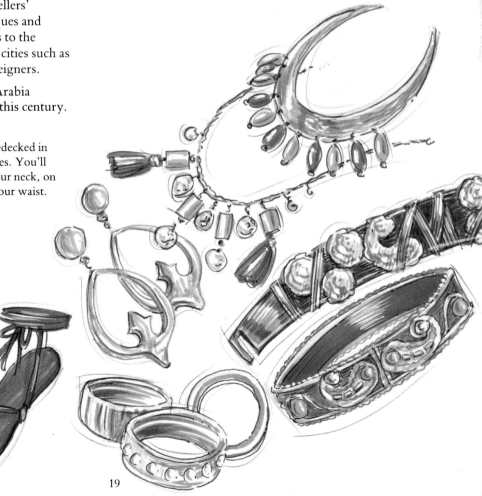

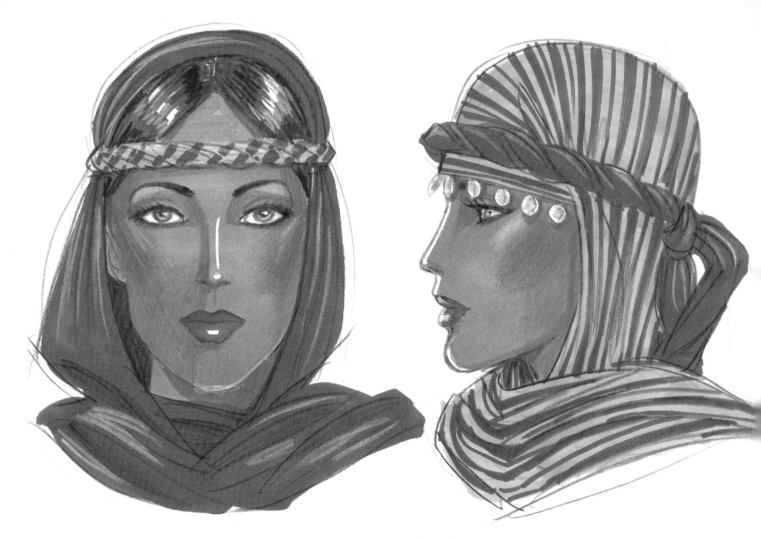

Above: Two ways of wearing your headdress. On the left, a length of fabric centred on the top of the head, the ends thrown over the shoulder, and a twisted band of contrasting cloth holding it in place; on the right, the scarf is brought down to just above the eyes, a pleat is formed at the crown and the wrapping is finished as above. To vary these treatments a little, wrap the securing headband with golden thread or sew coins or similar baubles to one end as shown.

women's own attitudes and men's attitudes towards them. Despite Western influence, however, most Arabian women still behave and dress much as their forebears did. In fact, the clothing styles which have evolved over the centuries for both men and women have changed little and are for the most part still in evidence today.

For women modesty, discretion and seclusion have always been paramount. Traditional apparel consequently includes long baggy underdrawers, a full-length long-sleeved dress of kaftan shape (a *djellabah*), an all-enveloping cloak (an *abaya*) and, of course, some kind of head covering and the essential face veil. This latter item is the most characteristic and immediate indicator of the truly authentic Arabian look; even the concubines and odalisques of the fabled harems are always depicted wearing veils – despite the often scanty covering of the rest of their bodies. In practice, the veil, which hides all of the face except the alluring eyes, often has the opposite effect to that of modesty!

THE LOOK

Like THE INDIAN and several other styles of ethnic inspiration, the Arabian look takes two distinct forms. Daytime wear is based on the Arabian woman's traditional covered-up apparel described in the previous section; by total contrast, evening wear takes its cue from the heroines of the Arabian Nights – it is uncovered, exotic and sensual.

To emerge as either the wife of a desert Bedouin chieftain or as the dancing girl of a harem, you will need to give some thought to the way you combine the components of the two versions of the Arabian look, albeit with a bit of Western artistic licence. Neither is a look for lovers of uncluttered line and pure colour; it's bold and big and very decorative.

The traditional Arabian crafts of dyeing, weaving and embroidery have exerted an enormous influence over the ornamental aspects of Arabian clothing. Decoration is concentrated in panels, yokes, hems and arm and sleeve bands, geometrically woven or embroidered with beads, seeds and mother-of-pearl.

Loose, roomy, comfortable shapes characterize the less exotic Bedouin version of the Arabian style, so if you favour this covered-up more practical look, the following components will be vital: a pair of gathered, baggy trousers, a long, loose tunic, collarless shirt, smock or ethnically-correct kaftan and a vast, all-enveloping cloak.

The trousers are the equivalent of the full-length brightly coloured baggy underdrawers worn by Arabian women; for your Arabian look, however, these can be used as a more obvious component of the outfit. Select those cut in a 'harem' shape (gathered into a waistband at the top and into widish cuffs at the ankle) in a supple, lightweight fabric. You could also opt for the zouave shape, voluminous above the knee and tight from there down (see also THE GYPSY). This latter style (named after the French light infantry corps of Algerians who wore such garments) is not a truly Arabian fashion, but a North African one; however, it is suitable in spirit for this look.

On top, choose from one of the alternatives suggested above and look for a full, widely cut shape. Your chosen garment should hang outside your trousers and can be sashed and belted. (see *Accessories*). It should certainly fall to mid-thigh, but can hang even lower than that – to the knee, mid-calf or ankle (if a kaftan and worn without the trousers underneath). On broiling days this loose shape will keep you cool but protected from the scorching rays, when the weather is a bit cooler, add another layer or two underneath – the effect will not be bulky since the top will be roomy enough to hide the insulation below.

The final layer of this version of the look is a voluminous cloak or wrap. Because of its loose shape, it can be draped over the shoulders or drawn up over the head and used to veil part of the face in true Arabian fashion. A softly woven blanket or vast serape (see THE LATIN) is an acceptable alternative.

When an invitation to an exotic extravaganza or a fancy dress event beckons, remember that there is nothing more eye-catching than a floaty shimmering harem girl outfit (though you may of course be called upon to live up to your inspiration and do a belly dance or perform the Dance of the Seven Veils!) If you decide to take the risk, however, you will certainly be the focus of attention.

Low-slung harem pants are essential; in floaty fabrics and exotic colours they should hang on your hips, allowing full view of the belly dancer's essential belly button; gather the billowing legs into neat ankle bands. If you are feeling ultra daring, wear only a sequinned strapless bra on top. However, if you blanch at the thought of this, wear instead either a short-sleeved, low-cut bodice, similar to those worn by Indian women under their saris, or a bodice with a low neck but billowing sleeves gathered into wrist bands. Whichever you choose, make sure the midriff is left entirely bare.

For fabrics, always select those which drape and hang well; silks, chiffons, voiles and any shot, shimmery materials are the obvious choices for evening. By day opt for soft and supple cottons, smooth silks, lightweight wools, such as challis, jerseys and even good quality slinky synthetics such as polyester. Make your selection according to the seasons in which you plan to adopt the Arabian look; there are many soft wools and jerseys available today which make the Arabian a definite possibility for autumn and winter wear, as well as summer. And remember that with the addition of extra jewellery and perhaps a fine silver belt, you can adopt the Bedouin version of the look for casual evening events if you prefer to give the exposed harem look a miss.

As far as colours go, stick to the traditional Arabian shades and naturally-dyed hues. All the warm desert tones look marvellous combined together: rich warm reds from cochineal, madder and henna, burgundys, burnt siennas, oranges, golds and deep yellows, all accented with crisp whites, sharp blacks and bitter browns. Beautiful blues are there too: indigo (for a long time grown in Arabia), turquoise (of Persian and Islamic ceramics) and a lighter mid-blue. Together with a limited range of moss greens, these are the colours used in Islamic geometric weaving and embroidery, so allow yourself to experiment with hand-woven stripes and simple patterns as well as plain colours.

ACCESSORIES

Jewellery is essential. Arabian women wear lots of it, and much is dramatic, intricate and noisy! Traditionally, they often carried their own wealth (from their dowries) and that of their husbands on them in the form of necklaces, belts, bracelets, rings and other items.

You may not be in a position to emulate their example, but you can at least create a similar visual impression. Silver is *the* metal to go for, and coral, turquoise and amber are the appropriate stones. Augment the latter with wooden or stone beads and a mass of medallions and large coins. Look for filigree work, embossing, relief designs and granulation, bells, baubles and layers of chains and silver mesh on chokers, necklaces, twisted bracelets, armbands, dangling earrings, finger, nose and toe rings, anklets and heavy intricate silver belts. And don't forget amulets or a hand of Fatima as a talisman to ward off the evil eye!

If you can't afford one of the impressive silver Arabian belts for your waist, there are alternatives. Should you feel that a belt of some description is essential over your baggy kaftan, try a tightly wound sash or cummerbund, worn with ends hanging free or wrapped round again and again. Alternatively, begin by wrapping your waist with a wide cummerbund of very soft leather or suede or a scarf or length of fabric. On top of this wrap thinner toning or contrasting belts; use rouleaux of fabric or leather, satin or cotton cording, metallic rope or lengths of satin ribbon, for a very opulently swathed effect.

To give your outfit the final touch of authenticity, you really should wear some sort of headdress and preferably a face veil! However, in this instance, the veil is really only appropriate for the harem look; add a veil and/or a headdress of the same gauzy fabric as your trousers and top. The veil can hang from below the eyes (on an elasticated headband or tie – see *Ideas*) to below your neck; alternatively, use a gauzy shawl: wrap it round the head and draw it over the front of the face.

For your Bedouin attire, use scarves wrapped in different ways around your head (see *Ideas*) or try the Arabian man's traditional *ghutra* or *kaffiya* worn under an *agal*. The *kaffiya* is a large piece of black or white cloth (or the well-known red and white or black and white checks available in many boutiques) secured in place on the head by the *agal*, a double coil of heavy cotton cording.

In hot weather wear nothing on your feet save anklets and toe rings. Alternatively, go for strappy ornamented sandals or those which lace up the leg. High heels are fine for evening but choose flat ones for day. In colder weather wear boots.

Bags are big by day and tiny by night; a carpet bag or a large woven satchel are ideal for the daylight hours, while a precious gilded leather purse or satin drawstring pouch is perfect for hours after twilight.

FACE AND HAIR

Give your face as tanned a look as possible unless you have real sultry colouring, by applying a darkish foundation, but avoid anything which will give a phoney appearance. Shadow lower eyelids with a dark khaki or russet shade and add a goldish tone just under the brow bone. In the outer corner of the lower lid, blend a very dark brown shadow bringing it around under the lower lashes, too. Smudge this lower line if necessary to avoid a hard look, then use a black kohl pencil inside the rim of both lower and upper lid, as close to the lashes as possible. If your eyebrows are pale, emphasize them with a brownish pencil. Finish by applying a rust blusher to the cheekbones and a medium rust or apricot shade to the lips, outlining them with a tan pencil if they are not full enough. A gold highlight in the centre of the lower lip will also aid the illusion of a luxurious mouth.

Don't fret too much about your hair, since ideally it should be hidden under a headdress, shawl or part of your cloak, though you can leave it loose and flowing if you wear only a face veil on your head with the harem outfit.

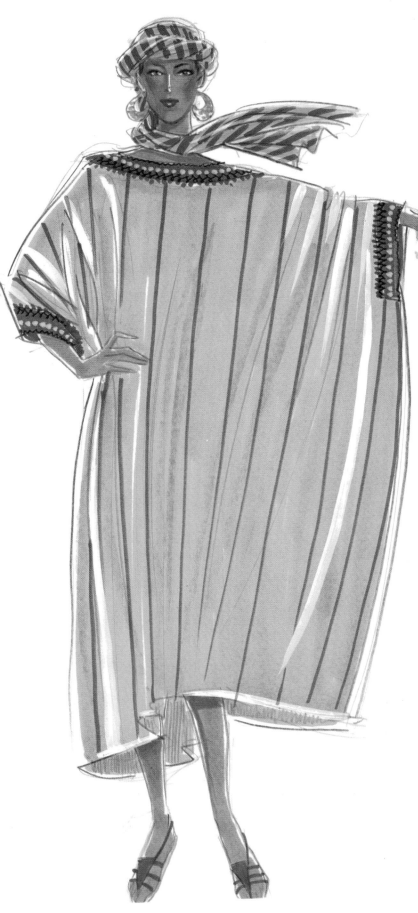

IDEAS

● Make a gauzy face veil to go with your harem outfit. Cut fabric into a 24 inch square; hem raw edges and gather top edge on to a thin elasticated headband. Decorate the headband and upper and lower edges of the veil with sequins, glittery braids or any decoration which matches your outfit.

● Attach coins, little bells and medallions to scarves, cummerbunds and headdresses to make them look more authentic.

● Wrap and tie scarves in different ways to give the impression of an Arabian headdress. Use one large flowing scarf as your *kaffiya* and another as the *agal*: place the first over your head and forehead with the ends hanging loose; on top twist the second scarf like a headband round the crown of your head and tie the ends at the back. Alternatively, use the first scarf as before, then place the second over the crown of your head down to the eyebrows; gather it together at the back and tie, tucking the ends in under the knot. In both instances the ends of the first flowing scarf can then be draped around your shoulders and neck.

● A simple kaftan can be made very easily: seam together two large rectangles of cloth, leaving slits for the arms and head; hem remaining raw edges. For a less basic alternative, cut a deeper neck opening and long, wide sleeves out of the rectangles; decorate neck opening and cuffs and even hemline with borders of embroidery, wide braid or contrasting fabric. Choose whatever length you desire.

● Create your own harem pants by gathering the ankles of widely-cut existing trousers in a supple fabric; those with a gathered waistline are best. Slip a length of elastic (as long as the circumference of your ankle) through the hemline of each leg; join the ends of the elastic with a few stitches and sew up the gap in each hem.

Left: Another look appropriate to **The Arabian**: a kaftan made from a rectangle of cloth as directed in *Ideas* above. Her turban is made from two scarves, with one twisted round and round her head, the ends left free to flow.

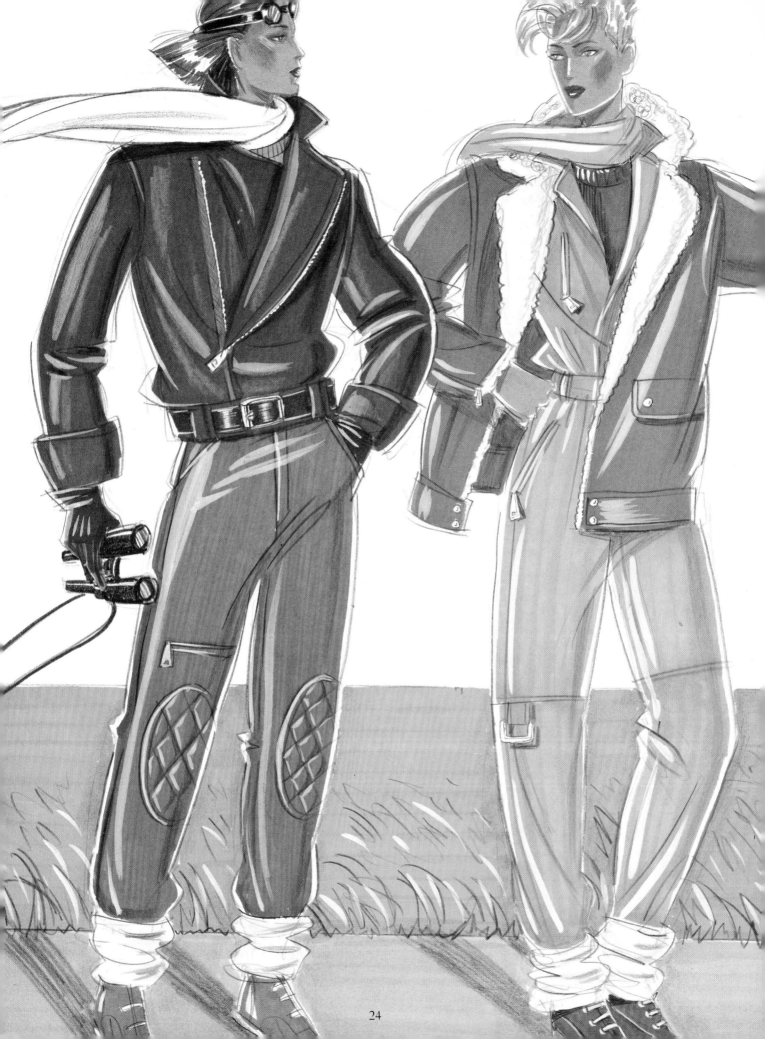

THE AVIATRESS

BACKGROUND

In 1932, Amelia Earhart became the first woman to complete a solo flight across the Atlantic. It took 15 hours 18 minutes in her small Lockheed plane and made her world-famous overnight. Amelia possessed rare courage; tragically she disappeared in 1937, somewhere over the Pacific, while attempting to fly around the world at the Equator. Photographs taken before her premature death show a striking woman with high cheek bones and short, tousled blonde hair. She was immortalized by Rosalind Russell in the film *Flight for Freedom* (1943). THE AVIATRIX symbolizes the rare freedom of courageous pioneers such as Amelia and Amy Johnson and is an appropriate inspiration to liberated women today.

Dressing like an aviatrix can be utterly practical or chic and elegant, worn summer and winter, even translated into luxury fabrics for special occasions. It is also a very simple look to achieve because the components are always the same: blouson jacket, one-piece flying suit, ankle-length boots and long, flowing scarf.

THE LOOK

Begin with the blouson jacket, sometimes referred to as a 'bomber jacket'. This can end either at the waist, or the hips. It is traditionally made of weathered brown leather, lined with fleecy sheepskin which also covers a large collar to pull up over the ears. Side pockets fasten with sturdy zips, straps adjust the waistband and sleeves, outer breast pockets with flaps hold goggles, a man-size handkerchief, and maybe a compass.

However, there are several alternatives to this traditional brown leather gear. The leather can be black, even tan, blue, red or green, provided the styling remains more or less the same as shown in the illustration. The collar may be small and it doesn't have to be fleecy. If you prefer not to wear leather, look for a less sturdy jacket in corduroy or wool, preferably in navy, brown or olive shades. For summer it can be of cotton or nylon cire – try white or pastel shades for a lighter effect.

Below: Stylish gear for an amazingly wearable look: leather-trimmed duffel or shoulder bags hold lots of gear; gauntlet gloves are sheepskin lined for warmth, watches are shock- and waterproof; a helmet-shaped hat with earflaps is a nice touch; and absolutely essential are aviator-style sunglasses.

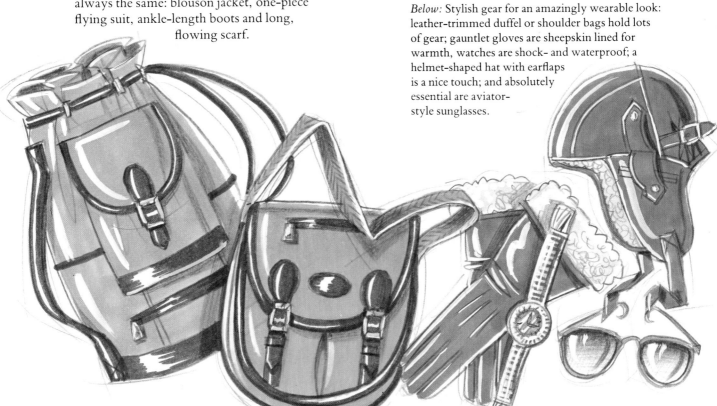

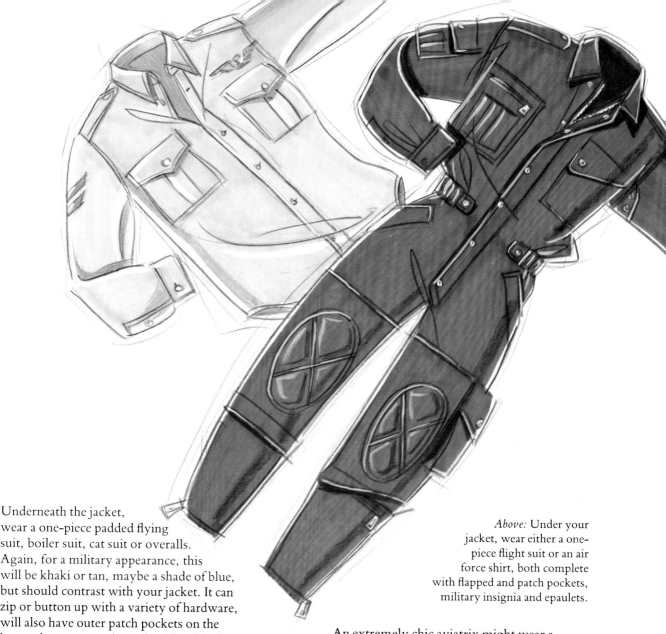

Underneath the jacket, wear a one-piece padded flying suit, boiler suit, cat suit or overalls. Again, for a military appearance, this will be khaki or tan, maybe a shade of blue, but should contrast with your jacket. It can zip or button up with a variety of hardware, will also have outer patch pockets on the breast, bottom, maybe at the side of the legs, and might have straps for adjusting sleeve and pant legs. The flying suit can be made of anything from canvas to cotton to wool: in summer it might be cotton or viscose; for evening satin, silk, even a glittery fabric. It can fit snugly or loosely – if it is roomy, wear a roll-neck sweater underneath in anything from thin cotton knit to thick wool depending on the weather and occasion. If you haven't got a flying suit, substitute a high-necked sweater(s) and a pair of baggy-topped trousers, even jodhpurs.

In really cold weather, finish the look with an outsize officer's coat from an army surplus store. Or add a down or leather waistcoat under the blouson jacket. (In fact, most of the components of this look can be found at army surplus outlets or second-hand clothing shops – the price will be far less than designer equivalents and the fabrics harder-wearing.)

Above: Under your jacket, wear either a one-piece flight suit or an air force shirt, both complete with flapped and patch pockets, military insignia and epaulets.

An extremely chic aviatrix might wear a sand-coloured suede jacket over a leather flying suit, her neck wrapped in a cashmere scarf and her feet well-heeled in designer boots. For evening, she might wear a pastel satin flying suit with a satin quilted bomber jacket and high-heeled boots. Whatever the fabric, whatever the colours, the clothes are the same. THE AVIATRIX is an amazingly simple look – the magic comes in the accessorizing.

ACCESSORIES
There are two critical accessories to this look – boots and scarf. First, boots. They may be any colour, though brown, black or variations on these dark neutrals are most versatile; they can be ankle- to calf-length; they should lace, buckle or zip up, and they should have crêpe or similar soles for comfort. (Avoid high heels unless you're wearing the look on a dressy occasion.) This same functional boot will also

work with other outdoor looks such as THE COWGIRL, THE FAIR ISLANDER, THE IMMIGRANT, THE SOLDIER, and THE OUTDOOR GIRL. Under the boots wear thick cotton or woollen socks – palest yellow or cream look good. Let these show a little by cuffing them over the top of fitted boots, or wear them pulled up over the bottom of your trouser leg.

The second essential accessory for THE AVIATRIX is her long, flowing, fringed scarf. It will wrap her neck and ears in cold weather and will add a much-needed touch of brightness to the airforce colour scheme. Traditionally, the scarf is of heavy creamy-white silk, but you may choose soft wool, cashmere, or acrylic, even polyester or viscose, though man-made fabrics don't feel so nice nor are they as warm. (If you like dressing like THE AVIATRIX but have chosen a more adventurous colour scheme, then the colour of the scarf may co-ordinate, but it should remain long and fringed).

To keep your hands warm, choose leather or leather-palmed gloves. Driving gloves are ideal, gauntlet styles will also look right, and string gloves in white, cream or tan will look good for summer. But the gloves should look rugged – no fine kid or lacy ones here.

On your wrist wear a chunky functional-looking watch – nothing dainty. Borrow a man's if you have to. Jewellery is inappropriate unless you have some stripes for glory or a good-luck charm. This is no look for glitter.

Your bag should be a satchel or shoulder bag,

Below: Add a military note to more prosaic clothes by a simple change of buttons – brass airplanes, stars and eagles look great.

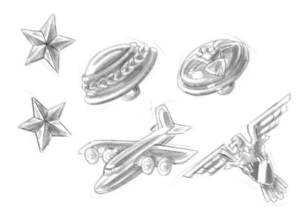

again in a neutral shade. Choose one with a sturdy zip and outside pockets. It can be leather or fabric, even a sailbag or old nose-bag will do.

Finally, if you plan to do a lot of cold-weather or high-altitude flying, get a fleece-lined hat with earflaps, or any army style that flatters. Alternatively, ear muffs are perfectly adequate for those staying at ground level!

FACE AND HAIR
Wear your hair short and tousled, à la Amelia. You might even make it stick out a little by massaging in a little setting lotion while wet, then blow-drying it. Bronze your face with tinted foundation; add rosy cheeks with a glistening blusher. Add a clear lip-gloss to prevent your lips chapping in the wind.

IDEAS
● Make your own fringed scarf for pennies. Buy 1½ yards (150 cms) of 36-inch width (95 cms) fabric. Make it heavy silk or fine wool if you want the best, otherwise soft acrylic, polyester or viscose. Fold the length in half, sew the long ends together, turn the length inside out, so the seam is on the inside. Sew matching silken fringes to each end, or create self fringe by unravelling an inch or so of the fabric using a thick needle or seam ripper to loosen threads.

● Create a more airborne impression by replacing buttons on your jacket or flight suit with metallic stars, silver airplanes, or simply bold and brassy buttons.

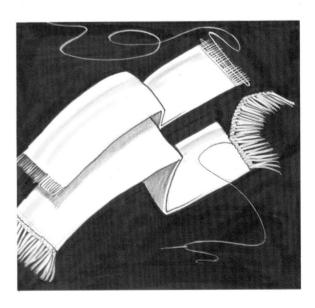

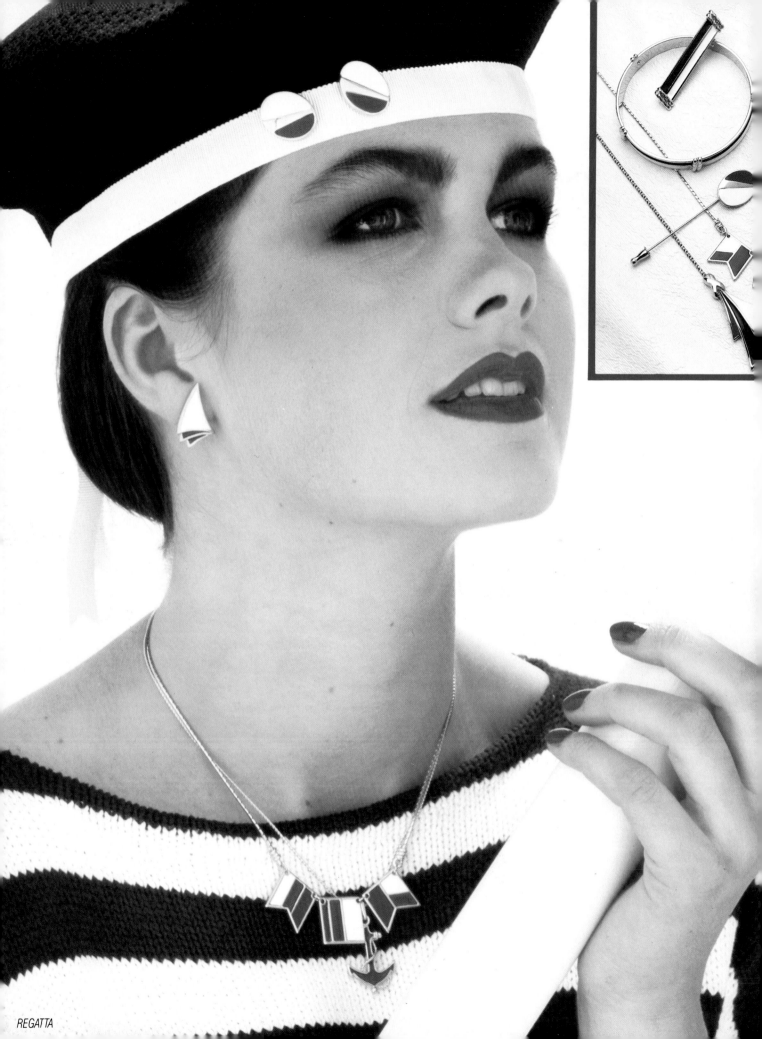

REGATTA

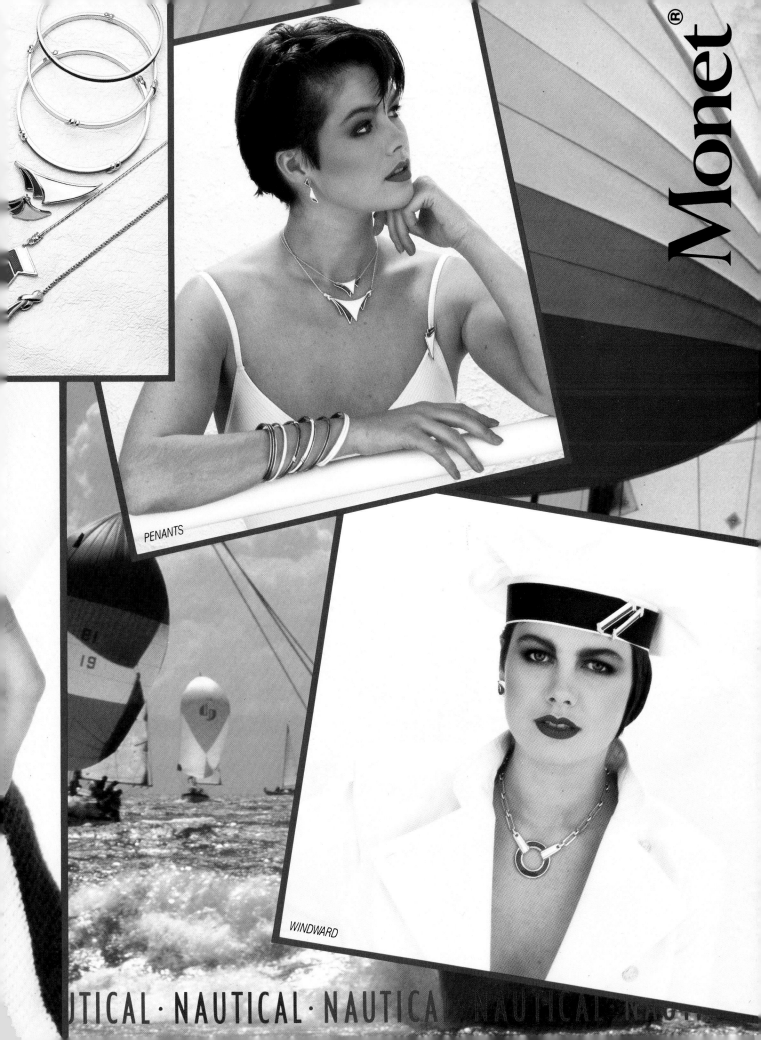

Monet®

PENANTS

WINDWARD

UTICAL · NAUTICAL · NAUTICA NAUTICAL · NAUT

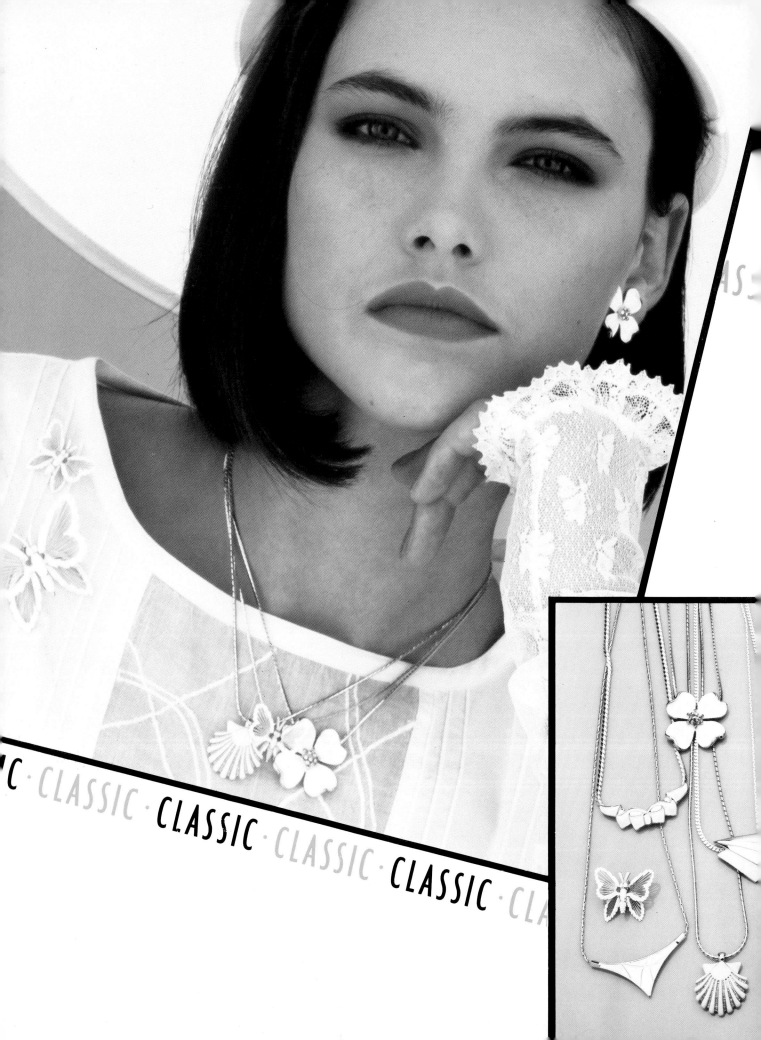

CLASSIC · CLASSIC · CLASSIC · CLASSIC · CLA

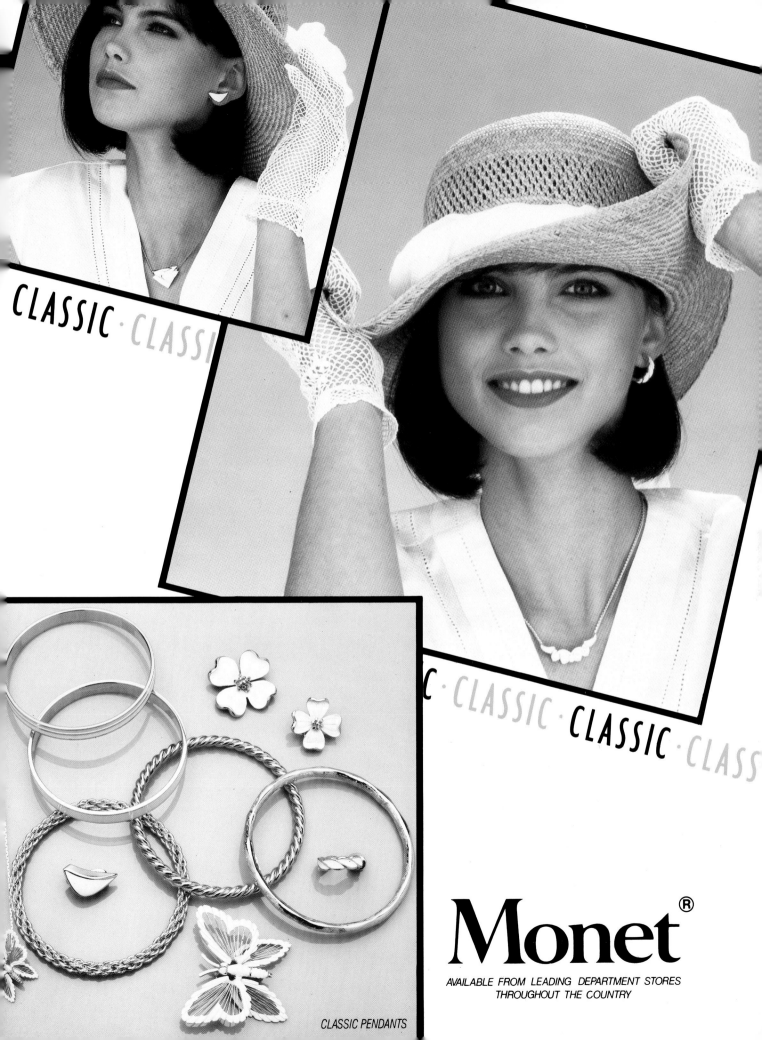

CLASSIC · CLASSI

C · CLASSIC · CLASSIC · CLASS

CLASSIC PENDANTS

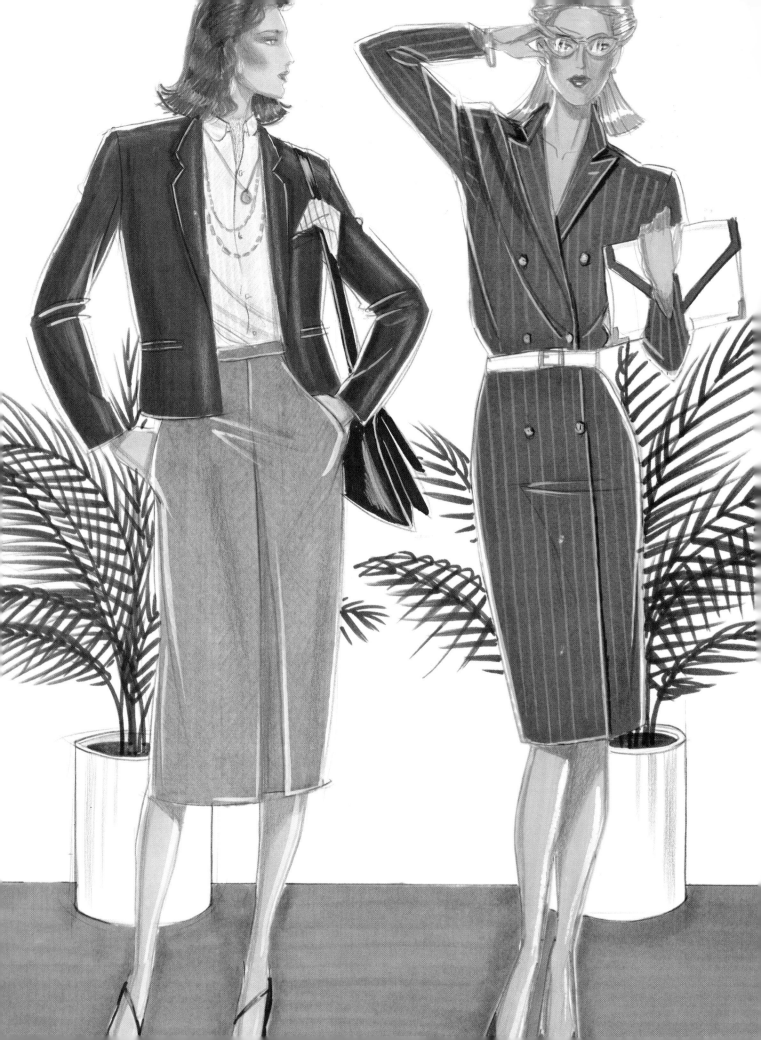

THE BUSINESSWOMAN

BACKGROUND

Every good businesswoman knows that in her struggle for equal recognition she has to look professional: the business world is no place for coquettish clothing or little-girl looks. While men have narrowed their costume down to a fairly rigid uniform of three piece suit, shirt, and tie, women are permitted a little more rein in terms of colour, variety of fabrics and styling of garments. At the same time however they must maintain the sensible, immaculate and unfussy example of their male colleagues.

The look is based on the suit and blouse combination, and dates from the early Forties when women began taking jobs and living more emancipated lives through necessity, since most of the men were away fighting the war. Most of them had very little money and often shared each other's clothes, but they still managed to look smart by using their imaginations.

THE LOOK

As with the THE GENTLEMAN, a well-cut suit is the basis of the look. It is therefore worth making as generous an investment as you can afford when buying this suit. On the other hand you may be lucky enough to find a good condition, beautifully-tailored version for much less in a secondhand clothes shop. The disadvantage of investing in expensive suits is that styles have an unnerving way of changing drastically every four years or so, and your once-stylish suits are suddenly no longer fashionable. However, good fabrics seldom wear out, so send them to a good tailor for alterations. If you find that you take to this way of dressing, invest in one suit per season to spread the cost and you'll never be out of fashion.

In terms of suiting fabrics, choose any hard-wearing fine-quality wool for winter – worsted, gabardine, challis, tweed; for summer wear linen, cotton and silk or mixtures of these. Avoid man-made fabrics, although a small percentage can help natural fibres keep their shape longer. Although man-mades are sometimes easier to care for they never stay fresh-looking for long, catch easily on jewellery and seem to harbour perspiration odours.

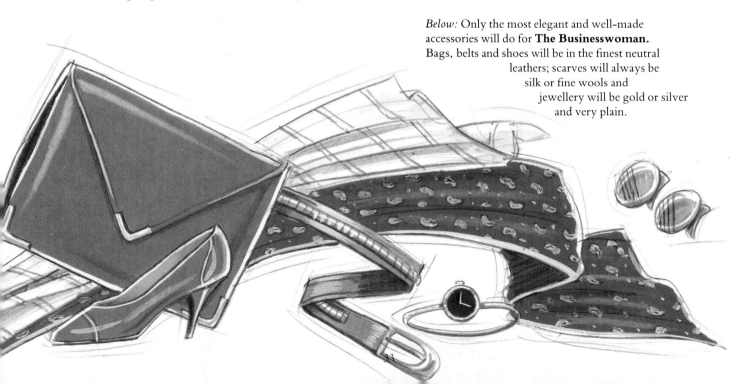

Below: Only the most elegant and well-made accessories will do for **The Businesswoman.** Bags, belts and shoes will be in the finest neutral leathers; scarves will always be silk or fine wools and jewellery will be gold or silver and very plain.

Choose a style of suit to complement your figure – try them on in front of a full-length mirror before buying to find the right proportions for you. Both skirt and jacket can be any shape from pencil-straight to very full. Generally speaking, the bigger and longer the jacket, the fuller the skirt and vice versa. For maximum versatility begin with suits in fairly conventional plain colours, such as navy, grey, burgundy or black. Wear paler versions of these shades in the summer.

Blouses must be in neat traditional shapes and patterns subtly enhancing the severity of the suit – pinstriped, dotted, plain, or with subtle prints – and well-tailored with a minimum of frill. For example, a striped shirt may have a lace collar or a foulard tie but avoid excessive ruffles and embroidery. Ideally they should be in pure cotton, or if you can afford the upkeep, invest in one or two good silk blouses to wear for special business lunches or to turn a day suit into a smart evening outfit when you don't have time to go home to change. Natural fabrics will always cost a little more, but they will reward you with many years' more wear and withstand frequent cleaning. If you despair over the prices of pure cotton shirts in women's shops, consider those that cater for young boys and men; although the shirts will button up left to right, the prices will be lower and the selection greater.

For extra warmth wear a sweater on top of your blouse. Begin by collecting classic styles like round and V-necks, progressing to Argyll plaids and lacy cable knits in wool, cotton, cashmere and silk. The sleeveless V-neck pullover, so popular today, is ideal for office environments and is available in a multitude of colours and designs.

For outerwear, choose a classic trenchcoat; for colder weather a good quality chesterfield, balmacaan or loden.

ACCESSORIES

Creative accessorizing for this look needs imagination, as the components (suit, shirt and sweater) are so predictable. Coats and jackets can be decorated with belts, scarves, shawls, even a simple piece of jewellery. Over shirt or sweater, a gold or silver chain, antique or otherwise, looks great, but avoid dangling initials or charms. Earrings, bracelets, rings need to be equally low-key. Traditionalists will choose simple gold or silver; more

Below, left to right: To personalize **The Business-woman**'s jacket tuck a lace-edged hankie into a breast pocket; add a fake or real flower to a lapel; cinch your waist with a fine leather belt; throw a silk or paisley shawl across your shoulders.

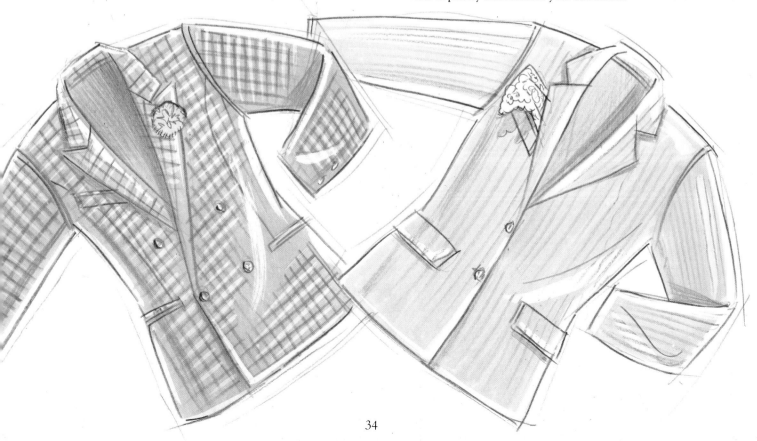

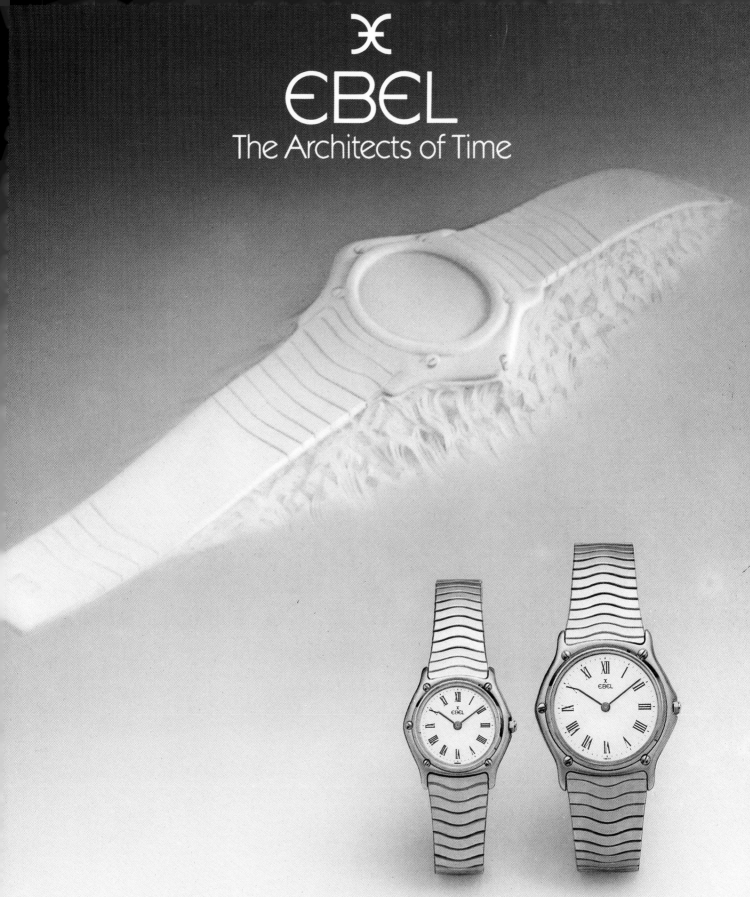

EBEL
The Architects of Time

Quartz. 18 ct Gold, Steel and 18 ct Gold, Steel; water resistant 30 m.

LIST OF EBEL AGENTS IN UNITED KINGDOM

adventurous businesswomen will opt for modern pieces. In any event, jewellery must be kept to a minimum. Your watch should be similarly plain and practical.

Shoes and handbags are probably more important to this look than any other group of accessories. They must be of excellent quality, and should ideally be in matching plain colours. All leather accessories should be of good quality; as they will get lots of use they must age gracefully. If you can afford only one pair of shoes and one bag to begin with, choose black or brown for both. Bags should be roomy, indeed briefcase and large envelope shapes are perfect if you carry a lot of papers; if you can get away with a smaller handbag, go for one with a shoulder strap. Shoes should have flattish heels, up to two inches high; save stilettos for evening and other looks. Classic court shoes are a useful option for summer and winter alike. Tights should be sheer or very slightly textured, but preferably co-ordinating tones.

Choose narrow belts in plain colours to co-ordinate with or match your shoes and handbag, or with classic fabric accents such as webbing stripes. Use belts not only through the belt loops of skirts and trousers, but also over sweaters and jackets to define a waist. Scarves and shawls of silk or fine wool, whatever their shape, are invaluable. Wear them cravat-style under blouses and sweaters, wrapped around your neck, tuck them into breast pockets of jackets, throw them over your shoulders or knot in front; try larger ones on top of coats and jackets to add interest. See THE CLASSICIST for ideas and techniques with scarves.

FACE AND HAIR

Gimmicky make-up and hairstyles have no place in this uncluttered look. Make-up and face powder should be natural; choose eye shadow shades to complement both your outfit and your colouring. Lips will be clear and precise with maybe a taupe outline but not too much colour.

Hair should be sleek and shiny, above shoulder length and not too curly or fussy. Alternatively, hold hair off the face with a headband or clasp, or pull it back into a chignon.

IDEAS
See THE GENTLEMAN

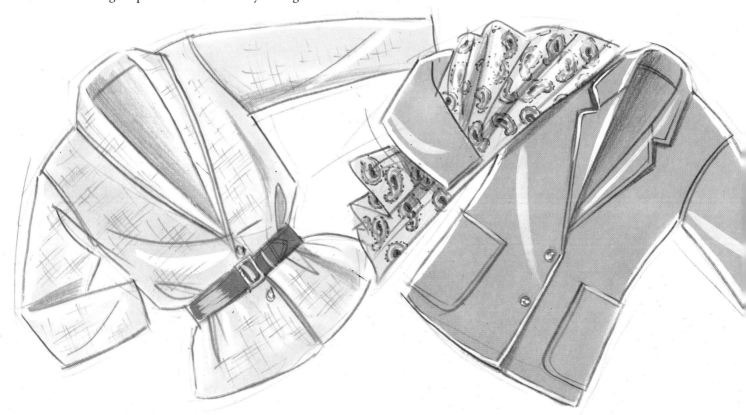

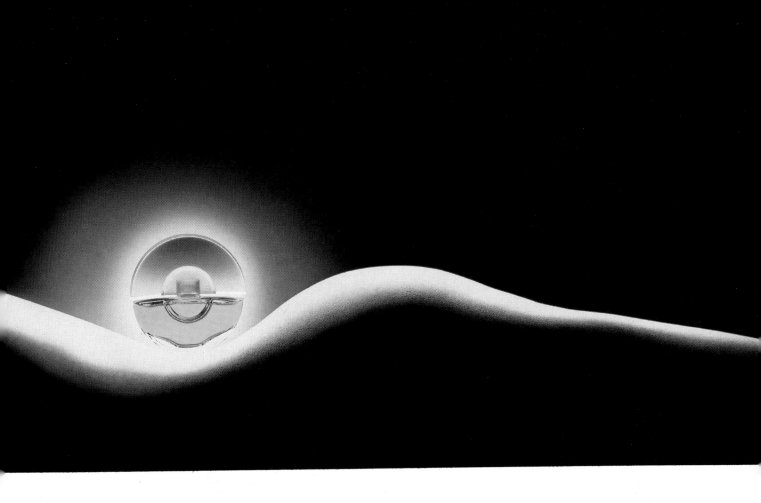

PARADOXE DE CARDIN. LA FEMME EST SON ECRIN.

Cool and passionate. Quiet and daring.
Innocent and mysterious. A woman is all these things.
A paradox. Paradoxe de Cardin.

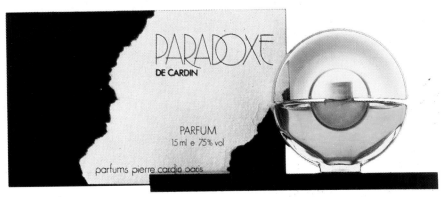

PARFUMS PIERRE CARDIN PARIS.

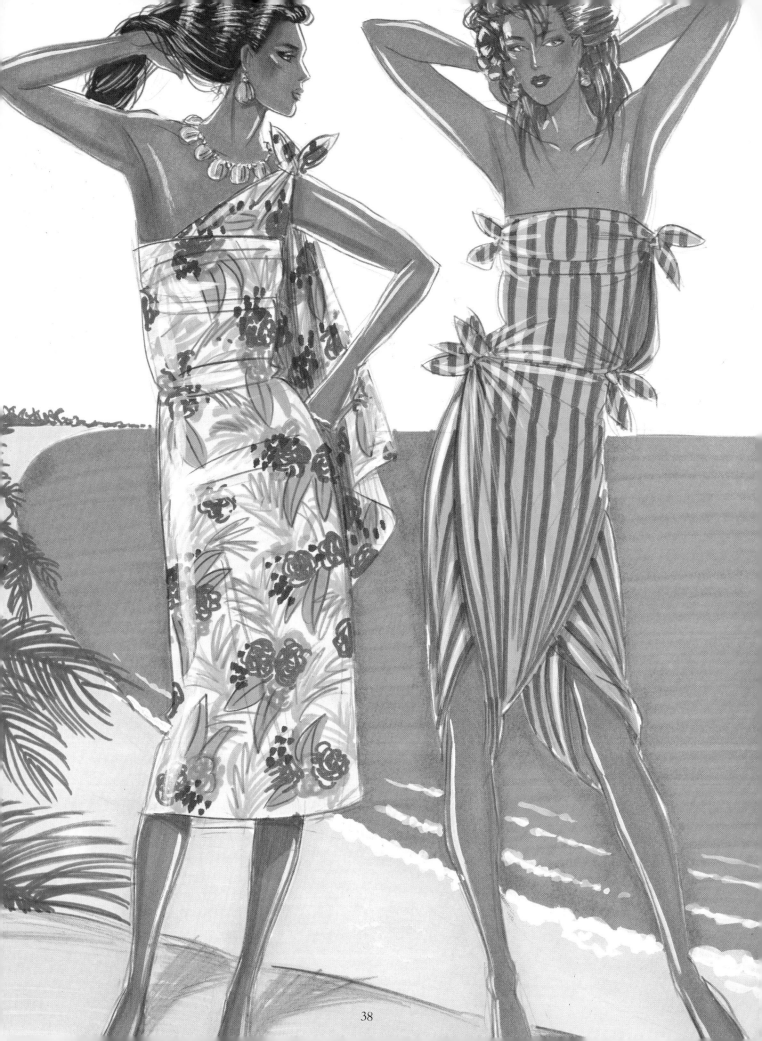

THE CASTAWAY

BACKGROUND

Washed up on a desert island? Haven't a thing to wear? Only a length or two of fabric and no sewing machine in sight? Then this is the look for you.

THE CASTAWAY is the ideal solution too for those seamstresses who buy yards of fabric, with all the best intentions, but somehow find themselves with trunks full of material and no clothes.

THE LOOK

To make these quick cover-ups, use only the softest, stretchiest or clingiest of fabrics – stretch towelling (terrycloth), gauzy cotton voile, lightweight or imitation silk, cotton or acrylic knits, satiny nylon, even sensual velvets. The flavour of the clothing will be determined by your choice of fabric – for example, in dark panne velvet any of the tops with the trousers or zouaves will look stunning with pale skin on a wintery evening, while in summer the same clothes in a zanily-dotted cotton jersey worn with bright jewellery will result in an entirely different effect.

For the most part, standard widths of 36-inch (90 cms) and 45-inch (115 cms) fabric, in lengths of 1 to 3 yards (metres) are used, but once you get the hang of knotting, tucking, folding, and bunching fabric into instant garments, you'll find yourself improvising.

Obviously, THE CASTAWAY is the ideal hot weather look. It is also a very practical and stylish way of dressing for similarly steamy places like pulsating discotheques and packed parties.

For the most part the tops are fashioned from smallish pieces of fabric or ready-made scarves. The Hawaiian-style halter with its knotted front is made from one length of fabric 18–24 inches (46–61 cms) wide × 36–45 inches (91–115 cms) long. Begin by wrapping the long end of the fabric just above your bust, knotting the top opposite corners at the centre of your bust, tucking the bottom corners into skirts or pants, finally decorating the central knot as suggested in *Accessories*.

To create the Polynesian-style top, use the same size fabric or scarf as described above, but place the knot at the side, and pin a huge fake flower over the centre of the knot. Should you have a longer length of fabric, say 45–60 inches (115–150 cms) in length, this top becomes a dress.

The Egyptian-style top is created from two matching or contrasting lengths of fabric, 18 × 36 inches (45 × 91 cms) or from a single

Left: The one-shouldered sarong and the Zouave outfit.

Below: **The Castaway**'s accessories are minimal – with that gorgeous tan what else do you need? Wear sandals of any style; jewellery can be made from shells, beads, coral; hats are big-brimmed or turban-styled.

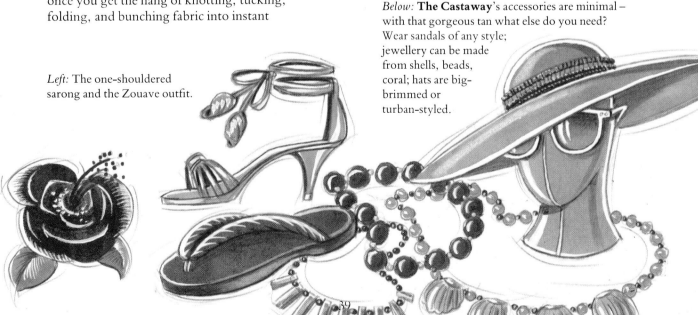

length 18 inches (46 cms) wide × 54 inches (136 cms) long. Centre the length or the lengths knotted together at the nape of your neck, bring each end round to your front, crossing them over your bust and expanding the fabric to cover each breast, finally knotting at your centre back. Or begin at your centre back, and end with a knot at your nape.

The Grecian-style halter is made from one or two lengths of fabric as described above. Centre the length of fabric at your upper back, bringing the ends forward and crossing them over each other at the centre bust. Finally, knot the ends at the nape.

Wear one of these tops with the time-honoured tropical island skirt – the sarong. The sarong skirt is made from a length 30–45 inches (75–115 cms) wide × 54–72 inches (136–180 cms) long. Position the long end of the fabric at your centre front. Holding on to the corner, wrap the rest of the fabric around you until meeting with the first corner, then knot the remaining

From left: **The Castaway**'s tops: the Egyptian, the Grecian, the Polyaesian and the Hawaiian.

end with the one you're holding. To make a mini version of the sarong, simply use fabric less than 36 inches (91 cms) wide. THE CASTAWAY can also use this sarong skirt as a dress: position the long edge of the fabric above the bust and wrap and knot as directed above.

For those castaways anxious to acquire maximum tan, a sunsuit or one-piece bathing suit can also be fashioned from less than two yards (metres) of material, ideally in a stretch fabric. Using a length 24–36 inches (61–91 cms) wide × 54–72 inches (136–180 cms) long, take the centre of the fabric through your legs, knotting the back and front corners at your shoulders. Pin at the waist with a safety pin (from your first aid kit, of course) and/or sash with a contrasting or co-ordinating scarf or remnant as directed under *Accessories*. To cover up, add the sarong skirt to the sunsuit.

Should you decide to dress a little more formally on your desert isle, you can also make a dress from a length of fabric 18–36 inches (61–91 cms) wide × 54–80 inches (136–200 cms) long. The width of the fabric will determine the length of the sleeves, although bear in mind that you don't have to

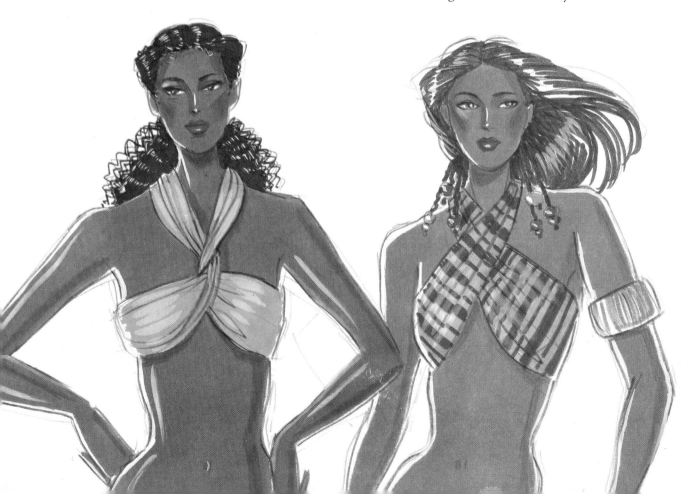

cut the fabric to achieve the cap sleeve effect as illustrated, merely turn under the width at each shoulder. The length of fabric will determine the length of the dress – vary it from mini-short (as a bathing suit cover-up) to ankle length.

To create this dress, fold the length of fabric in half and make a slit 10–12 inches (25–30 cms) long along the fold for your head to go through; use pinking scissors to prevent fraying or simply fold and press the raw edges under and if time permits hem round. Place the front panel of the dress over the back panel at your sides, securing with a small safety pin on the inside and/or a sash at the waist.

For something a little more revealing, there's the one-shouldered sarong. Using a length of fabric 36 inches (91 cms) wide and 72–90 inches (182–230 cms) long, hold one corner of the long end of the fabric at your shoulder. Wrap the rest around your body at bust level, finishing by knotting the remaining corner with the one you are holding. The dress can be sashed as above and/or worn with the trousers that follow.

To create instant castaway pants, use two lengths of fabric, 30–36 inches (76–91 cms) wide × 36–45 inches (91–115 cms) long.

Knot the short side of one length at the waist or slightly below, tying it at your side. Create the ankle by crossing the lower corners twice before knotting, rolling up to adjust the length if necessary. Repeat for the other leg, positioning the second piece of fabric just under the first waist knot. Inner legs will be slightly exposed; close the gap with two safety pins on each leg if you like.

For the briefest halter, take one length of fabric 14–18 inches (35–46 cms) wide, 36 inches (91 cms) long, folding it in half or thirds so it is wide enough to completely cover your bust. Knot the ends at your back, then, using ribboning, a strip of fabric, string or twine, loop around the fabric at the centre of your bust, finally taking each end of this over each shoulder and knotting them together at your nape.

To make the zouave trouser outfit, begin with the top which is fashioned from two pieces of fabric, 20–24 inches (51–61 cms) square. Knot the squares together at the top and bottom corners, securing them to fit above the bustline and at the waistline. For the zouaves, use one length of fabric 36 inches (91 cms) wide × 54–72 inches (137–182 cms) long. Knot the short ends of the fabric at the side of your waist; bring the rest of the length through your legs, knotting the remaining short end at the other side of your waist. Adjust length of fabric for length of zouave.

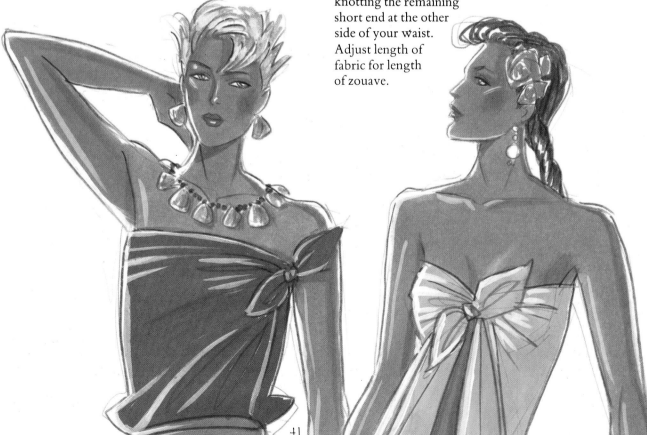

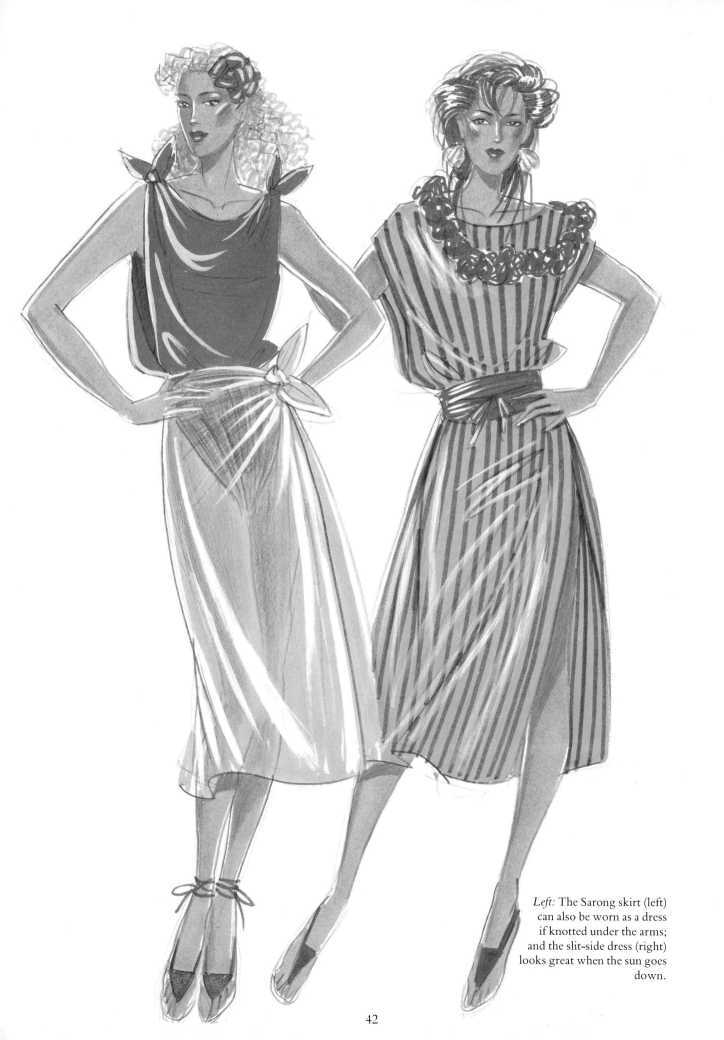

Left: The Sarong skirt (left) can also be worn as a dress if knotted under the arms; and the slit-side dress (right) looks great when the sun goes down.

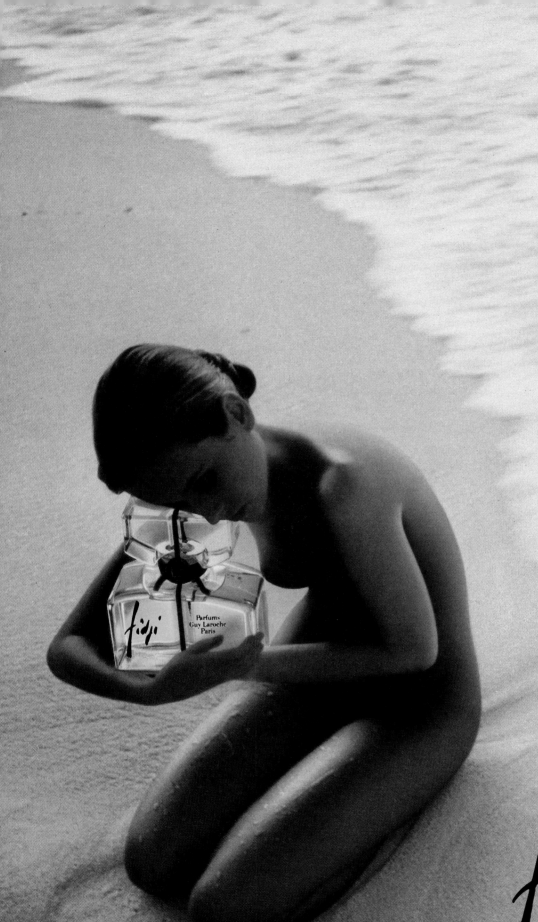

Guy Laroche

Paris

Fidji

La femme est une île,
Fidji est son parfum.

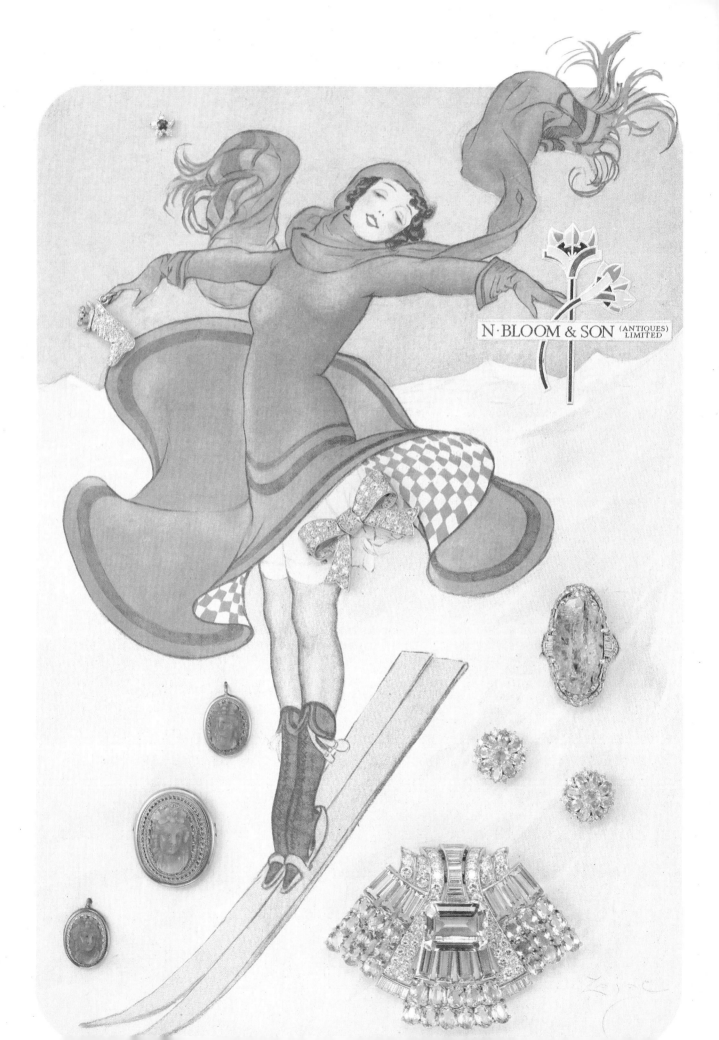

ACCESSORIES

To give THE CASTAWAY a tropical paradise effect, decorate any of the knots with blowsy fake exotic flowers in silk or organza or similar gauzy materials. Alternatively, create a different effect with chunky ethnic brooches in semi-precious stones, carved wood, silver or bronze, pinning them to the knots.

At your neck and ears, wear jewellery made from the things you'd find on the beach – seashells, seeds, coins, small bits of glass, or more precious items like coral or jade. Simple metallic bands will also look striking with a tan and this carefree clothing.

For belts, use lengths of fabric to create sashes, or scarves which work with the main fabric you've chosen for the garment in question. Use, too, double belting techniques described in THE INDIAN or THE GYPSY.

On your feet wear sandals. Let the form follow the function – if you are lounging by a pool choose styles which you can easily pop on and off; if you're about to be rescued and whisked off to the nearest party, choose something higher and jazzier, maybe decked with fruit, or created from metallic strips of leather. Ideally, avoid wearing tights. Fake tanned legs with instant tanning lotion or get the real thing.

Sunglasses are, of course, essential and can be as tame or as wild as you like. Straw hats complete the look – wear them as big as sombreros or as small as cloches, but don't forget to decorate them with a strip of fabric to match your clothes, a fake flower, or a string of seashells, or beads.

FACE AND HAIR

Make-up will be absolutely minimal if used at all – after all, with your gorgeous tan all you need is a lick of mascara on upper and lower lashes and maybe a dash of blue or green eyeliner to echo the colour of those deep lagoons, close to your lower lashes.

For styling hair, use any of the tricks established in working with wet hair. Twist, braid, or wrap it with rags for ringlets later. Secure it into a chignon or bun, tie it, pull it into a ponytail or two, anything to expose your beautifully healthy face. Hair too can be decorated like hats see *Accessories*.

Right: **The Castaway**'s pants and briefest halter top.

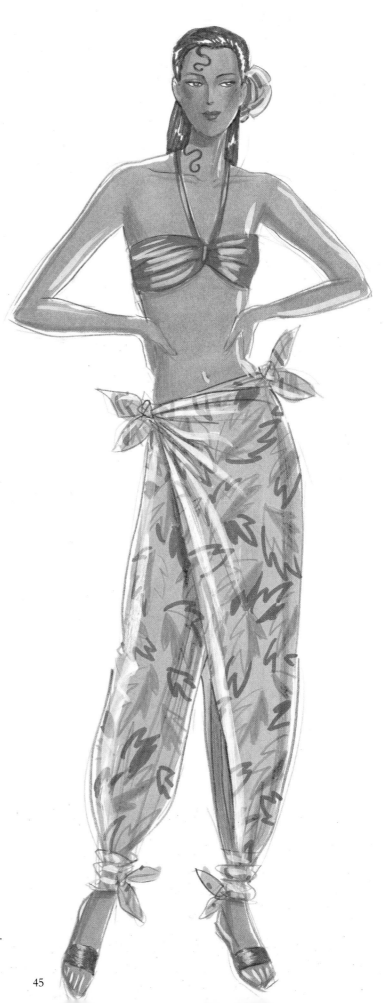

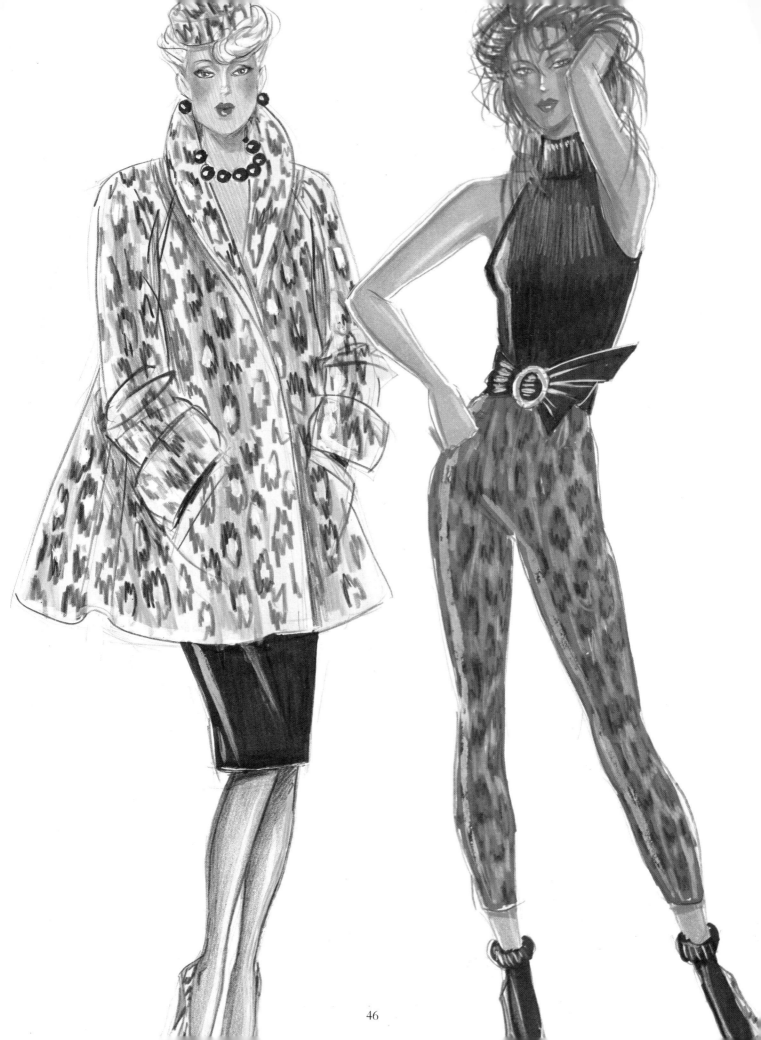

THE CAT WOMAN

BACKGROUND

Purr, stretch, scratch, claw. Become the feline huntress you secretly are. If one of your fantasies is to dress like a cat, don't hesitate. Although THE CAT WOMAN is not a look for the timid, it is very adaptable and easily-achieved – wear it discreetly by day or tease your victims with its seductive powers by night.

As a fashion style THE CAT WOMAN originally comes from the super hero characters of American comic books of the late Fifties. During the Sixties the immensely popular *Avengers* series on British television established a particularly slinky and deadly version of the look in the public's imagination. Most recently, cats have stolen the show in Andrew Lloyd Webber's hit musical *Cats*, based on T.S. Eliot's poems.

THE LOOK

More than any other look in this book, THE CAT WOMAN depends on style and temperament. It's no good being meek in cat's clothing. If you have got a streak of the huntress in you, whether it be jungle cat or alley prowler, then explore your nature with clothing printed with big feline patterns: leopard spots, tiger stripes, ocelot dots. This and accentuated cat-like eyes are the basic requirements of this look, and just one piece of clothing in any of these distinctive designs is enough to convey the idea. It is ideal for

cold weather because of the textures, but can also be pared down for summer.

Feline clothing – for human purposes – is of a furry or stretchy variety. Mix and match the two. For winter choose coats and sweaters in mohair, shag or fake fur. Under-sweaters, trousers and tights are best in black. Wear them tight and slinky if your figure allows. You can also find some wonderful crazy knits in synthetic fibre printed with cat's paw motifs or wild-game stripes; even if the stripes are zebra, the feline image is still successfully conveyed. The colour scheme of the big cats tends to be black or dark brown spots and stripes on buff or creamy ground, but they have very adventurous imitators – you'll find unusual combinations such as black stripes or spots on bright blue, yellow or red. If you like the look, amass the 'skins' in whatever colour combinations flatter you. They will usually co-ordinate with the more authentic colorations, adding a nice dash of kittenish fun.

By day prowl the streets in a fur coat. Not the luxury length and deep fur of the MOVIE STAR but the now classic, boxy-cut numbers of the Fifties and Sixties. These three-quarter or 'fingertip' length coats (as fashion writers of the time described them) came in ocelot, cheetah or leopard. You may still come across

Below: For instant effect, choose cat-printed accessories with leopard spots, ocelot dots and tiger stripes to set off plainer clothes. In terms of style, go for fifties' shapes such as high stiletto heels, wide belts, jangly jewellery and clutch bags.

a real fur from the period (before most of the big wild cats became protected species), but it is more ecologically sound to wear a good imitation. Look for a squarish shape with big, baggy sleeves and either large patch pockets or inset pockets; the collar should ideally be mandarin or Peter Pan and the fastening invisible or fur-covered buttons.

With your spotty coat wear basic black as the ladies of the Fifties did. Choose a 'little black dress' or black polo- or round-necked sweaters and a straight skirt. These items don't have to be period perfect; just remember that the essence is streamlining and an understated, downbeat slinkiness. Trousers likewise are stretch and look best just above the ankle.

Alternatively, be a little more daring. For example, wear white, off-white and camel-coloured clothes with the spotty coat; even add a dash of bright red. A skirt of fake fur, printed wool, cotton knit, or stretchy jersey, in any style from rara to pencil could match or co-ordinate with the jacket.

Below: An unmistakably leonine face is essential for **The Cat Woman.** To transform your own, see the instructions under *Face and Hair*.

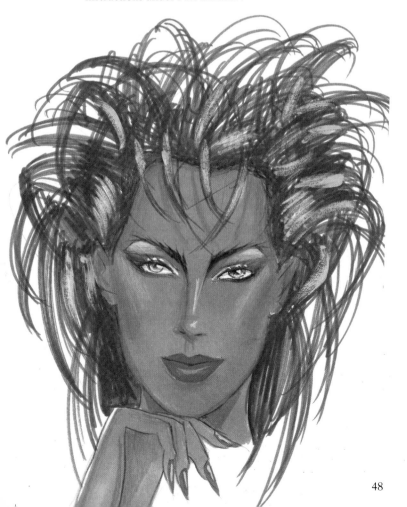

If you prefer to be a kitten rather than a wild cat opt for the softest and fluffiest sweaters around. They can be voluminous or fitted, in stretchy fabrics, in fine wool yarns such as mohair or angora, or in man-made alternatives. The top can be any style as long as it works with what you are wearing on your lower half, but if you do opt for a patterned sweater, wear a neutral colour below. Don't overdo a good thing.

For those of a predatory nature wear this look at night, vamped up for parties – a sort of Jungle Jane look. To achieve this, you need a lithe, tanned body and a sense of daring. The clothing is minimal: a short, one-shoulder sarong made of animal-motif-printed skins, (as the illustration shows) often found in off-beat designer shops. (See also *Ideas*). Team it with the highest heels or the barest sandals you can find and go out into the night and prowl.

Another way to achieve a party version of THE CAT WOMAN without the bother of sewing is to team a big-cat printed body stocking or leotard with a ultra-short black or neutral mini skirt and black or cat-printed shoes.

ACCESSORIES

There's no limit to cat-printed accessories. You'll be able to find everything you could possibly dream of – umbrellas, wallets, socks, shoes, jewellery, belts, bags, gloves, hats, all covered with spots or stripes. You'll find left-overs from the Fifties, cheap junk store imitations and wonderfully awful plastic articles printed with 'catty' skins. Collect them all.

Track down cat-printed shoes. They look marvellous with the plain neutral shades of more classic clothes and are a perfect finish to this look. Get them with high or flat heels – in court or sandal styles.

Choose sheer black stockings or the palest buff colour, unless your legs are nicely tanned. With more informal clothes, tiger socks look great with plain black shoes. Bags can match or co-ordinate, as can hats and belts, but don't overdo it. Avoid mixing too many patterns and too many colours.

If you like lots of jewellery, opt for simple gold pieces – thick armbands and chokers look just right.

A world of beauty lies at your fingertips when you train with . . .

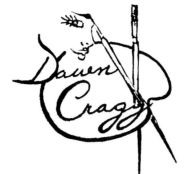

THE DAWN CRAGG SCHOOL OF FILM AND TV MAKE-UP, HAIR DESIGN AND WIGMAKING, ONE YEAR DIPLOMA COURSE.

THE PARK SCHOOL OF BEAUTY THERAPY — ONE YEAR, TWO TERM AND ONE TERM COURSES IN ALL ASPECTS OF FACIAL AND BODY TREATMENTS AND ELECTROLYSIS. ALL MAJOR INTERNATIONAL AND NATIONAL EXAMINATIONS CAN BE TAKEN.

INTERNATIONAL MAKE-UP ARTIST
STORCROFT HOUSE, LONDON ROAD, RETFORD, NOTTS, DN22 7EB, ENGLAND. TEL: 0777-707371

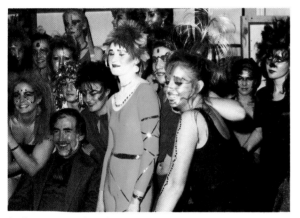

Students preparing for a show in fantasy make-up, under the direction of guest make-up artist Mario Montalvo from California, USA.

The only school in the world to offer the DAWN CRAGG DIPLOMA IN FILM AND TELEVISION MAKE-UP, HAIR DESIGN AND WIGMAKING. All aspects of make-up are covered including: Mannequin, Photographic, Fantasy, Body Painting, Character and Animal Make-Up. Film and Stage techniques include: taking impressions, making moulds, colouring latex pieces, making foam appliances (noses, chins, ears, limbs etc), the creation of a whole face from latex, ageing skin and hands, the design of wounds and scars, the use of theatrical blood and collodion, the making of bald caps, designing and making false teeth, etc. The students also study the history of the theatre, special lighting effects for photography and the stage, costume design, colour co-ordination and the hairdressing and head dress design. Wigmaking is taught with the co-operation of the local college of art, and students will take the City and Guilds examination in Wig-making. Artistic ability and a pleasing personality are considered to be of more importance on this course rather than high academic achievement.

INTERESTED? Then send us your name and address, and a postage stamp and we will send you full details by return.

An International and family run school, offering day or residential places to students from 16 years onwards. Both male and female students are accepted on most courses. The School has its own Self Catering Accommodation for older students, and also a Hall of Residence with a Matron and meals provided for younger students. Retford is only $1\frac{1}{2}$ hours direct by train from London King's Cross. The town has a sports centre, and riding facilities within a short distance from the School.

Students are accepted at the Park School from 16 years and courses range from one to three terms in length. The school is recognised by the principle independent Beauty Therapy examining boards and the school tutors will help to choose the examinations appropriate to the background personality and needs of the individual student. The school has a fully equipped beauty and hairdressing salon at which students are taught client care and reception duties as part of their course.

In addition to the main examination courses several specialist courses are held and there is a one term finishing course for young ladies, which includes deportment, grooming, advice for interviews, general etiquette, etc.

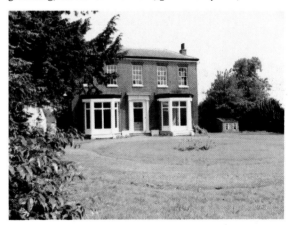

The School is housed in a beautiful Georgian building set in the heart of the Nottinghamshire countryside.

"If you don't have the foresight to train with DAWN CRAGG for the rest of your life you may wish that you had!"

PRINCIPAL: DAWN CRAGG **DIRECTOR OF STUDIES: JOHN M CRAGG**

FACE AND HAIR

Begin with a foundation and a light dusting of powder to match your own colouring. Then concentrate on the eyes: apply dark gold or khaki shadow to the lower lid, and a frosted gold just under the eyebrow. Use a dark grey or nearly brown shadow in the inner corner, bringing it up to the eyebrow, keeping it along the line of the nose. Next apply a very dark shadow in the outer corners and along the crease, bringing this up to the outer end of the brow and just along the outer edges of the lower lashes. Emphasize eyes even more with an application of black kohl pencil along the inside rim of the eye, keeping as close to the lashes as possible. Apply dark brown or black pencil to the eyebrow, keeping the shape very defined.

Give yourself high cheekbones with an application of tawny blusher just under the bones, and apply a dot of ivory highlighter to the tip of the nose to make it look as if it tilts up. Finally, outline lips with a brownish-pink shade, making the line well inside the natural shape as you want the lips to look as small as possible. Colour lips with a natural brownish pink lipstick. Hair can be as wild as you like – back-comb your entire head, spray with a soft-hold hair spray and leave it.

IDEAS

● Should you get carried away with big game, go all the way and replace buttons on sweaters and blouses with cat-printed ones. They may be covered in fake ocelot or plastic printed with tiger stripes. Use shanked ones to decorate the ends of long hair pins, as in THE DANDY.

● It is easy to make a sexy feline sarong. Purchase three or four pieces of inexpensive chamois; experiment with draping the skins to find out which are the best where; then sew them in place using an upholsterer's, or leather-worker's or similar heavy-duty needle, and string or thin leather shoelaces, etc. Never mind tidy seams and hems; your 'dress' should look primitive. When complete, wear it 'natural' with 'catty' accessories or paint on big cat stripes or spots with fabric leather dye.

Right: For the ultimate party look, create a feline sarong as suggested under *Ideas*. Finish the effect by wearing jewellery made in the primitive mode – using ivory, bone, feathers, leather and fur.

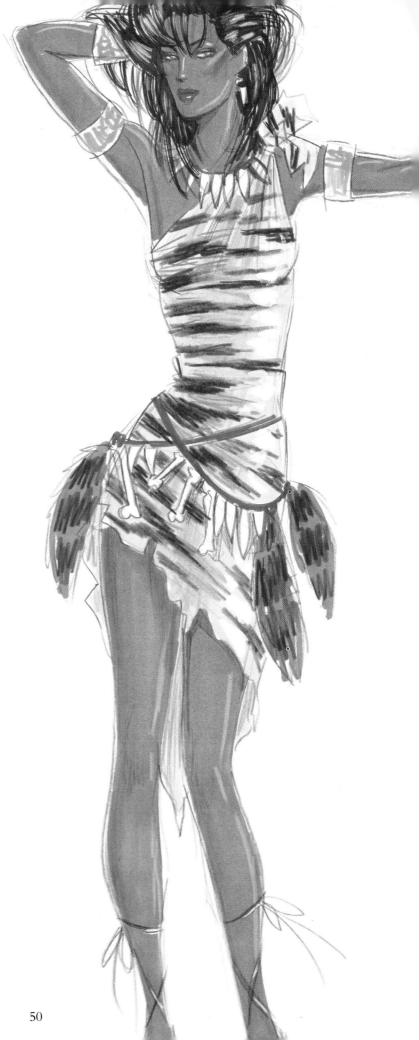

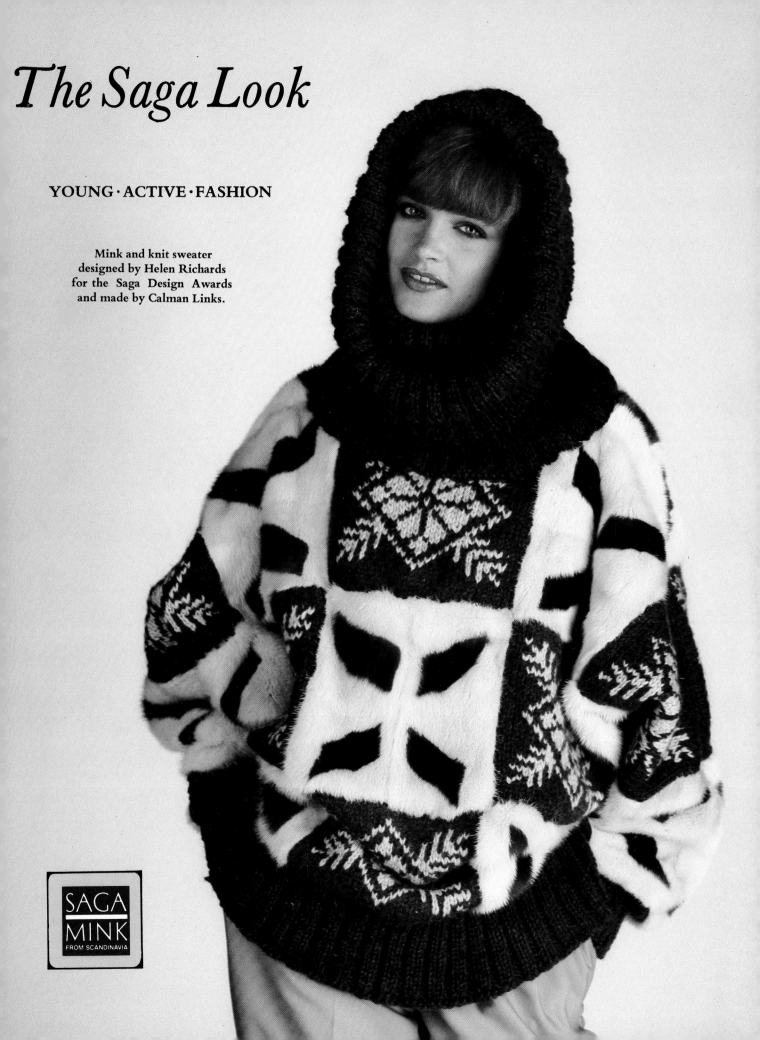

The Saga Look

YOUNG · ACTIVE · FASHION

Mink and knit sweater
designed by Helen Richards
for the Saga Design Awards
and made by Calman Links.

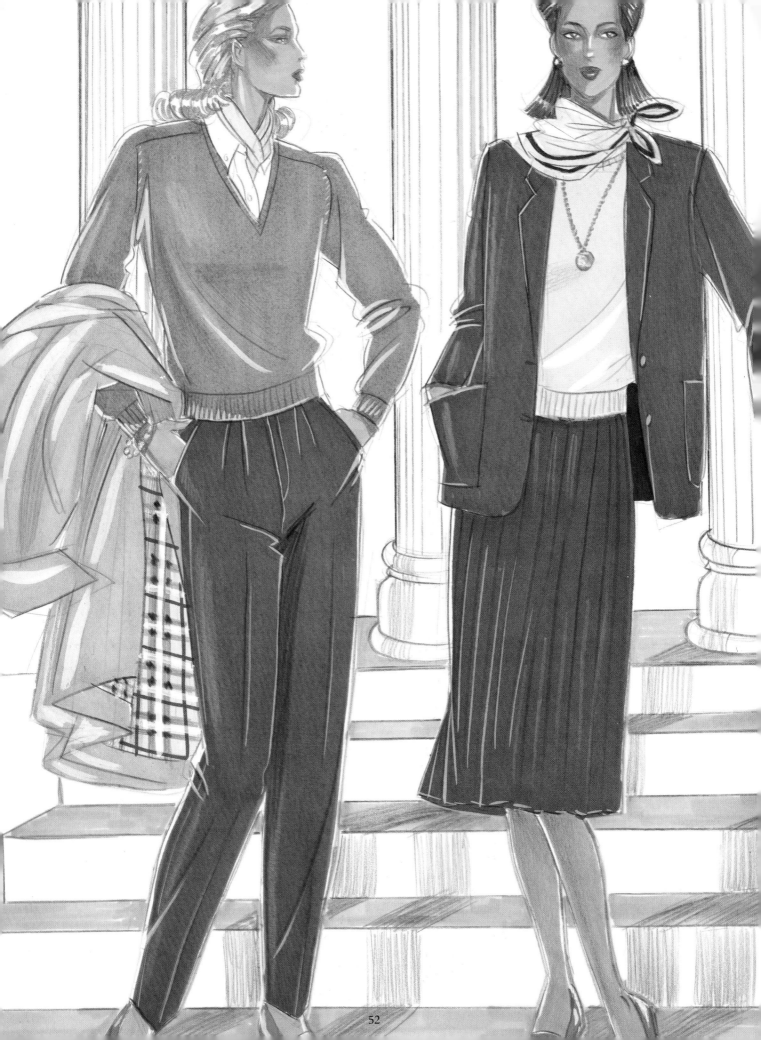

THE CLASSICIST

THE PREPPY GROWS UP

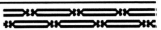

BACKGROUND

Take a stroll down London's elegant Bond Street, New York's fashionable Fifth Avenue or Paris's chic Faubourg St Honoré and see what the ladies who throng such thorough-fares have in common: all of them are Classicists.

The true CLASSICIST follows a well-defined code in her choice of cut, cloth and colour. The rules to which she adheres are generations old and it is more than likely that her mother and her grandmother followed them too.

THE LOOK

THE CLASSICIST aims for a well-groomed, elegant appearance – not over-formal but *never* scruffy. To achieve this, she bears the following factors in mind when choosing her wardrobe: the clothes which are the most classic are also those which are simple in style and barely affected by fashion's swinging pendulum; proportions rely on pure, uncluttered line, though lengths might change very slightly; cut is generous – never skimpy – and there are no petty economies on cloth.

Below: **The Classicist**'s accessories will always be the height of good taste – very well made with a minimum of ornament. Handbags will be clutch or shoulder styles, belts with plain buckles, shoes have sensible heels and jewellery is mainly gold, silver, or pearl.

Understatement is the order of the day; fuss and frills are not to be seen. Manufacture and finish are of the highest quality: linings are essential, seams and buttonholes are immaculate, hemlines even. Additionally, only the best natural fabrics are used: wools, worsteds, gabardine, linen, silk, cotton and of course, cashmere. Colours, too, are kept pure and simple; pattern is for the most part avoided. Neutrals – beige, cream, camel and so on – are the most favoured tones, closely followed by grey, navy and burgundy; brighter hues such as scarlet or emerald are used for accents. Such well-made clothes are expensive, but to THE CLASSICIST they are essential investments.

However, don't panic at the thought of such regulations, for the code is a basic one, and the resulting look has a great many advantages. Firstly, it is safe – as a way of dressing it is never out of place on any occasion; it may not be imaginative, but it will never be wrong. It is also totally international; a French or Italian Classicist would look and feel at home in New York and be virtually indistinguishable from her American counterpart. It is ageless, a look that can be

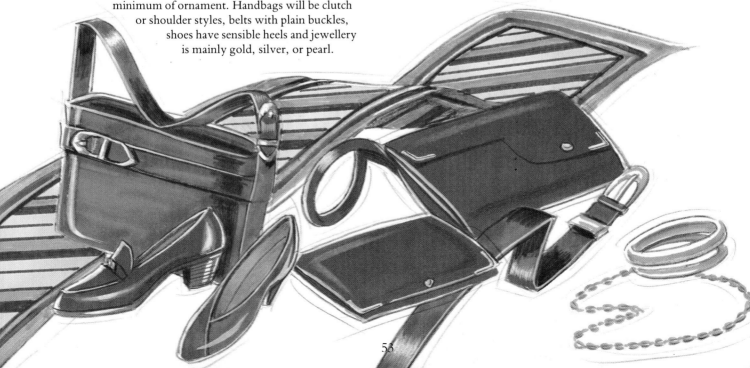

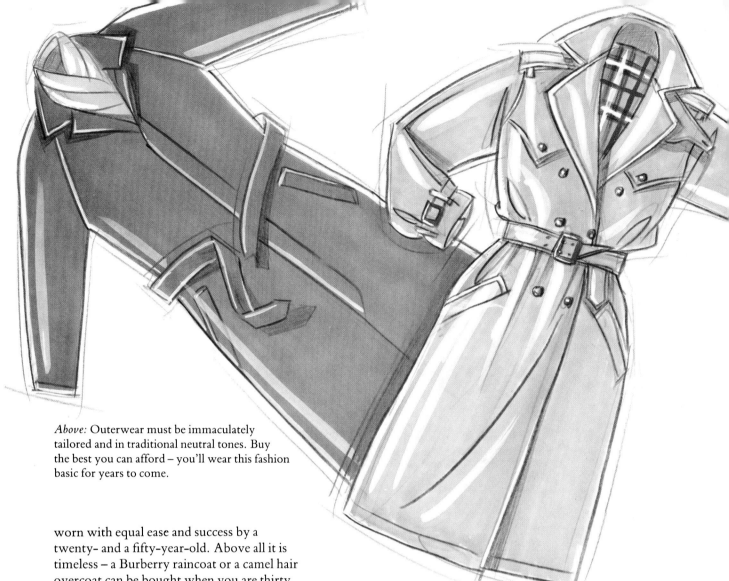

Above: Outerwear must be immaculately tailored and in traditional neutral tones. Buy the best you can afford – you'll wear this fashion basic for years to come.

worn with equal ease and success by a twenty- and a fifty-year-old. Above all it is timeless – a Burberry raincoat or a camel hair overcoat can be bought when you are thirty and worn for the following thirty years.

Choose separates for the components of the look. Beautifully-cut, French-style, gabardine or flannel wool trousers, gently pleated at the waist, or immaculately pleated skirts (narrow-pleated navy being *de rigeur*).

Shirts must also be tailored in style. Look for those made of silk or pure cotton in plain colours such as white, pink, blue or pale yellow, or those with thin stripes; collars and cuffs should be small and neat. Alternatively try a blouse with a soft bow tie at the neck or a striped shirt with white collar and cuffs.

In an ideal world, all THE CLASSICIST's sweaters would be made of cashmere; a cashmere and wool mix or those in the softest lambswool are good alternatives. Again, choose unadorned styles polo-necked, round-necked or V-necked – in colours which match or co-ordinate with skirts and trousers. THE LADY's twin-set is also suitable, as is the longer hip-length cardigan from THE OCEAN VOYAGER.

A suit is ideal for more formal daytime events. Opt for a navy, grey or burgundy blazer for all the year round, perhaps oatmeal or beige shantung silk for warmer days. Jackets and skirts can match or co-ordinate. Alternatively, the shirtwaist dress, beloved by THE LADY and THE DEBUTANTE, will fit THE CLASSICIST's bill admirably.

For outerwear choose either a Burberry raincoat (or a well-made copy), a classic camel coat or a blazer. The trench coat shape of the raincoat epitomizes THE CLASSICIST's principles of a neat but chic appearance. Wear it over every outfit from informal trousers and sweater to the smartest silk shirtwaister dress. On days too cold for the raincoat, choose a camel coat in either a wrap-around style with tie belt, or with single- or double-breasted buttons shape. A blazer in worsted or velvet is an extraordinarily useful garment to wear over all the THE CLASSICIST's clothes on warmer days and more formal indoor occasions in place of a jumper or cardigan.

Jemima Jones
B Nº 27509
Eaton Square
London SW1
Red Patterned
Silk Kimono

Jemima Jones
B Nº 27538
Eaton Square
London SW1
Black Satin
Jumpsuit

Jerome Jones
B Nº 27566
Eaton Square
London SW1
Cream
Linen
Suit.

Jemima Jones
B Nº 27534
Eaton Square
London SW1
Green
Embroidered
Kaftan.

Jerome Jones
B Nº 27517
Eaton Square
London SW1
Khaki
Safari
Suit.

Jemima and
Jerome
Jones
B Nº 27524
Eaton Square London SW1
2 Blue and Red
Towelling
Track Suits.

In January, June and July, Jerome and Jemima Jumped Jets to Japan, Jived in Jamaica, Jazzed it up in Java, Joked in Jerricho, Juggled in the Jungle and then Jogged back to JEEVES!

Jeeves Valet Shop Hand finished dry cleaning
Jeeves Laundry Shop Shirt and fine linen service
Jeeves Snob Shop Fine quality shoe menders

LONDON NEW YORK

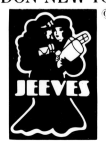

Jeeves Valet Shop
8 & 10 Pont Street
Belgravia
SW1.
Tel: 235 1101

Jeeves Snob Shop
7 Pont Street
Belgravia
SW1.
Tel: 235 1101

Jeeves Laundry Shop
9 Pont Street
Belgravia
SW1.
Tel: 235 1101

Jeeves Hampstead Shop
11 Heath Street
Hampstead
NW3.
Tel: 794 4100

Jeeves Marble Arch Shop
59 Connaught Street
Marble arch
W2.
Tel: 262 0200

Jeeves Mayfair Shop
54 South Audley Street
Mayfair
W1.
Tel: 491 8885

© 1974 Jeeves of Belgravia Limited Jeeves Logotype is a trademark

ACCESSORIES

If you have just inherited a small fortune, pop into Gucci, Hermès, Céline or Louis Vuitton and buy all your 'classic' accessories in one sweep! These are the luxurious establishments where the international Classicists acquire all their acroutrements: shoes, bags, belts, headscarves plus little niceties from keyrings to wallets, each item emblazoned with the logo and the colours of the house.

You may not, however, be attracted to the status symbol angle of such accessories. In that case, simply emulate the styling and perfect finish of the big names. Shoes must be restrained: court-shoes or moccasins in plain colours with medium heels, perhaps with some sort of subtle decoration – usually a gold snaffle, buckle or chain apparatus or a striped band emulating the Gucci stripe. Boots follow the same restrictions: plain, simple and no snazz. Neutral or navy tights are THE CLASSICIST's staple choice of legwear.

Bags should match your shoes (and gloves). Look for a small, neat shape with a well-finished shoulder strap; or try the thinner envelope shape in navy or black with a long, gold chain. Similarly, well-made and matching belts add to the well-groomed look. Look for narrow styles with a gold clasp or detailing to match those on your shoes or handbag.

As the final touch, most Classicists have a drawer full of silk scarves in all sizes. Indeed, this square of silk is often the only place for pattern and brighter colours. Once again, use the Gucci or Hermès originals as inspiration and choose those scarves with a wide, plain-coloured border and a pattern or design in the middle. See *Ideas* for hints on ways to integrate this silk square into your outfit.

Jewellery is discreet and always genuine, preferably gold, which, of course, works well with all the other gold accents on your accessories. Wear several chains of different lengths around your neck, or choose a plain pendant, locket or fob watch on a long gold chain. Alternatively, bring out your pearls. Add a couple of gold chain bracelets, or a ring and earrings, plus the essential gold wrist watch.

FACE AND HAIR

For a flawless finish, choose a cream-coloured foundation, followed by a dusting of loose powder. Subtly shadow eyes in a pearly soft stone shade over the lower lid, blending into a soft shell or off-white colour under the brow. For just a little more definition, you might add a touch of navy blue or grey liner in the outer corner of the lower lid and into the crease line; bring this also just under the lower lashes. Use soft dusty pink blusher on the cheeks and a rosy lipstick to give the mouth a slight colour.

IDEAS

● Tie your silk scarf as you like: around the head with a knot tied under the chin; as a cravat tucked inside a shirt collar or sweater neck; folded on the diagonal and worn over sweaters with the knot at the side; tied in a knot on the handle of your bag.

● If designer silk squares seem outrageously expensive, opt for acetate or polyester imitations in classic colours or look for silk remnants. Make sure the remnant is square, then hand roll and hem the edges with tiny stitches for your own version of the classy scarf.

Below: Ways with a triangular scarf or square scarf folded on the diagonal: over the head with a knot under or on the chin; tied at the nape for a soft effect under blouses and/or sweaters; around the neck over a plain sweater with knot worn at the side; and tied onto a handle of your bag.

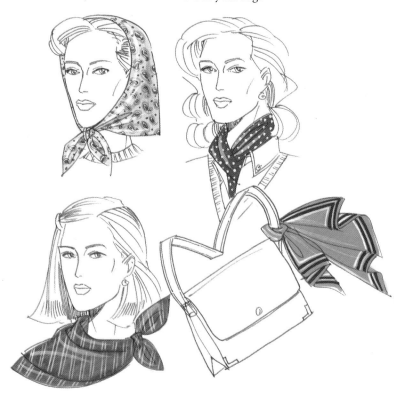

CRS

Who tried to shave closer than the Philips Ladyshave?

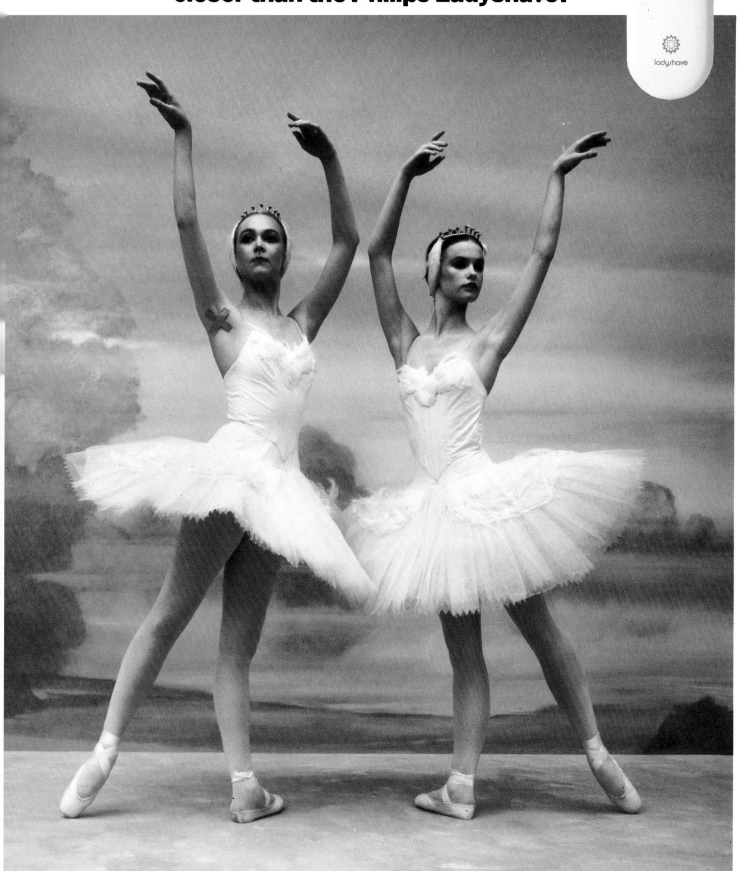

It seems silly to use a razor with all its snags. Especially since the Philips Ladyshave now leaves your delicate skin as smooth as you could possibly wish.
Any closer could be too close for comfort. **The Philips Ladyshave. The smoothest Ladyshave yet.**

 PHILIPS

PHILIPS

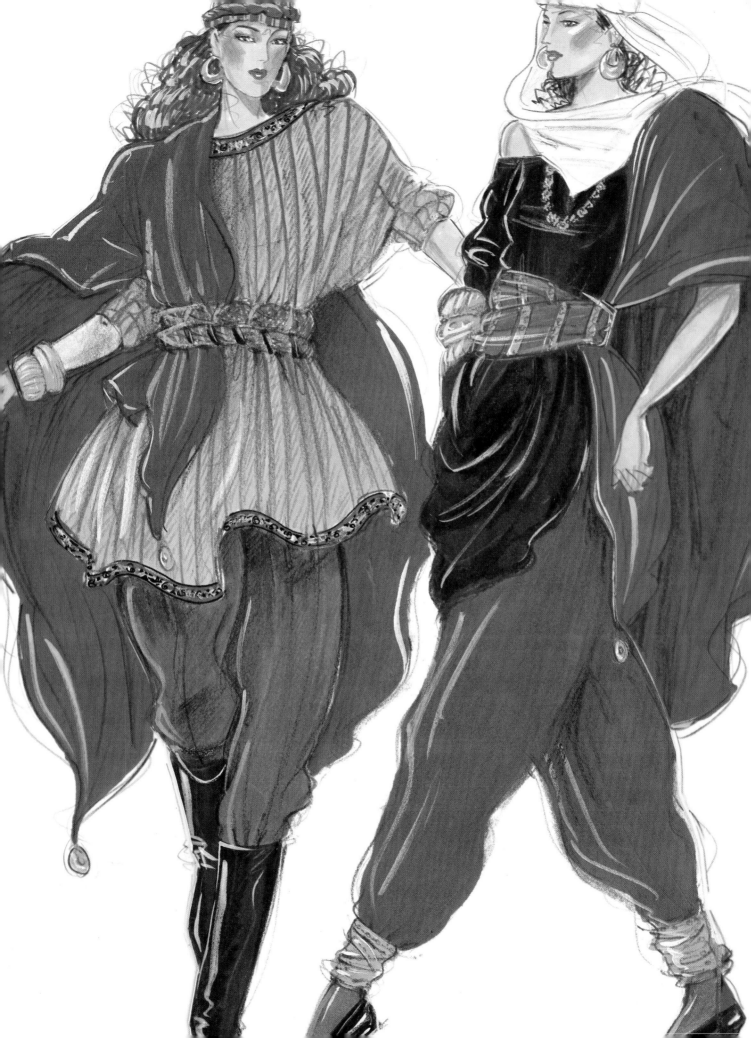

THE COSSACK

BACKGROUND

THE COSSACK comes straight from the windswept steppes of Russia. The landscape is vast and dramatic, the winter long and bitter, and the clothing reflects both. The Slavs are an expansive people: their garments dramatic in lush, rich colourings and bright embroidery against backgrounds of browns and blacks.

THE COSSACK is an intensely romantic look despite its practicality. It comes to the West via such films as *Anna Karenina* with Greta Garbo swathed in long furs, and *Dr Zhivago* with its careful reproduction of period and national detail. But a more exotic, theatrical version of the look has been beloved in Europe since the early years of this century when Diaghilev brought his Ballets Russes to Paris. Although wildly romantic, it is also supremely wearable for every day. Its layered effect, however, is most effective as winter wear.

THE LOOK

For the day choose skirts that are gathered or softly pleated from a wide waistband in thick woven fabrics like challis and wool, brushed cotton and felt; corduroy is not so effective but if soft and the skirt generously cut it can work too. Trousers are likewise cut for volume, although fabrics will have to be lighter than for the skirt to ensure free-flowing lines – materials with a small percentage of synthetic fibre in them, such as cotton viscose, work well.

The most characteristic garment is the cossack shirt. This is full and generously cut, with voluminous sleeves ending in a small buttoned cuff. It has a neat stand-up collar fastened by a row of buttons running at an angle from the collar down the side of the shoulder. These blouses can be worn by day

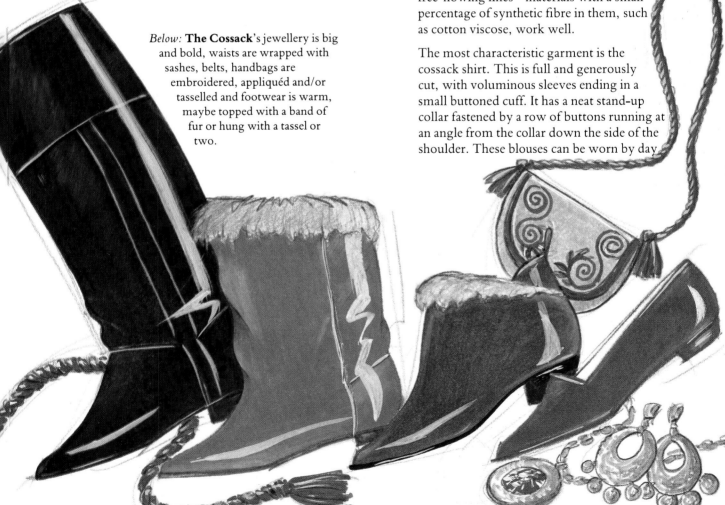

Below: **The Cossack**'s jewellery is big and bold, waists are wrapped with sashes, belts, handbags are embroidered, appliquéd and/or tasselled and footwear is warm, maybe topped with a band of fur or hung with a tassel or two.

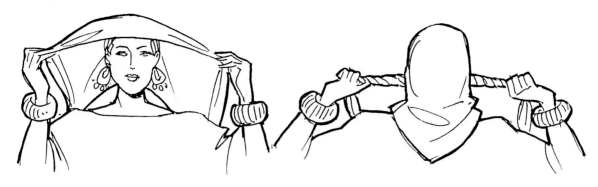

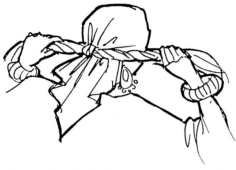

Make a turban by folding a large (24 ins/61 cms) square of fabric on the diagonal and centre the long end over your forehead. Twist the ends in back and bring them forward to tie in front, or even better, take another length of twisted fabric, place that on top of the first square. Take both ends to your nape, knot and bring them around again if long enough.

and by night, for the business meeting or the dinner party, to lunch or a dance, and can be in any supple fabric from brushed cotton to silk, wool or satin.

Over this billowing garment wear a box-cut waistcoat, embroidered or plain, in fabric or leather. Alternatively add another layer for extra warmth in the shape of a tunic, sleeveless, cap-sleeved or with three-quarter length, straight wide sleeves, under which the contrasting cuffs of your blouse can peep out.

Coats and jackets can be loose or fitted but look best when securely belted. Fur trimming on cuffs and hem is, of course, perfect. Add a large fur or fur-edged hat to go with the coat. For a final layer add a huge shawl – even two – in fine wool, challis, paisley or even suede. Wrap it around and around your shoulders right up to your nose for a romantic but mysterious look or, for a more practical effect, cross it over in front and tuck the ends firmly into your belt – as shown in the illustration. (See also THE GYPSY.)

The variations to this look are many, since the essence is layering. Always choose sensuous materials and flowing lines, fabrics that drape and envelop; nothing should create a rigid form or sharp edge. For evening the style is identical, but there are fewer layers and the materials are suitably special – satins, silks and velvets with brocade and rich embroidery.

Allow your imagination to range when thinking of embroidery (see *Ideas*). The overall effect should be a riot of glorious colour.

ACCESSORIES
Boots are THE COSSACK's most essential accessories. They can have flat or high heels, depending on the occasion, but they should be wide enough at the top to enable you to tuck

Right: Lengths of fabric or scarves can be twisted into rolls and bound with satin cording to make belts, head-bands, ties, or turbans.

Right: Two ways of wrapping your head regardless of the length of your hair.

trousers in and have baggy folding ankles. Ideally, they'd be of lush suede or leather in colours such as burgundy and emerald.

Your handbag should be large and squashy, similarly in leather or suede or even go for a carpet bag. Or choose a luxurious embroidered or braid-trimmed pouch or shoulder bag.

Belts can be made from an assortment of materials, and are ideally composed of two layers – first, a wide cummerbund of scarves, remnants, lengths of hide, indeed anything which will wrap your waist once or twice. Over the top, tie leather thongs, ribbons, satin curtain cording, braiding, in fact any thin binding material to hold the cummerbund in place. (See below for specific instructions.)

Jewellery should be intricate yet bold: chunky metallic pieces inlaid with semi-precious or imitation stones. Chains can be hung with oriental medallions, or perhaps a scent bottle filled with an essence such as jasmine.

Hair ornamentation is a must. Cover your locks with a fur-trimmed hat or a headscarf with folksy designs. Tie the scarf as the illustration shows, ornamenting it if you like as suggested in *Ideas* below. Alternatively, roll a scarf or remnant into a headband and wear it around the crown of your head or over your ears. As a final touch of ornament, thread a few beads on to a lock of your hair or wrap a strand or two at the front with some bright embroidery silk. The ultimate accessory for THE COSSACK is the fur muff.

FACE AND HAIR
Hair should be worn free, decorated or coaxed into waves with rag curls as in THE IMMIGRANT. Making up requires a little effort if the correct, smoky, oriental eyes are to be achieved. Follow the instructions for applying

eye shadow in THE VAMP, but use colours such as burnt orange, russet, deep mauve or steel blues. Define eyes with a line of kohl pencil along the inner rims, as close to the lashes as possible. Emphasize cheeks with a wine or sienna blusher under the bones to imitate high oriental cheekbones. Gloss lips in a deep burgundy or bronzed orange.

IDEAS
● Use leather thongs, thin belts, strips of suede, satin curtain cording, braiding or bindings to decorate the cummerbunds and headbands. Twist two of these strips together, plait three or twine them as the illustration shows. Knot the ends in together with the fabric they bind, then knot as required at your waist or at the back or side of your head.

● Trim knitted accessories with a band of fake or real fur.

● Use flowery embroidered tapes to trim cuffs of blouses, edges of pockets, hems, etc.

Below: Bold and brassy necklace made from eight brass curtain rings and a length of satin cording. Make two or three to co-ordinate with your **Cossack** clothes.

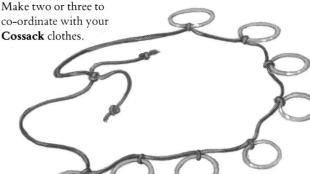

61

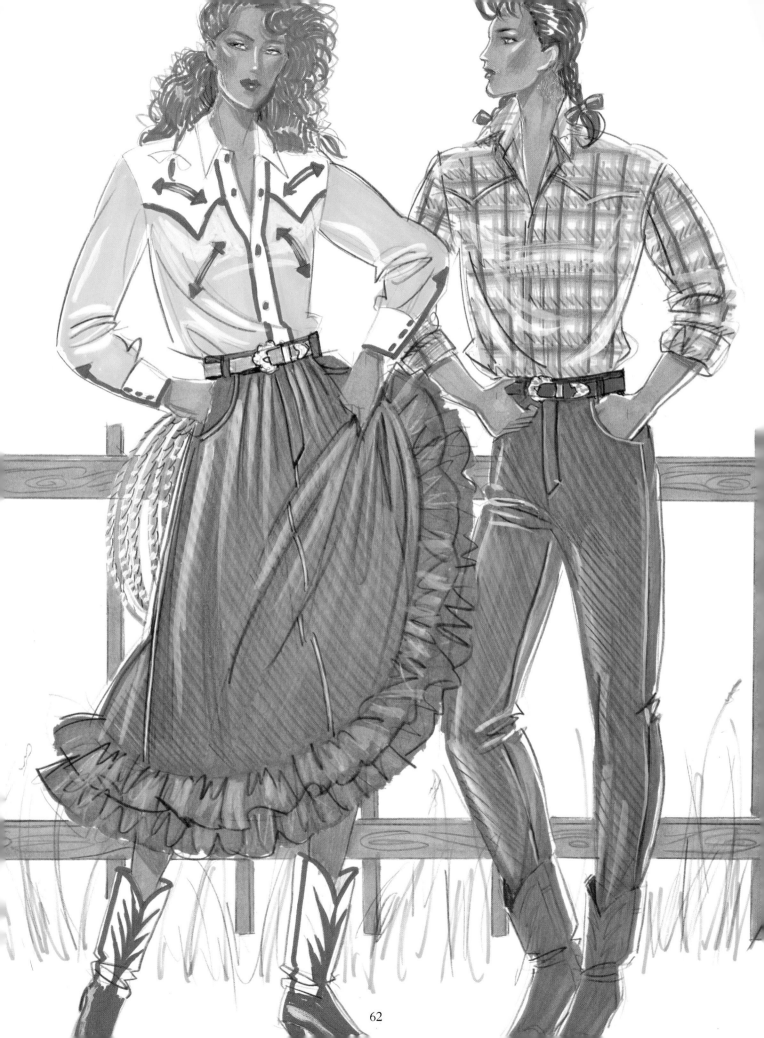

THE COWGIRL

BACKGROUND

Ride wild horses or the downtown bus in this eternally fashionable look. Born on the backs of men who drove immense herds of cattle across hundreds of dusty miles to the meat markets of mid-America, the rugged romance of this 'uniform' of the range and the Hollywood Western has captured the imagination of recent generations and spread like wildfire during the last few decades. Today, denim jeans are a global currency and the basis of the cowgirl look. Their popularity comes as no surprise when you consider the hard-wearing practicality of denim – made to be worn in the saddle for weeks on end, it is the only natural-fibre fabric which can be washed in the hottest tub, dried in the scorching sun and worn with no ironing at all.

THE LOOK

There are two versions of the cowgirl look. The authentic version consists of blue denim jeans, warm, long-sleeved shirts and the sensible boot with the two- to three-inch heel that is designed to stay in the stirrup. But with the advent of Dolly Parton the cowgirl has gone slick. Country-and-western singers and their fans wear their jeans lavishly embroidered and studded with rhinestones. Top designers (like Ralph Lauren and Calvin Klein) have followed suit in their attempt to get in on the action and bring the ubiquitous blue jean up-market into the realms of *haute couture*. Their particular personalization touch is usually to slap their signature across the back pocket – and then treble the price. Other fashion variations include different coloured denims, knee patches and fancy stitching. But when all is said and done there's nothing like a good-fitting pair of well-worn blue denim jeans.

Everyone's wardrobe should have a pair of the original blues, but since the basic design is such a perfect example of functional form – with its sturdy double seaming, sensible fastenings and extensive range of styles and

Below: Home on the range requires several specific accessories: cowboy boots, tall or small, plain cow-hide or beautifully appliquéd; a silver-decorated belt, maybe with some turquoise too; gauntlet-style, fringed gloves; a lariat and, of course, a cowboy hat.

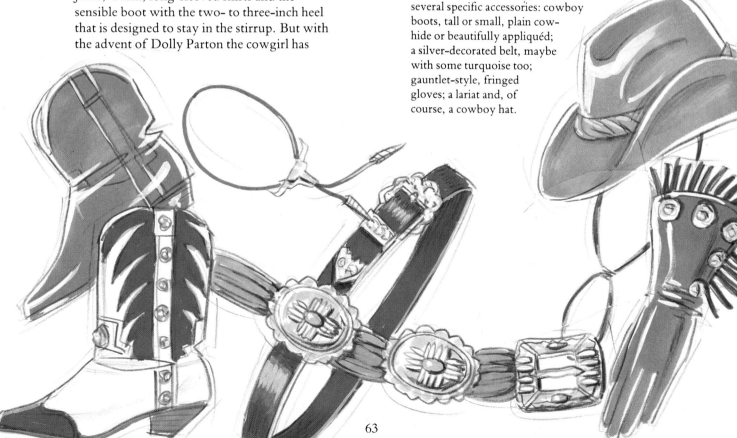

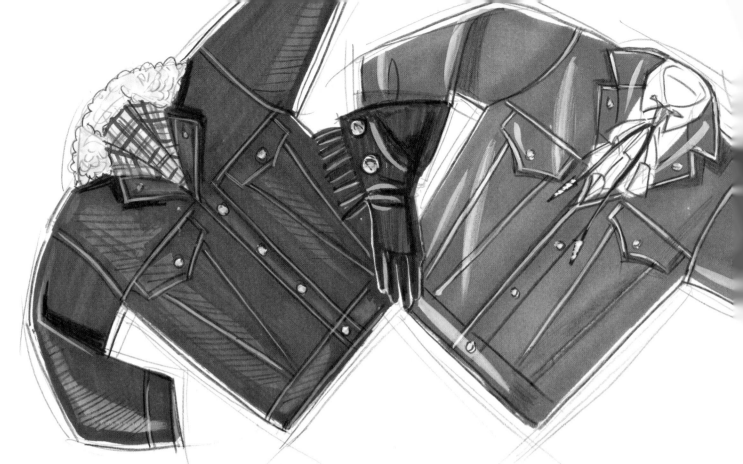

sizes – there is no reason why you shouldn't have several pairs of jeans in various fabrics and styles. Everything and more has been done to the blue jean since its birth. The traditional yellow stitching has been replaced by white, red, even green; the blue denim has been stone-washed, bleached, over-dyed or faded; and you can find the same wonderful design has been replicated in corduroy, wool, cotton, cire – be they bell-bottomed, baggy-topped, straight-legged or drainpipes.

Apart from jeans, denim has been made into virtually every type of garment imaginable – mini-skirts, longer, flounced skirts, dresses, waistcoats, and of course, jackets. The range of denim outerwear starts with the simple waistcoat – sometimes fleece- or flannel-lined for warmth – proceeds to the short-waisted long-sleeved jacket with the traditional copper-coloured fastening buttons, and ends with the hip-length blouson jacket sometimes patch-pocketed and accented with corduroy or leather collars, cuffs and elbow patches. The jacket, like the jeans, is a wonderful classic, and you'll find that you wear it with more than just jeans.

For winter, wear thick warm woollen sweaters with your denims; for summer, switch to short denim skirts or pastel cotton jeans. For authenticity, wear denims with plain or plaid shirts with Western details such

Above: To keep out the prairie winds, **Cowgirls** have few choices: a denim jacket with or without a flannel lining *or* a corduroy or suede jacket, ideally with characteristic top-stitching, yoke pockets and maybe lined with plaid or sheepskin.

as pearl-topped snap fasteners, a V-yoke in front, swirly embroidery, deep cuffs and pointed collars. Wear these shirts tucked into jeans or skirts of any style topped by a denim jacket or larger denim shirt. You can of course wear denims with Shetland sweaters and tennis shoes, but for an authentic cowgirl look, go the whole hog and add cowboy boots and range-riding accessories.

ACCESSORIES
Boots are essential to this look, and far from being a frivolous extra they can become a staple worn with other rough-and-ready styles like THE AMERICAN INDIAN, THE FAIR ISLANDER, THE HORSEWOMAN, THE GYPSY and THE OUTDOOR GIRL. Cowboy boots come in several lengths, dozens of colours and at any price – you can pay hundreds of pounds for a hand-made, heavily appliquéd pair, or well under £100 for a fascimile from Spain. For starters, try a tan pair with the characteristic highish heel and a little top-stitching. (Boots which are leather-lined are best for comfort and warmth.) Get a silver-buckled belt to

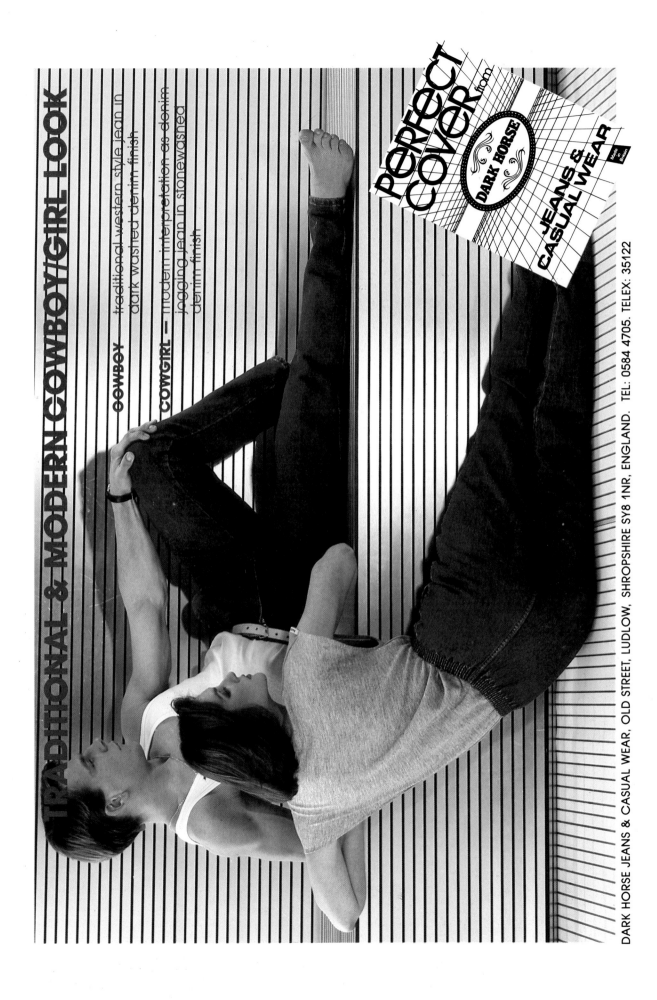

TRADITIONAL & MODERN COWBOY/GIRL LOOK

COWBOY — traditional western style jean in dark washed denim finish

COWGIRL — modern interpretation as denim jogging jean in stonewashed denim finish

PERFECT COVER from DARK HORSE

JEANS & CASUAL WEAR

match or co-ordinate. If you discover that you love this way of dressing, buy a more ornate pair of boots and matching belt later. Cowboy boots can be worn with skirts of any length and trousers can be worn outside the boot or tucked in.

Wear a top-stitched and/or tooled leather silver-buckled belt at the waist of jeans and skirts, or loosely on top of over-shirts, or around your hips holster-style. Wear two or three belts if you like, at various levels about your hips.

Unless you opt for the glittery country-and-western singing star look, avoid too much jewellery. At your neck, wear a lariat (thin satiny strands with silver pointed ends and a centre clasp) or a bandana, red or blue polka-dotted or with a white paisley design tied choker-style. (These same red or blue kerchiefs will also double as small handbags. Tie opposite corners together and wrap up your belongings.)

In cold weather, wear gauntlet-style gloves. These are often found with deep-fringed cuffs and etched silver decorations – they look great and because of their length are warm and practical. If you tend to carry a lot of gear around with you, use tooled saddle or shoulder bags or cheaper, softer versions in denim, suede or canvas.

Should you get completely carried away with your cowgirl image, you can buy chaps to protect your legs from the sagebrush. Usually in buff-coloured suede or leather, often with silver detailing, they are expensive and only for real devotees. As a final touch add a cowboy hat.

FACE AND HAIR
Wear an absolute minimum of make-up unless you're after the Dolly Parton gloss-

and-glitter style. A slight suntan and rosy cheeks are ideal – apply a little blusher across the bridge of the nose for a sun-kissed look. Wear hair in plaits or ringlets – see THE AMERICAN INDIAN for ideas with plaits, THE IMMIGRANT for making rag curls. Use twisted bandanas or leather strips to keep the hair out of your eyes – see instructions below.

IDEAS
● Pin on a cheap sheriff's badge from a toy store for a touch of authentic fun.

● Fold a bandana diagonally, then roll into a rope twist, and tie around neck or forehead, leaving the ends free. If you have two bandanas, or a complementary length of fabric, twist the two rolled fabrics together and knot.

● Sew suede or leather elbow patches to worn-out areas of shirts, trousers and jackets. Use thick thread such as buttonhole thread and a large-eyed needle to make the job easier.

● Twist leather thongs or shoelaces together for belts and headbands – you could even wrap a twisted bandana with the leather thong to secure the twists.

Below: For a few inexpensive finishing touches, wear a bandana in traditional red, navy or any of the newer shades and a cheap sheriff's badge as suggested in *Ideas* above. For a quick headband, roll the bandana along the diagonal, wrap it with a leather shoelace, and tie it around your forehead.

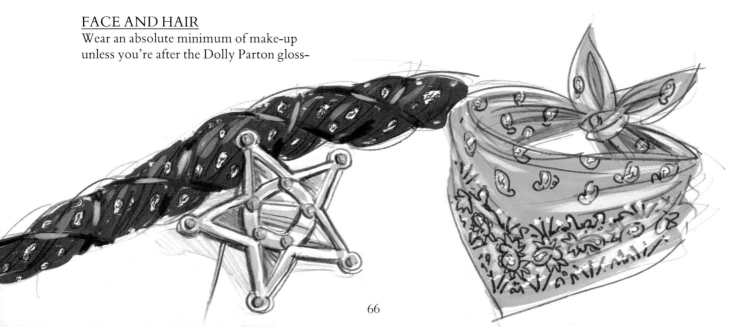

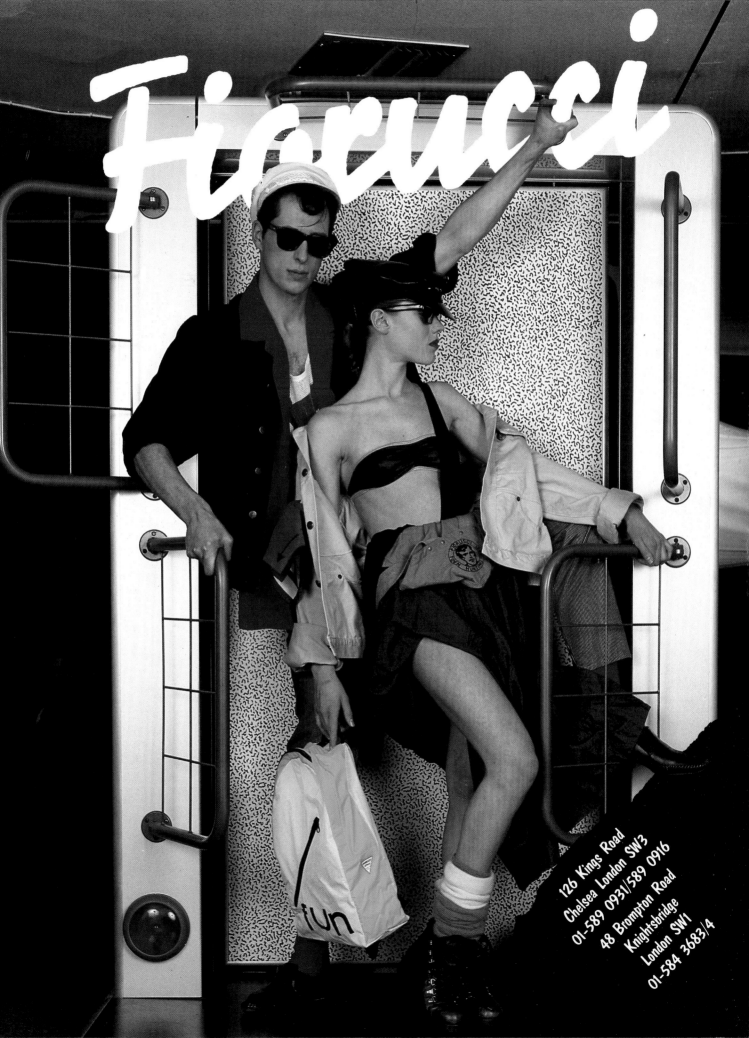

Fiorucci

126 Kings Road
Chelsea London SW3
01-589 0931/589 0916
48 Brompton Road
Knightsbridge
London SW1
01-584 3683/4

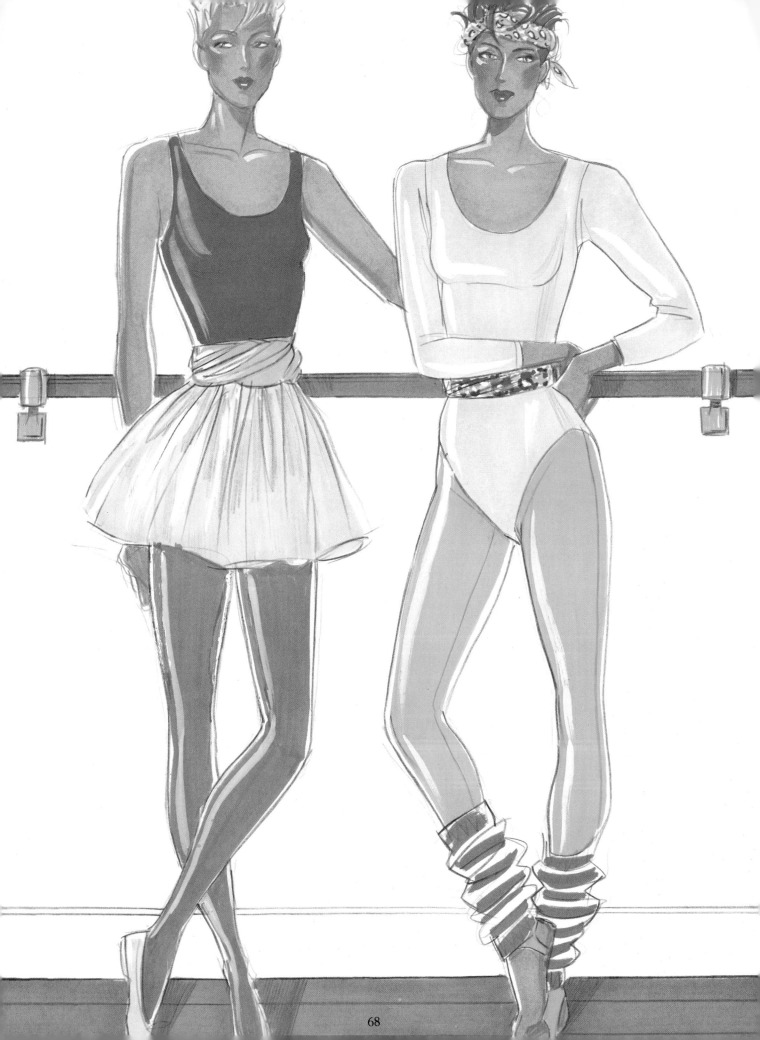

THE DANCER

BACKGROUND

When Jane Fonda published her *Workout Book* she gave the ultimate boost to the keep-fit craze which began round about the mid-Seventies when thousands of young and old took to the streets to jog their way to health and fitness. Our cities are now alive with the neon brightness of peppermint greens and electric blues, of shocking pinks and blazing yellows – colours which epitomize energy, movement, fun and a new physical awareness.

THE LOOK

The clothes for THE DANCER are primarily functional and made for comfort rather than to show off a pretty figure or disguise an unfashionable one. The basic component of this look, the leotard, is the ultimate figure-hugging garment and should not be worn on its own by those without the streamlined figure that it was designed for. However, the rest of the gear that goes to create THE DANCER is wonderfully loose and comfortable and ideal for a casual, active lifestyle. Furthermore since fitness has

Below: There are very few accessories which typify **The Dancer**, except, of course, ballet slippers, tap shoes and ballroom pumps. However, any flat style will do for street wear. For the studio, choose leg warmers in plain shades or zappy patterns.

become so socially desirable, dance clothes can be worn almost anywhere and for almost every informal occasion from doing the shopping to prancing at discos and parties. To dress like THE DANCER, begin with a leotard. They're in eternally stretchy synthetic fabrics such as lycra, sometimes shiny, sometimes matt. Usually plain, occasionally patterned and always available in dozens of wonderful colours. They come sleeveless, long or cap-sleeved, scoop-necked or high-necked, even one-shouldered and backless, and you can find them anywhere from bona fide dance shops to inexpensive boutiques. Collect leotards for their other uses also: the sleeved version is a first layer under other outfits; the sleeveless one doubles as a one-piece bathing suit. Experiment with different colours and patterns.

With the leotard, wear tights, sometimes called leggings. Traditionally, they are footless or have a stirrup for the dancer's instep, but if you're not wearing them for dancing, this is not so important. The only requisite is that the fabric is not too sheer and will withstand a fair amount of activity – lycra and similar synthetics are ideal, but any opaque, stretchy material will do. Don't hesitate to have several pairs as they are a wardrobe essential and can be incorporated into many of the other looks. Colourwise, tights can either match or co-ordinate with the leotard. Off-beat colour combinations such as hot pink with bright blue or clear red with violet are quite in keeping.

As an alternative to the two-piece leotard and tights combination, there is the one-piece

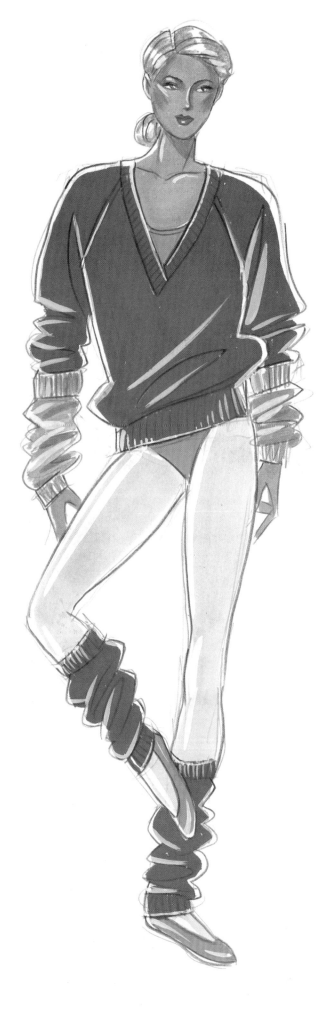

body stocking. The disadvantage is that when it's damaged, you have to toss the entire thing away but they are ideal with *really* short skirts.

On top of this underlayer, you have several alternatives. If the weather is warm, choose a short, floppy skirt – make it rara style or cut on the bias; even an old mini will do. Again, be imaginative: the skirt can match or contrast with the underlayer. Professional short skirts come in the same stretch fabrics as leotards, but are also found in stretchy cotton and acrylic knits. The other outer layer – every dancer's staple in fact – is a pair of jogging pants with elasticated cuffs and a drawstring waist (see THE SPORTSWOMAN).

When the weather is cold, add a big chunky sweater (mohair and bouclé yarns provide a nice contrast to the smooth texture of tights and leotards) on top of the underlayer (a very popular solution in dance studios during chilly spells). The sweater ought to be a generous fit and thigh-length, but no longer as it would restrict movement.

Alternatively, the traditional dancer's wrap-around cardigan looks pretty with the leotard combination. This has a deep V-neck, comes just to the waist and has long knitted tabs that tie in front. Since it is fitted, it looks best with a skirt rather than jogging pants.

Leg warmers provide warmth for legs and are a vital part of this look. Wear them like knee socks, or pulled over the knee over tights, bare legs or trousers. They should co-ordinate with some part of your ensemble.

ACCESSORIES
With such a fun and youthful look as THE DANCER, accessories are really secondary, although they can add a stamp of individuality.

Footwear is probably the most important. For shoes, choose flat ballet-type slippers or lace-up ghillies. Running or tennis shoes can also be worn with this look – in pastels or bright colours rather than stark white. Socks can be ankle- or knee-length, but ought to be fairly thick knit. Wear them rolled down around the ankle or pulled up to the knee. Leg warmers are worn over socks or over tights, when the weather's cold. Layer as much as you like.

Left: Leg warmers worn as arm warmers plus a big sweater over a leotard and tights for a great cold weather look. To make it more street-worthy, substitute tight pants for the tights, but keep the leg warmers.

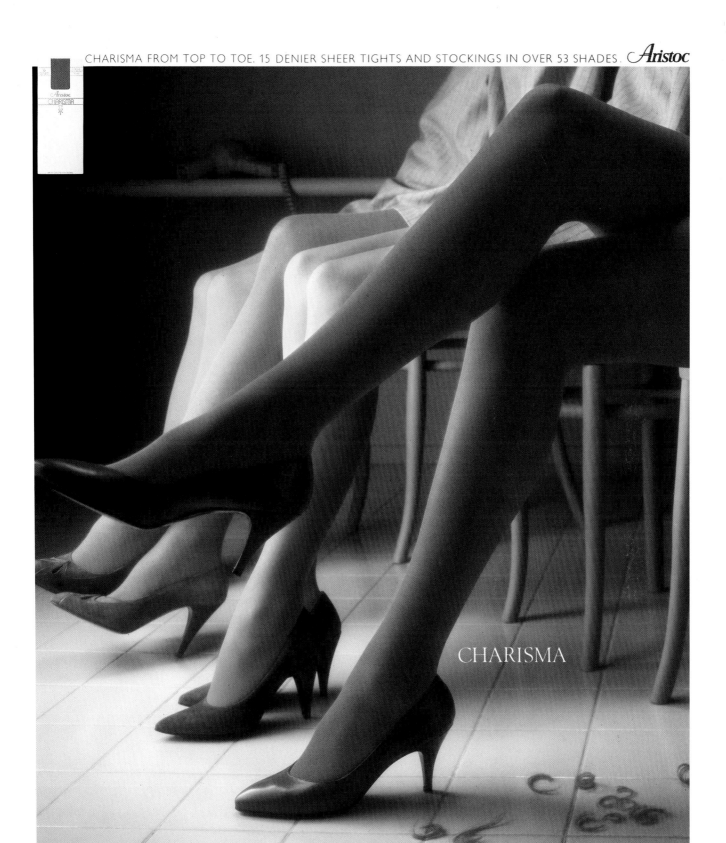

CHARISMA FROM TOP TO TOE. 15 DENIER SHEER TIGHTS AND STOCKINGS IN OVER 53 SHADES. *Aristoc*

CHARISMA

ARISTOC

BECAUSE LEGS SHOULD BE MORE THAN JUST PRETTY

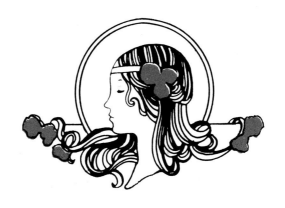

Chelsea Studio & Suntan Centre

TELEPHONE 01-581 3705

Excessive jewellery is not practical. Thin gold or silver chains at the neck, wrist or ankle are fine provided they aren't too loose. However, if you are wearing this look to a party, and have chosen jazzy colours, you might bend the rules and opt for big and arty jewellery to enhance your colour scheme.

With so few trinkets, THE DANCER can afford to ornament her waist. Twisted lengths of silky or woolly fabric look great knotted at the waist – twist two or more contrasting colours together as the illustration shows.

FACE AND HAIR

As this is a supremely healthy look, THE DANCER cannot wear much make-up as it might streak and run when she perspires. Classical ballet dancers whiten their faces, but a tinted moisturizer might be more appropriate for the street or studio. In terms of shadow, work with the colours in your clothing; for example, if you are dressed in pink and turquoise, use a pinkish shadow on the inside corner of the eye, blending it into a turquoise shadow on the outside corner. Define the eyes with a line of navy or brown pencil along the lower rim, and under the cheekbones blush with fuschia blusher, and finish with a pink or plum-coloured lipstick. The overall effect should be soft for the studio but more dramatic for discos and parties.

Long hair should be tied back in a chignon or ponytail. Alternatively plait it and bring the plaits up over your head securing them on top like THE IMMIGRANT. Short hair can be wild and spiked – gelled for a dazzling party look. Or wrap a band around your forehead like THE SPORTSWOMAN.

IDEAS

● If you're dressing for the disco, add some glitter to your leotard and/or skirt: sequins, beads, braiding can be purchased by the yard and stitched to the edges of your clothing.

● If you haven't time to sew on glitter, and are wearing THE DANCER for a festive occasion, sprinkle glitter in your hair.

● Freezing weather? Wear leg warmers as arm warmers on top of your leotard.

Right: Simple leotard and short full skirt transformed with strands of sequins for a disco look. Here the Fifties motif of a double note was used, but any simple pattern will work.

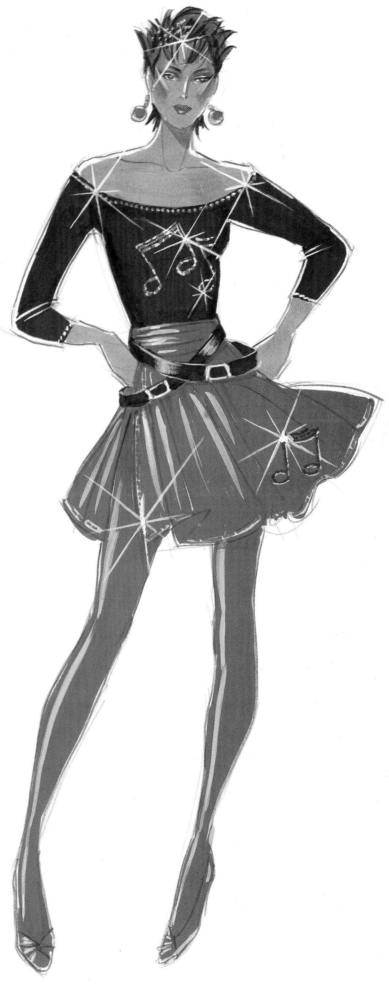

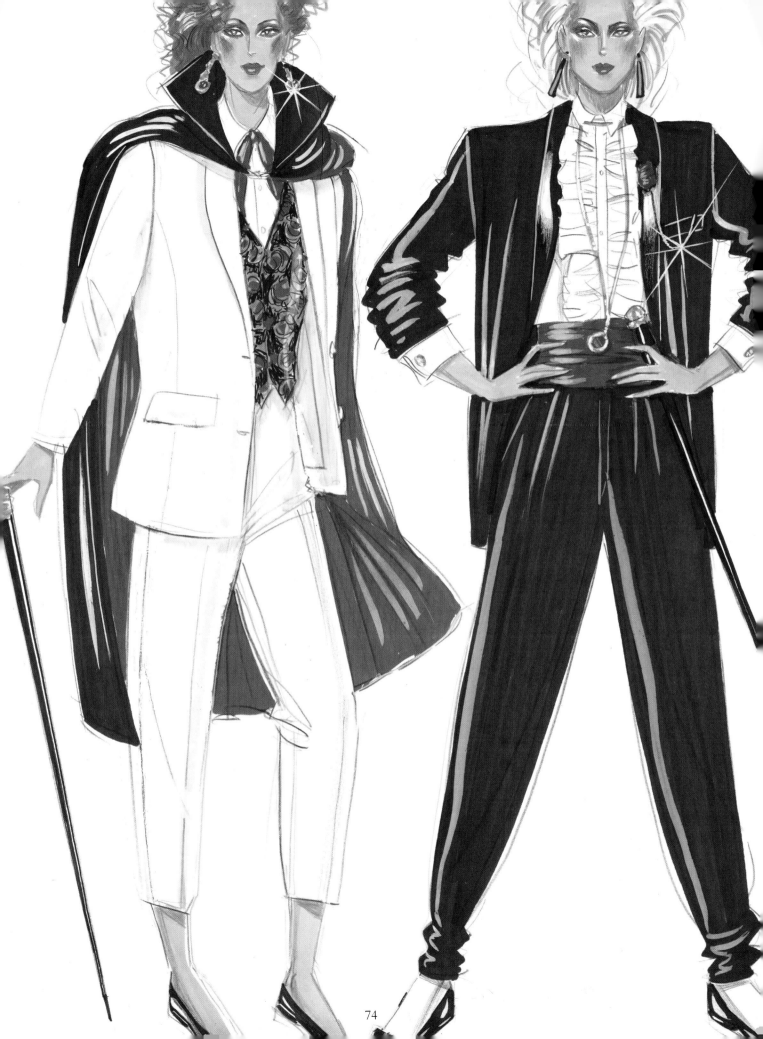

THE DANDY

BACKGROUND

Beau Brummell; Oscar Wilde; Jean-Paul Goude;Baudelaire; David Bowie: all decadent dandies, concerned with sartorial matters and immaculate style. Dressing like a dandy is a trifle flashy for day, but perfect for a night life of clubs, concerts, casinos and dinner parties.

Although based entirely on men's evening clothes, this look is nonetheless luxurious. No detail is spared, no fabric too rich, no accessory too fine. It is a look for perfectionists, and a great favourite of the designer Yves St Laurent who has incorporated it in collection after collection.

Moreover, if you cannot afford to invest in the rather costly ingredients of this look, they are relatively easy to hire. There are a host of dress hire firms catering for weddings, black-tie dinners and other formal events, providing clothes in a wide range of sizes, so you should have little trouble finding one to fit. As an alternative, borrow a man's dinner-suit or tuxedo, or rummage through secondhand clothing shops.

THE LOOK

The colour scheme is essentially severe and bold, with black as the base and one, or at most two, other strong colours – burgundy, red, or emerald – concentrated in one area. If, however, you find this too heavy, soften the look by having a pastel shade, such as a cool lemon yellow or icing sugar pink, as your note of colour. Begin with a black dinner jacket or white tuxedo in fine wool (perhaps linen or silk for summer), maybe with satin lapels. It can be any length, from the short waiter's style to the longer three-quarter length, but choose a jacket with well-fitting rather than outsize shoulders. Wear the jacket with either a white, pastel or a deep-coloured ruffled or pin-tucked evening shirt. Alternatively wear it buttoned up with nothing at all underneath, or substitute the shirt for an evening sweater in angora, cashmere or similar luxury yarn for a softer effect. Should you get completely carried away, wear a velvet or brocade waistcoat under your jacket, or choose a smoking jacket with a lustrous sheen to it.

Add matching or contrasting evening trousers in black or white, usually accented by a satin ribbon running down the outside leg seam – although this is not obligatory. The trousers can be cut to fit, or slightly large so that you have to cinch the waist (as directed under

Below: No accessory is too fine for **The Dandy.** Choose shoes or spats in black patent, cuff links or collar studs in gold or set with fake stones, neckties and cummerbunds in silk, satin or brocade, all set off with a silver-topped cane and top hat.

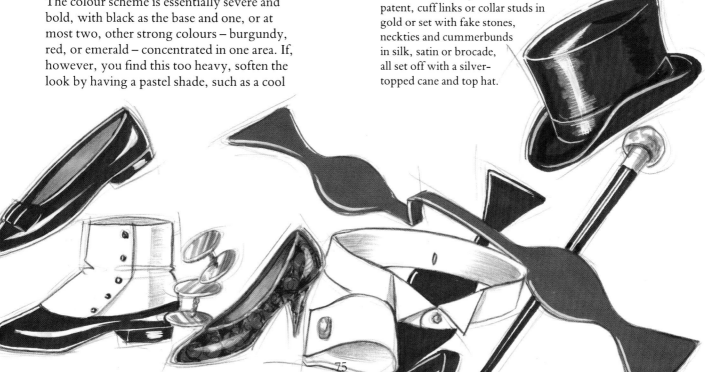

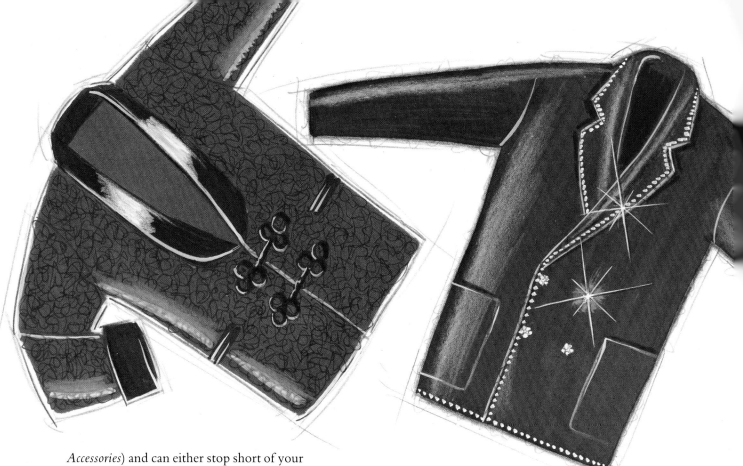

Accessories) and can either stop short of your ankle bone or rest on your shoes.

As an outer layer, don an opera cape with the traditional scarlet satin lining. A fur coat would also do for a touch of ultimate luxury.

ACCESSORIES

First concentrate on the neck of your dress shirt. It may come with detachable collar, cuffs and studs, in which case decide whether you can either wear it collarless, fastening the neck with a round brooch or single sparkly stud, or attach a collar with traditional collar studs and don a black bow tie. Alternatively, hold the collar with a gold pin, a ribbon of silk, satin or velvet, tied in a bow at the neck or just below, or even a cream or paisley satin cravat. Stick to the basic black and white scheme with just a dash of colour as highlights in the form of a silk handkerchief, silk evening socks, a cummerbund, a purse or fine silk or kid gloves.

Round your waist wear a belt or cummerbund. Belts should be of patent or other fine leathers, although cheaper alternatives can work well, too, such as satin curtain cording or thick ribboning (see *Ideas*). Cummerbunds should be wide and in a colour to set off the jacket and trousers, perhaps matching your bow tie. Men's braces in black or opera red worn over your white shirt will also look great.

Above: If you tire of wearing your black or white tuxedo all the time, consider the smoking jacket (left) or the evening sweater (right). Evening jackets in brocade, fastened with outsize frogs, look great with satin pants, while evening sweaters can be shaped like jackets, too – get them in luxury yarns like angora, mohair or silk, perhaps with some glittery detail.

On your feet you can wear shoes of virtually any style from high heels to flat slippers or pumps, depending on the length and cut of your trousers. They may be patent, kid or even spats, but black is most appropriate. If you like this look and plan to wear it often, consider evening slippers in satin, lace, velvet, peau de soir or any dressy fabric (a good investment anyway as they can be worn with many other dressy looks such as THE DEBUTANTE, THE LATIN and THE GYPSY). Fancy footwear may sport a neat pageboy bow or even glittery details such as stitching, ornament or appliqué.

Strictly speaking, any jewellery will be masculine – cufflinks, tie or stick pins, lorgnette chains, a fob watch. Carry an antique cigarette case or moiré silk purse to hold lipstick and coins for the hat-check girl. As a final touch wear a top hat on your head and carry a silver-topped cane.

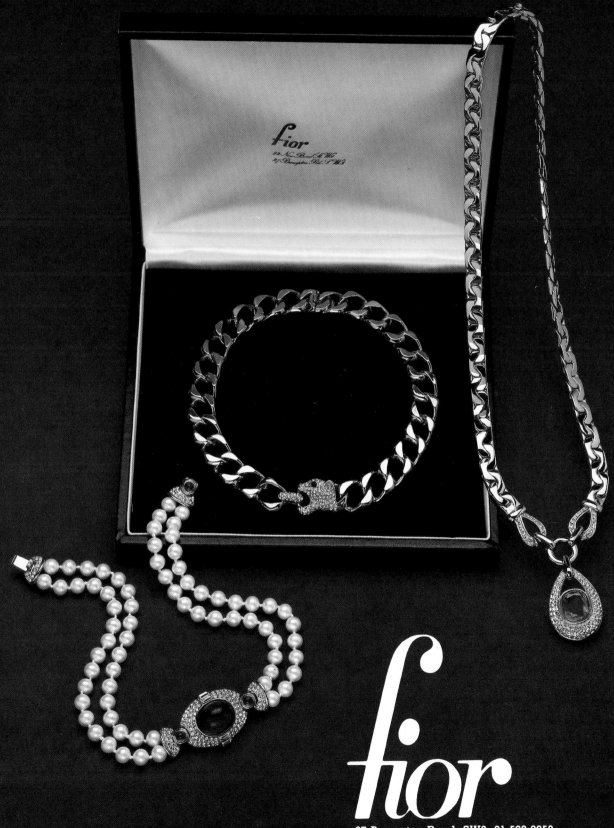

FACE AND HAIR

Ideally, hair should be short and slicked back with gel; if long, wear it very straight or tuck it up into a chignon or ponytail. Secure with ornamented hair-pins, but keep the effect simple. If you do wear a top hat, simply tuck your hair inside and let your glossy mane tumble down when you remove it.

Make-up will be simple but dramatic: a pale and powdered face with dark charcoal or brown eye shadow and black mascara for intensity. Remember that the famous dandies of the turn of the century – the 'flaneurs' of Paris, such as the poet, Baudelaire – cultivated the consumptive-as-chic style: drawn, wan and coolly aloof. Hollow your cheeks with dark rose blusher. Finally, add a red lipstick to contrast with the starkness of the black and white outfit.

IDEAS

● For instant evening trousers sew grosgrain or satin ribbon to the outside seam of a straight-legged pair. Use matching thread and a large running stitch so you can remove the ribbon later.

● For dressy cufflinks and hair-pins use shanked buttons with faceted or rhinestone heads. For cufflinks, join two buttons with a 1½-inch loop of elastic thread; for a hair ornament, slip the button to the curved end of a long hair-pin.

● Use ribbons of your choice for headbands or belts or to match a ribbon belt or cummerbund. For ribbons choose burgundy or black velvet, scarlet or emerald satin, cream, pink or pale yellow silk. Thread 6 inches of ribbon through the buttonholes in each cuff and tie a small bow on the outside cuff. Use ribbons with restraint as overdoing it can all too easily turn the striking but restrained dandy into the over-dressed fop.

Below: Transform a pair of tailored pants with a strip of sequins or satin ribbon sewn to each outside leg. Use the same ribbon to make cuff links too, or join two shanked buttons with elastic thread. For adorning your locks, slide another shanked button onto a hair-pin, as directed in *Ideas* above.

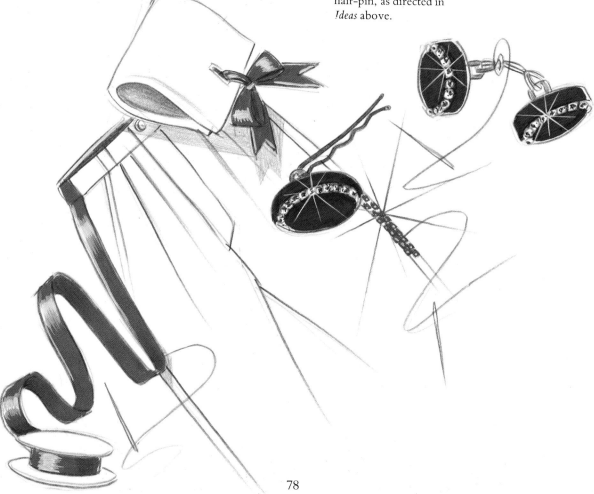

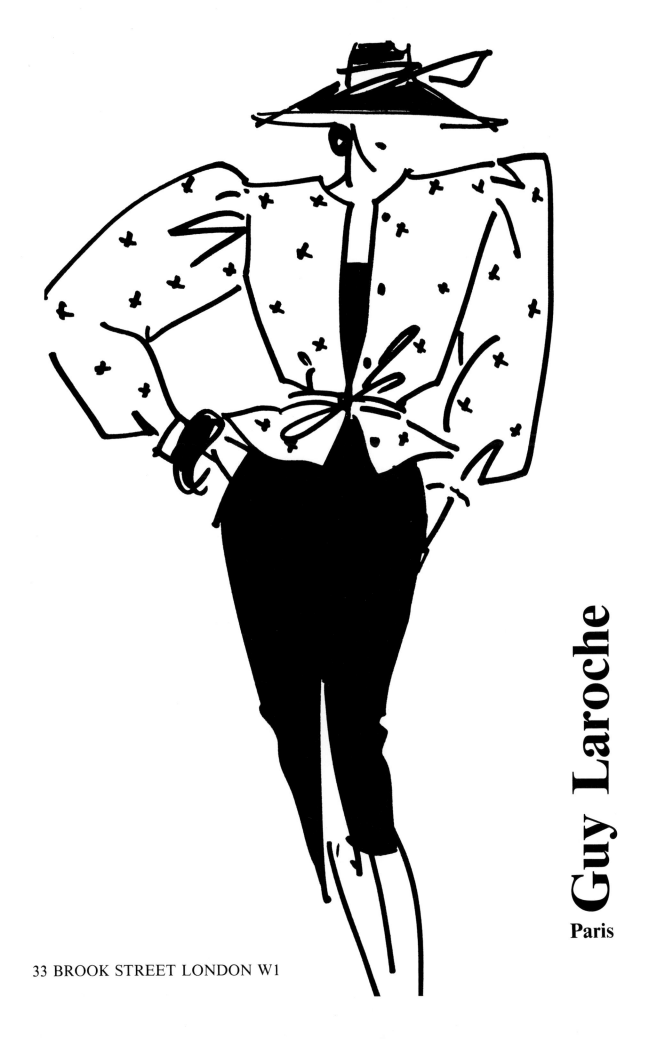

Guy Laroche

Paris

33 BROOK STREET LONDON W1

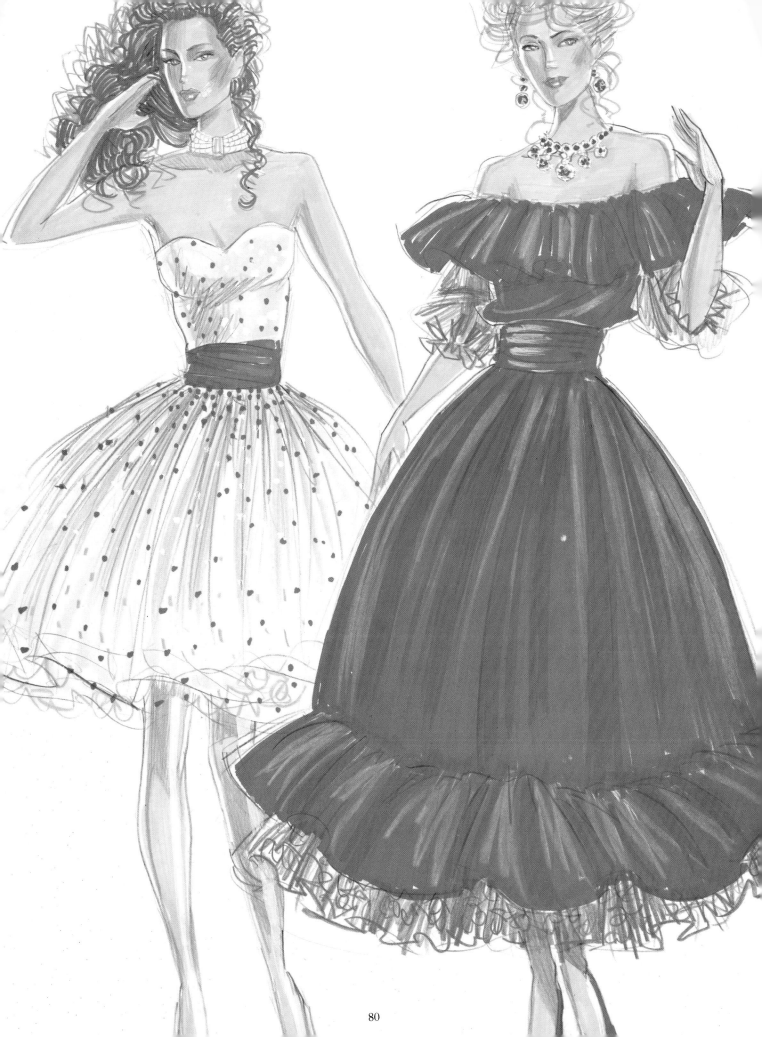

THE DEBUTANTE

BACKGROUND

Float down a Georgian staircase to the strains of the string orchestra below, dressed in your taffeta ballgown, white-gloved and satin-slippered, dance card in hand, to be swept on to the arm of your white-tied and black-tailed escort, the dashing and eminently eligible heir to the title and fortunes of.... Should you be so lucky to attend a very grand ball, think of THE DEBUTANTE, now a nearly extinct creature.

'Coming out' marked the deb's debut, and 'doing the season' was her *raison d'être*. Traditionally, young ladies of class were kept closeted in the schoolroom or at home until their late teens, being groomed in the social graces. Finally the day came for them to be launched into 'society'. Off they flocked to the balls, the parties, the society events of the Season.

THE LOOK

In the good old days before inflation and the demise of the butler, Mummy and Daddy threw a large and extravagant dance at which the deb made her debut. This was the occasion for the ballgown – stunningly and romantically beautiful, but not too sexy (no need for a bad reputation at such an early age).

Choose ballgowns in luxurious fabrics such as taffeta, organza, raw silk and moiré in gentle pastels or deeper jewel-like shades. Fresh and innocent, white is *the* traditional deb's colour. The ballgown skirt must be long and full, supported by layers of petticoats and the bodice fitted with a tiny nipped-in waist (just like the crinolines of the 1850s). Frills and flounces are important features of the dress; sleeves can be off the shoulders, puffed and frilled at elbows or wrists, shoulders discreetly hidden under a large floppy frill of lace or the fabric of the dress, and hemlines flounced. A broad sash with tapered ends can be tied in a large bow at the front or back. A cloak of black velvet or satin will protect this magnificent creation as you step from the Rolls or limousine.

Most of us cannot aspire to the ownership of a real couture crinoline, but the popularity of

Below: **The Deb**'s accessories are as traditional as her lifestyle – evening party pumps with low heels for dancing, long white gloves in white cotton or kid, and, of course, the family jewels.

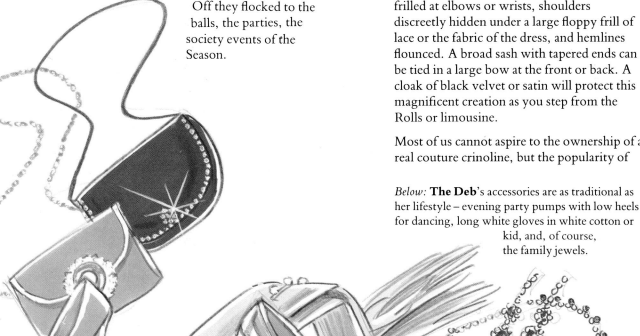

81

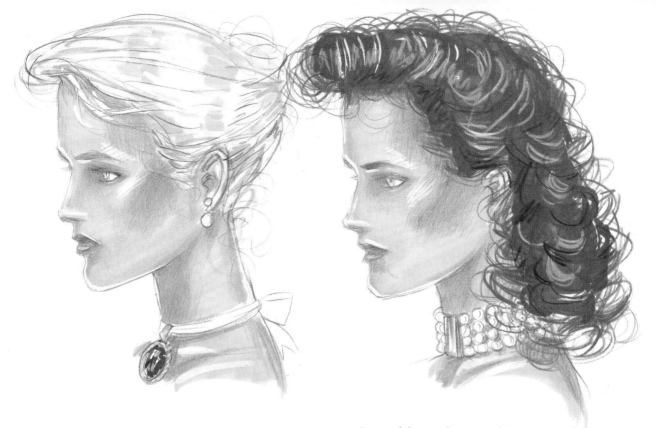

Above: Two sweet styles for **The Debutante**, both relying on hair with lots of body – see instructions in *Face and Hair* opposite.

this style has recently been revitalized by designers such as Belville Sassoon, Zandra Rhodes and the Emanuels. This revolution of the fashion cycle means that copies of such designers' originals are readily available in high street shops. You can even try the theatrical costumiers.

Today's deb may love the idea of dressing up in crinoline and cloak for the very grandest party of the season, but she's more likely to opt for a shorter version of the evening dress for most occasions. This look is not so formal but just as stylish and quite acceptable at even the smartest parties. And what's more, you have a very good chance of acquiring an example in the local charity shop or market since it's a classic style. The strapless or fine-strapped boned bodice, cut straight across the bosom or perhaps in a heart shape, tapers into a neat waist, from which a slightly gathered or very full skirt falls to the knee or mid-calf. Best in the same shades and fabrics as the crinoline, it is easy to wear and less cumbersome than a ballgown. Since it is a stunning shape, it really needs no further adornment, but you can get the skirt to stand out more with the addition of a full net petticoat, or try a sash in a contrasting colour as the introductory illustration shows.

A true deb spends most of her season with a champagne glass in her hand and that charming, social smile gracing her face at all times; but her social life is not conducted exclusively after dark. The champagne glass sparkles during the day, too – at society race meetings, weddings and garden parties. For the equivalents of these occasions in your life you will need some dressy daywear. A silk suit or dress is best, in a plain colour or a small print. Suit skirts are loosely gathered and worn with co-ordinating lawn or silk blouses, ideally with a pussycat bow. Dresses can be the classic shirtwaister variety of THE LADY, or more full and flouncy like THE GIBSON GIRL.

For winter, a good well-cut classic coat of camel, cashmere or wool/cashmere mix is essential. Those used by THE CLASSICIST or THE LADY are ideal – as is the velvet blazer of THE WOMAN and THE CLASSICIST.

ACCESSORIES

Choice of jewellery is what sets the true deb apart from her imitators. Strings of pearls, pearl chokers and pearl studs are deb classics and will always be acceptable. Alternatively, you can get the family diamonds out of the bank for the ball, but they must not be too ostentatious. If the real thing is still eluding you, go for paste imitations and the better contemporary fakes. Keep bracelets and rings to a minimum – a few perfectly chosen examples are in far better taste than a jangly clutter of everything you own.

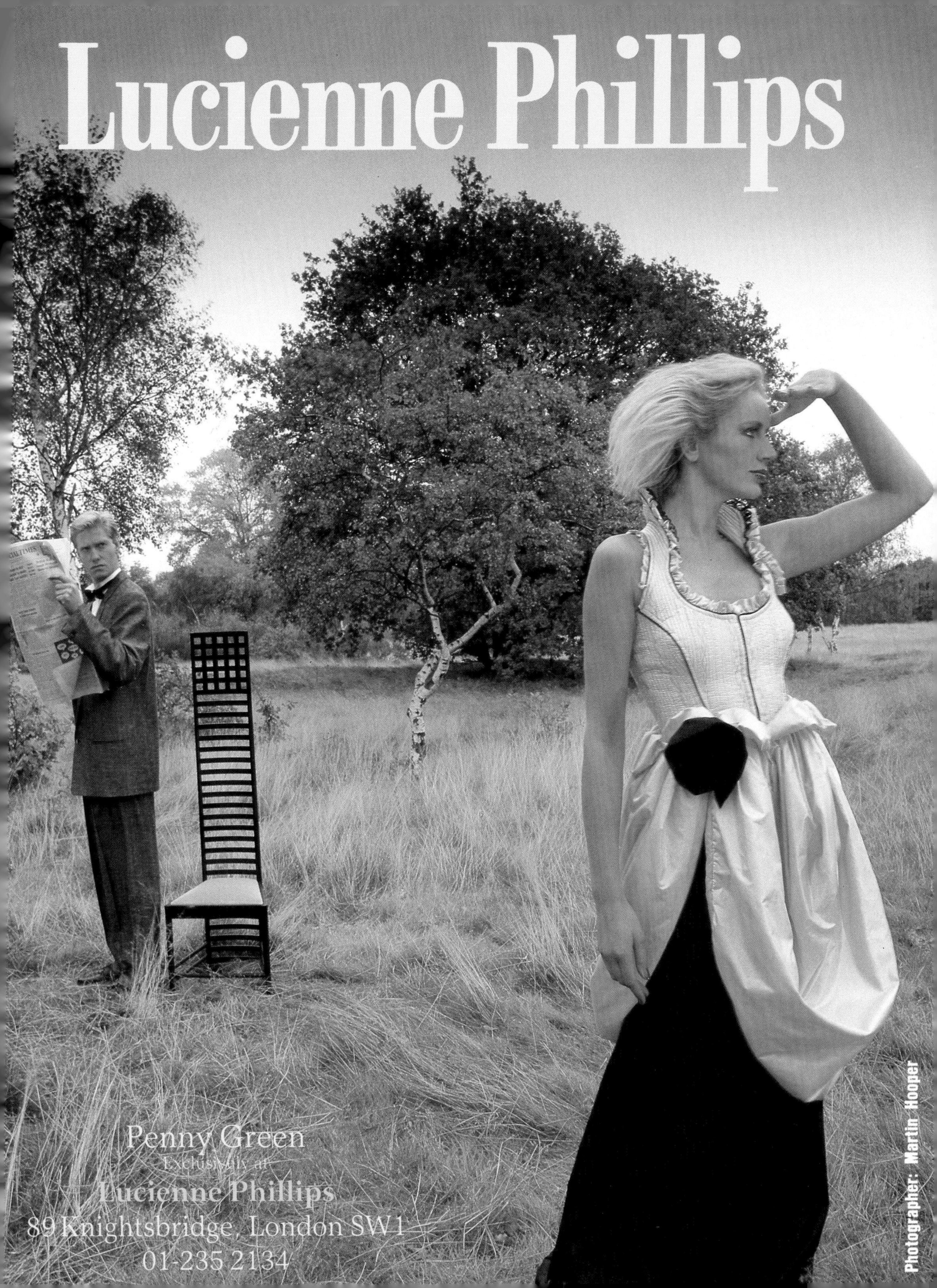

Lucienne Phillips

Penny Green
Exclusively at
Lucienne Phillips
89 Knightsbridge, London SW1
01-235 2134

Photographer: Martin Hooper

Evening shoes will be put through their paces with all that dancing, but they will not be given the constant daily punishment of most footwear. So allow yourself to be indulgent and search out the very prettiest and daintiest slippers to complement those perfectly turned ankles. Medium to low heeled slippers or pumps look lovely in satin, silk, moiré, brocade and embroidered fabrics; link them to your ballgown by the addition of paste buckles, moiré bows, and delicate seed pearl and lace appliques. For the totally traditional look, flounced and frilled in an all-white ballgown, white pumps are the rule. For day, select the same basic pump shapes, but keep them simple and uncluttered, except for the occasional flat grosgrain bow.

Every deb knows that in her day Mummy *never* left the house without her gloves, handbag and hat, though she's not so strict now. If you don't want to wear gloves, you can always carry them: long white kid with tiny pearl buttons on the inside of the wrists for evening, above the wrist in conventional shades of suede or leather by day. A small neat leather clutch bag or a black patent shoulder bag with a gold shoulder chain is correct during the day; at night an evening bag that matches your evening pumps. If you opt for a hat (for weddings for example), select an elegant brimmed fine straw with grosgrain band and a couple of large silk tea roses, or a neat pillbox.

FACE AND HAIR
After all those years closeted in the schoolroom, the deb is at last allowed to behave like an adult and put her hair up in the evenings, so take full advantage of this. Every kind of chignon is possible; make it as formal and elegant or as loose and romantic as you like. Curls can froth on the top and ringlets escape down the nape of the neck or be tucked up with long pronged tortoiseshell or paste combs, or ribbons and bows. Whatever style you go for, keep your long and elegant neck on view; the neckline of your ballgown and your necklace and earrings will enhance it. If your hair is short, try a soft full style with a wave or two for a less severe look.

A 'peaches and cream' complexion is one of the hallmarks of the deb. Be creative with your make-up palette to give a well-bred 'English rose' impression of innocence; invent some aristocratic cheekbones with the aid of a taupe blusher under the bones and gently highlight those fresh young sparkling eyes with blue eyeliner. Mouths follow suit and should be coloured and glossed in soft apricot or pink tones.

IDEAS
● If (not surprisingly!) your jewellery box does not contain ropes of diamonds, Victorian or Edwardian paste jewellery can be just as effective and sparkly. Search out pendants and earrings in antique markets, polish them up with jeweller's rouge or toothpaste on an old toothbrush and no-one will spot the difference. Alternatively, add a brooch or small paste buckle to a satin, velvet or moiré ribbon, which matches your dress or accessories, and wear it as a choker.

● A wide evening sash can be decorated by threading it through a large and glittery paste buckle, positioned in the middle, at one side or at the back of your waist.

● Decorate evening slippers or pumps with satin ribbons, bows or buckles, tacking them in place with tiny stitches or a dab of glue. Evening bags can be similarly adorned.

Below: Take ordinary shoes and bedeck them for dancing. From the top: flat pumps with grosgrain or velvet satin ribbon, glued or stitched in place; in the middle a paste buckle glued or stapled on; at the bottom, heels and toes adorned with a row of individual pearls glued in place.

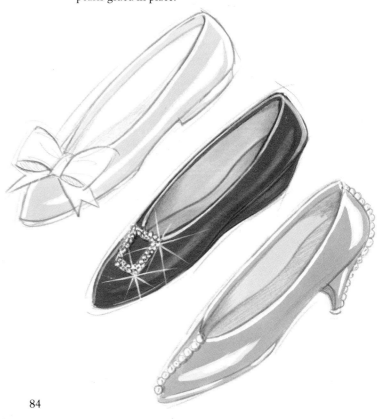

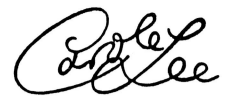

CAROLE LEE — Fantasy Evening Wear

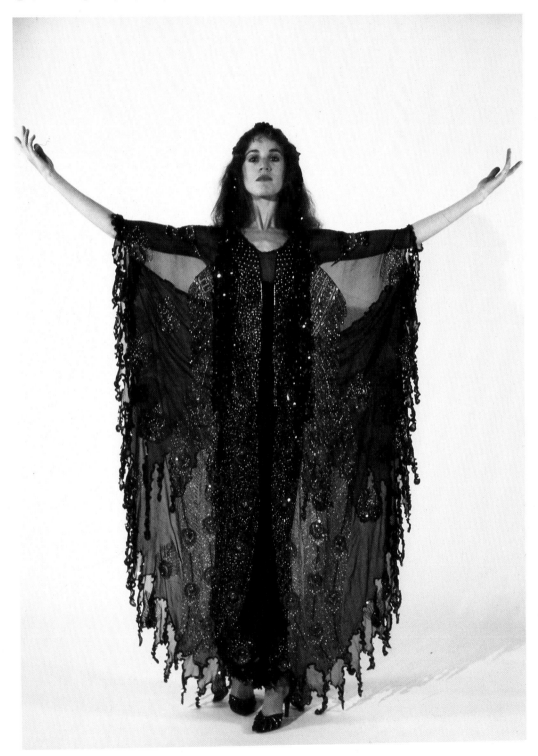

MODELLED BY BRYONY BRIND OF THE ROYAL BALLET. PHOTOGRAPH © LESLIE E. SPATT.

OONBEAM COTTAGE, 80 CHURCH STREET, LONG BENNINGTON, NEWARK, NOTTS. TEL: 0400 81739.

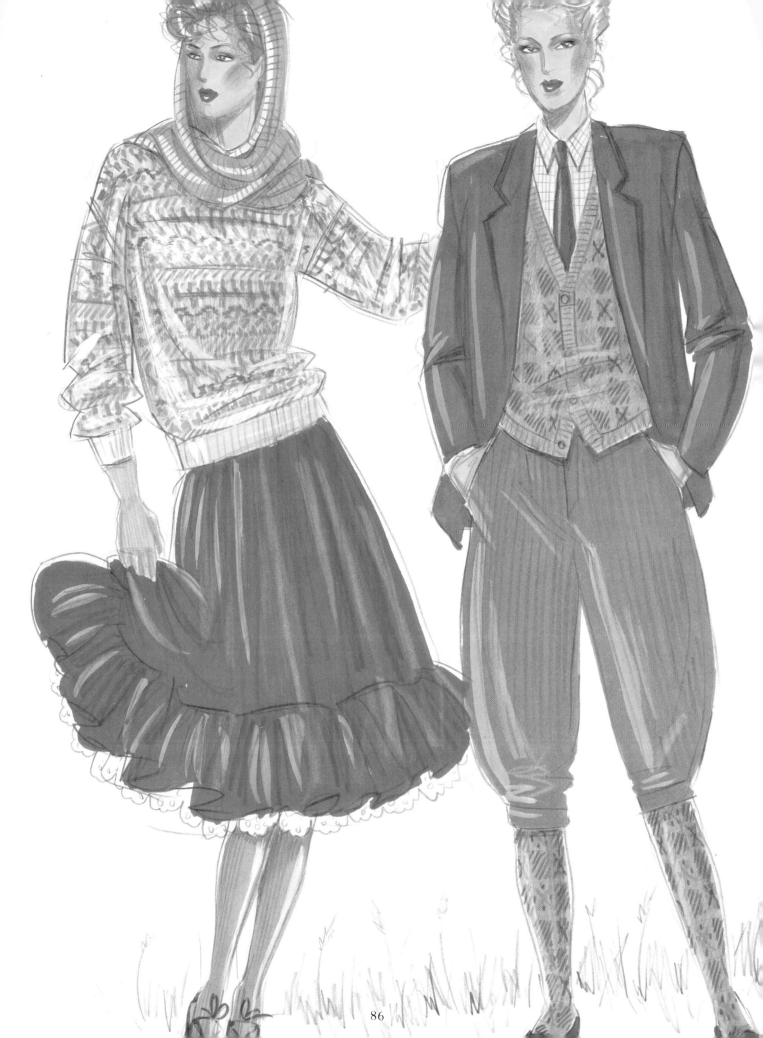

THE FAIR ISLANDER

BACKGROUND

Soft beige, cream and brown of grazing sheep, grey of stone walls and craggy cliffs, sludgy green of moss and field, slatey blue of sea and scudding skies, dusky pinks and heathery purples: these are the traditional colours of the hand-knitter's palette on Fair Isle, a remote and rugged outpost far to the north of Scotland. The now-famous intricate patterns of symbolic, geometric and natural inspiration are their brushstrokes. Colour and pattern, echoing the life, the culture and the changing seasons of the island combine to provide the canvas from which come the components of one of the warmest, most practical and comfortable of fashion looks.

Amazingly, the Fair Isle style is over 300 years old. For most of that time, however, the islanders' unique craft of hand knitting existed in relative isolation, supplying primarily the needs of its local inhabitants: scarves, hats, mittens, socks and stockings, and most importantly jerseys, the traditional working garment of fisherman and crofter. It was only in the early years of this century that the attractions of the look became recognized. Soon it became acceptable wear for everyone and was popularized by the Prince of Wales (Edward VIII), who wore a boldly patterned Fair Isle sweater to play golf at St Andrews in Scotland in 1921. Thus, the royal seal of approval secured a place in fashion both for the sweater and for the centuries-old knitwear traditions of the Fair Islanders.

Since the Twenties shapes have changed, colours and yarns varied, and stylistic emphasis altered, but the appeal of this classical and decorative look lives on. A truly British look, it can be dressed up or down, and adapted to suit the harshest or gentlest of climates. What's more, THE FAIR ISLANDER look will suit almost any type of figure; the layers characteristic of the style can conceal unwanted pounds or add dimension where needed.

THE LOOK

The Fair Isle sweater (or pullover, cardigan or waistcoat) with its decorative patterning and wonderful mix of colours is the focus of the look. Use it as the basis on which to build up toning colour schemes for skirts, trousers and jackets in compatible natural fabrics. Try traditional tweeds, wide- or narrow-wale corduroys, soft wools like challis, classic plaids, crisp cottons and floppy silks – even cashmere and leather for luxury lovers. To set off the Fair Isle design avoid too many other patterns; opt instead for plain but textured fabrics. Whatever you choose, the tones should be those of nature's own glowing

Below: Choose scarves, gloves, mittens and hats with a Fair Isle pattern that goes with your sweater. For footwear, choose sensible shoes or boots for walking miles across moors or tramping down city streets.

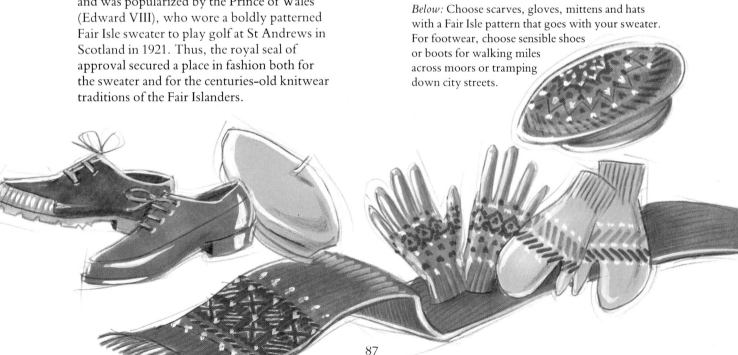

colours at their best – do not allow sharp synthetic hues to interrupt the harmony of such time-tested colour schemes.

With so much knitwear it goes without saying that this is essentially (but not solely) a winter look. For chilly days wear a softly gathered wool skirt, with perhaps a hint of petticoat peeping out, or knickerbockers or trousers, gently pleated at the waist, in tweed or corduroy. Top with a cotton and/or wool checked shirt, perhaps with a ribbon tied around the neck under the collar. Add your favourite Fair Isle, a cosy cardigan in a plain colour or a soft, slightly baggy jerkin, and then for the final layer, a tweed or corduroy hacking jacket or a too-big man's overcoat. Although not authentic, the mossy green loden coats, originally from the Tyrol but now available in every city, co-ordinate wonderfully well with the natural, muted colours of Fair Isle and Shetland sweaters

Fair Isle knits will keep you extra cosy in winter because of the stranded technique of double knitting used in their manufacture. The same air pockets will keep you cool in summer, so keep the lines and components of the look the same in warmer seasons, but exchange the wools for silks, linens and cottons.

ACCESSORIES
Scarves, gloves, mittens and a variety of hat styles all come in Fair Isle patterns, but don't overdo a good thing – either mittens or a beret in the same or similar knit as your sweater will be quite enough. If you wear a pattern on your head and hands, for example, go for plain colours for other accessories, and choose from the same colour range as the rest of your outfit.

Soften the line of your coat or jacket with a large, fringed cashmere or wool shawl or scarf (See *Ideas*). Or turn up your collar and add a muffler or two in toning colours. Try a silk scarf tied in a floppy bow or foulard at the neck of your blouse or tied in your hair.

For the coldest weather, and indeed to complete the winter look, a hat will be essential. Choose a neat tammie in a soft angora and wool mix, or if you feel a bit more dashing, a man's tweed cloche or trilby. Wool felt berets look good too, and they're inexpensive and come in a multitude of colours. Gloves or mittens, perhaps with Fair Isle borders, should be in wool, or in ecru cotton for milder days.

Protect legs with ribbed wool tights; add socks, possibly rolled down at the ankles, on

Below: Don't abandon this classic look in the summer – simple change the fibre composition of the sweater to a mix of cotton, linen and/or silk in pale shades and build your wardrobe around it.

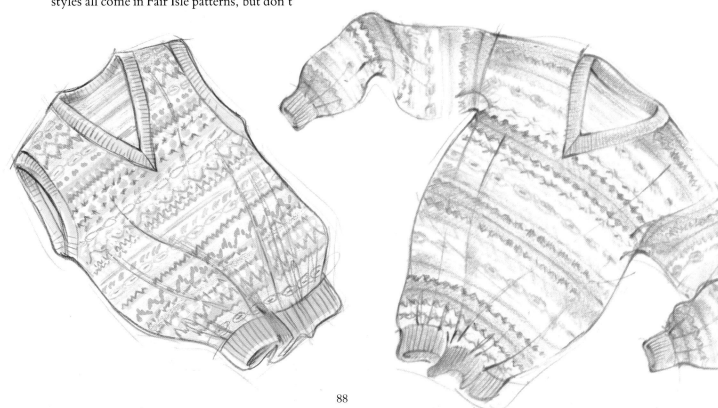

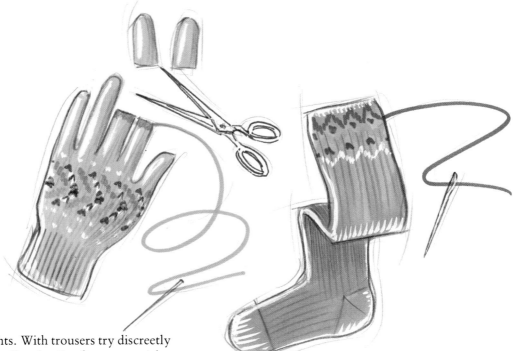

top of the tights. With trousers try discreetly patterned Argyll socks. For footwear, stick to the low-heeled classics: brogues, ghillies or loafers, ankle boots or leather or canvas riding boots. Olive green rubber boots also work well with this country look. (See THE LANDOWNER AND THE FISHERWOMAN). For summer, choose the same styles, but in lighter, even pastel, shades.

Finally, a neat webbing or thin leather belt over your sweater and a squashy leather or canvas bag will add the finishing touches to your outfit. THE FAIR ISLANDER is really a fresh, unadorned look but classic jewellery, such as simple ear-studs of pearl or another semi-precious stone, is in keeping. Amethysts, jade or coral tone with the muted shades of the sweaters and look extremely pretty, but the pieces should be discreet and unfussy.

FACE AND HAIR
Glistening and glowing, both face and hair of THE FAIR ISLANDER will radiate health and naturalness. Ideally go without make-up, but if you can't, use a translucent peaches-and-cream foundation followed by a soft dusting of blusher. Accentuate eyes just a little with shadow in subtle, earthy shades and add a hint of mascara. A touch of lip gloss and you're finished.

If your hair is long, leave it loose and natural and as windswept as you like. Alternatively, scoop it up into a full, soft tortoiseshell chignon kept in place with a comb or two or try a single plait at the back. Two locks taken from the sides of your forehead can be pulled back around the rest of your mane.

If you don't want to wear a hat, a woollen muffler or scarf pulled round and knotted at

Above: Take gloves with worn-out fingers, snip them all off, and use a needle threaded with contrasting yarn to tidy the cut edges. Secure the edges and you'll have a fingerless pair of hand-warming gloves – so useful when shopping. Complete your Fair Isle outfit by decorating a plain ankle or knee sock as shown. Pick out a simple pattern from your sweater, and repeat it in embroidery thread at the top of the sock.

the side of your head will look right, as will a wide ribbon in velvet or grosgrain tied at the top country-girl style.

IDEAS
● If you're a knitter, or can inveigle a friend or relation to knit for you, design your own Fair Isle sweater or search out traditional knitting patterns. But mix colours carefully. Use extra yarn for matching muffler, socks or mittens. If you are really do-it-yourself orientated and love the whole process of crafts, try hand-dying your own wools. Without going quite so far, you can knit your own sweater using hand-dyed wools from a specialist yarn shop.

● Soft wool scarves and shawls are economically made from remnants of tweed or other woolly fabrics; fringe each side by unravelling the raw edges an inch or so with the help of a safety pin.

● Extend the life of favourite wool gloves with worn-through fingertips: cut off fingers to the second knuckle and finish the ragged edge with matching or toning yarn.

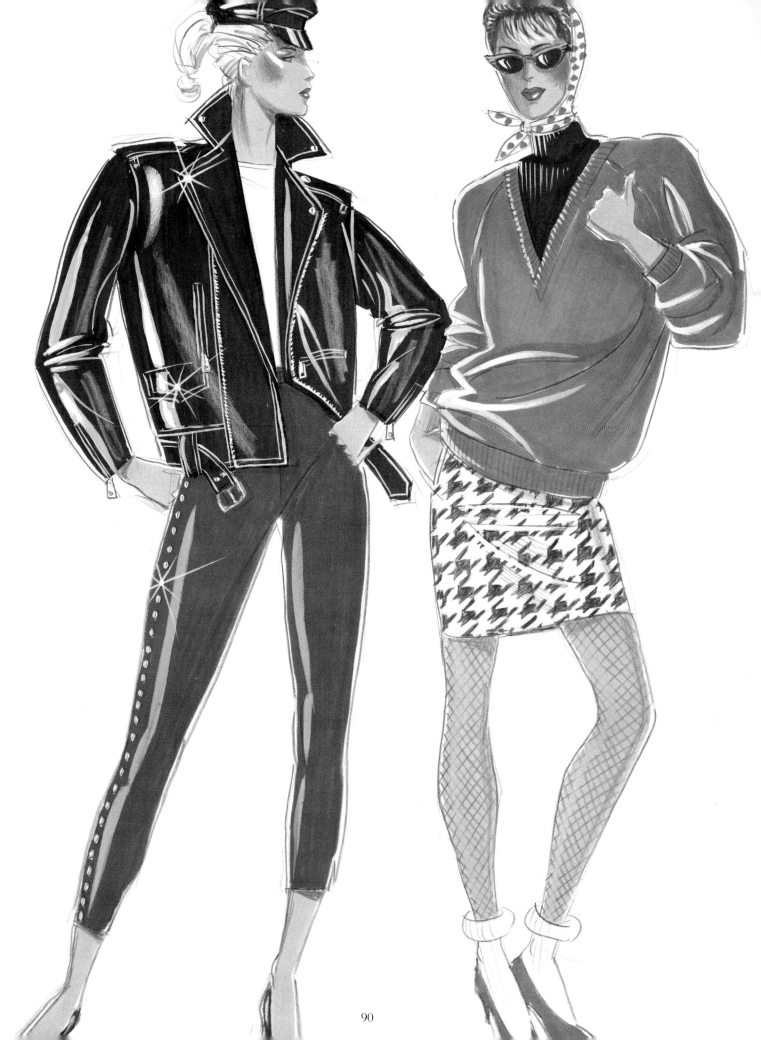

THE FIFTIES FASHIONABLE

BACKGROUND

The first nuclear bomb had been dropped and the West was beginning to recover from the Second World War. Styles in the arts were undergoing radical changes – rock 'n' roll was born. These were the Fifties. It was jive versus bop, big cars versus big cycles, crew cuts versus dove tails, Elvis Presley versus Buddy Holly. Young people were in real conflict with their parents' generation in particular and with society in general, as reflected in Elia Kazan's film *Rebel Without a Cause* (1955) with James Dean and Natalie Wood.

The new emphasis on youth culture, now an integral part of society was just beginning. Fashion designers responded enthusiastically to the new market created by the post-war baby boom, and began designing clothes specifically for this new species, the teenager.

THE LOOK

The Fifties look is with us again in the early Eighties, although the revival is overlayed with the influence of punk.

To dress like a time transplant from the Fifties, think black – it's the basis for almost everything you wear. Accent with a raw red, dead white, jaundiced yellow, brazen blue, wicked purple and the occasional wild print to offset this deepest black.

Trousers should be *very* tight. Stretch pants with under-foot straps are the perfect style, as are toreador trousers or pedal-pushers. Figure-hugging jeans should again be black or faded denim.

There are two alternative skirts: the first is characteristic of the beatniks, the 'intellectuals' of the period, who wore straight, short, black skirts with black tights and flat black shoes and read 'beat' poetry in seedy dives. But for jiving, be-bopping, rocking and rolling, wear a very full, cotton skirt (dirndl, gathered or circular) printed with gaudy floral patterns, French poodles, Hawaiian scenes or similar kitschy motifs. For winter, the skirt can be felt or wool, but again it must be full (give extra volume by wearing several nylon net petticoats underneath). The full skirt should be calf-length; the tight beatnik skirt, well above the knee.

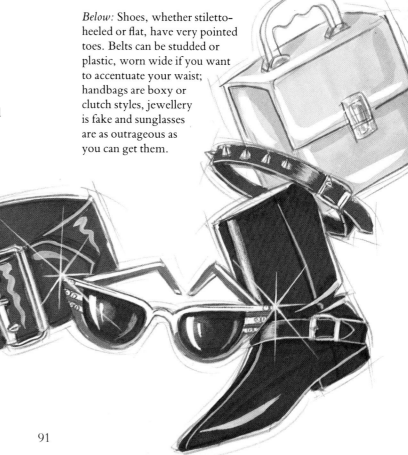

Below: Shoes, whether stiletto-heeled or flat, have very pointed toes. Belts can be studded or plastic, worn wide if you want to accentuate your waist; handbags are boxy or clutch styles, jewellery is fake and sunglasses are as outrageous as you can get them.

With trousers or full skirts, wear a short-sleeved white blouse. In hot weather, steal a trick from the boys: don a short-sleeved T-shirt, and roll the sleeves up for extra muscle. Garishly flowered short-sleeve shirts look marvellous in the summer with white pants or skirts. Beatnik women favoured fitted roll-neck sweaters in cotton or wool knits – usually black (or red to contrast with the straight black skirt). On top of a turtleneck or blouse, wear a mohair sweater. Shag is *de riguer*. It can be a loose, cowl-necked pullover or a chunky cardigan style with huge buttons, but it must be fuzzy. Colours can either be strong or off-key; sometimes primaries, even pastels.

Should you want to dress like THE FIFTIES FASHIONABLE there is no shortage of the dressy versions of the Fifties style available in secondhand clothes shops. Choose a full-skirted dress with a fitted perhaps boned, bodice strapless or with a wide V-neck. It might be in a garish print or chiffon and lace, but the proportion of neat fitted bodice to outsize skirt always holds good, and is even more exaggerated for evening wear – see THE DEBUTANTE. For an evening wrap a stole will do, or a lavishly embroidered cardigan. The prettiest are cream or pastel pinks and blues with intricate panels of tiny pearlized beads in flower patterns down the front.

Outerwear can be an overcoat in tweed, check or plain wool or your black leather aviator or motorcycle jacket.

ACCESSORIES

A pair of sunglasses was by far the most important accessory in the Fifties. THE FIFTIES FASHIONABLE will probably have several pairs since she wears them day or night, rain or shine, inside or out. They can be the dark-rimmed, wrap-around styles favoured by the local motorcycle gang, or the more exotic version with coloured 'winged' frames in a pearlized finish and maybe ornamented by a few rhinestones. (The lenses will always be very dark, the frames small in comparison with modern varieties). Collect these in junk shops. The more outrageous your glasses the better.

The second most essential accessory to the look is a pair of thick white socks. These are worn rolled down at the ankle, with two-tone lace-up or plain slip-on shoes. Yes, wear shoes and socks with trousers *and* full skirts. With the short straight skirt, wear matching tights,

Below: Nothing beats a full-skirted dress in a wild, floral print. Wear an embroidered-front cardigan and you'll be the perfect **Fifties Fashionable.**

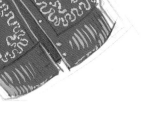

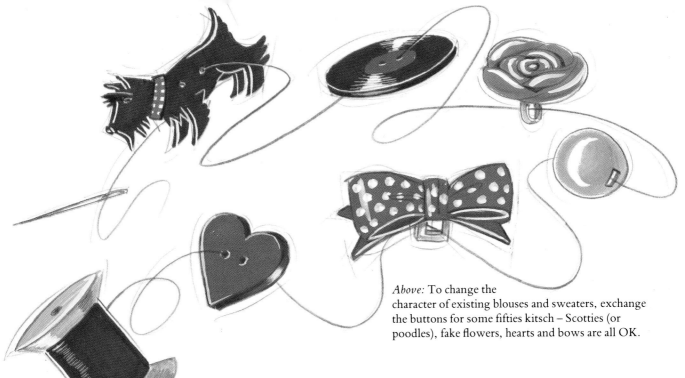

Above: To change the character of existing blouses and sweaters, exchange the buttons for some fifties kitsch – Scotties (or poodles), fake flowers, hearts and bows are all OK.

even under ankle socks. For evening dances and proms though, wear nylon stockings and a garter belt for an authentic flirtatious touch.

Shoes will be pointed and flattish, the sculptured stiletto heel featuring on special occasions. (Patent or pearlized leathers are ideal for dressy wear, and white for daytime). With trousers, you might also wear an ankle-high boot with a cuban heel, but whatever the style, all shoes must have pointed toes.

Hangbags should match shoes. Look for clutch styles with no handles or box-bags in tough plastic. Belts are wide. Wear them over mohair sweaters if your waist stands up to definition; otherwise over blouses with skirts and pants. Elasticized cinch belts are perfect and inexpensive and come in a multitude of colours. If you're into the black leather aspect of this look, wear belts with dog-collar-style studs on them.

Authentic pieces of jewellery are signet rings, charm bracelets, lockets, and necklaces of huge round beads. In addition, wear the most outlandish earrings you can find: big hoops and discs will do, but go for plastic flowers and fake metals too.

Rockers wore scarves to keep their hair in place. Tie as is shown in THE MOVIE STAR, or knot it under your chin or at the back of your head.

FACE AND HAIR
Hair can be worn in several ways – long and straight, short with 'kiss' curls, or softly permed. Best of all, wear hair in a single pony-tail at the back of your head, decorating it with a ribbon or two if you like.

Make-up starts with a natural or pale foundation, but eyes should be shadowed with a pale blue or green with a tint of grey so it doesn't look too hard. Apply liquid liner near the upper lashes, extend it into a wing shape at the end of the eye. Liner can also be applied underneath the lashes, but you need a deft touch so that the effect isn't too heavy. Finally blush cheeks with a soft pink shade and cover lips in a pale frosted pink. Finish the effect by applying whitish or very pale frosted nail polish.

IDEAS
● Decorate large-framed sunglasses by glueing small rhinestones, sea shells, plastic toys, plastic flowers, buttons, etc. to the ends of the frames.

● Invest in a bag of silver studs and a hand-operated punching machine for applying them. Decorate the seams on your jeans, your leather jacket, maybe even your shoes, instantly.

● Replace the tasteful buttons on your new cardigan with clashing, kitsch or plastic ones from the Fifties. These can still be found in old haberdashery or secondhand clothing stores – pink puppies and apricot flamingos are just the thing, as are the biggest, most faceted ones you can find.

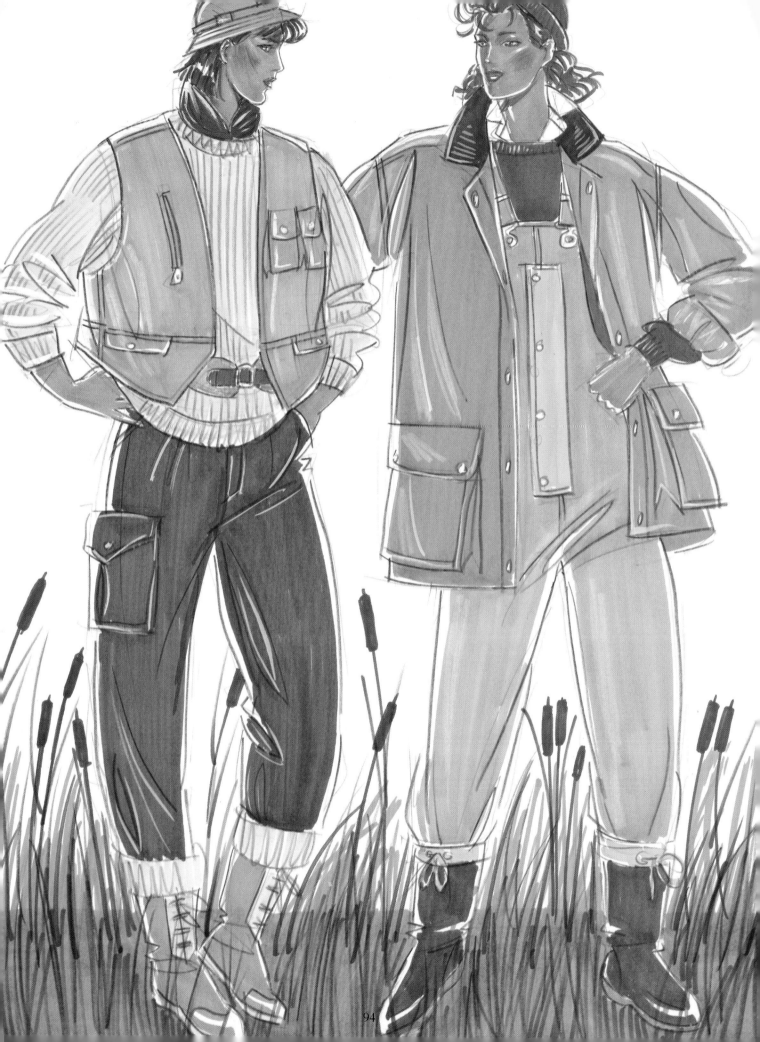

THE FISHERWOMAN

BACKGROUND

There's nothing more pleasant than taking fishing line and picnic lunch, camp stool and big umbrella down to the edge of a secluded river bank. Then cast your line and idle the rest of the day peacefully contemplating the occasional ripple on the water's surface. If this kind of outdoor lifestyle appeals to you – and most of us hanker after it – swallow the bait and fall hook, line and sinker for THE FISHERWOMAN's wardrobe. Even if you haven't the opportunity to take to the water's edge yourself, this is a perfect look for many outdoor activities, such as walking, camping or cycling and is also ideal for rainy days in town and country alike.

THE LOOK

Though THE FISHERWOMAN is one of the healthy, outdoor looks, unlike THE HORSEWOMAN or THE LANDOWNER it is not a style governed by rigid rules. By sticking to the right colours and having a few key garments and accessories at hand, you will not only be able to look the part but also feel wonderfully comfortable dressed in minimum effort clothes.

Because THE FISHERWOMAN spends her life in, near or on the water, clothing obviously must be waterproof. Heavy, proofed cotton, oiled

Below: Accessories for **The Fisherwoman** are inspired by the colours of woodland streams – natural straw, olive green, sludgy green, dirty brown, allowing a dash of yellow for sou'wester and shoelaces. The rubber and canvas boots work well in any wet conditions, whether washing the car or fishing for trout; the hats keep drizzle or glare from your eyes, and the bags are roomy enough to hold everything and free your arms with their shoulder straps.

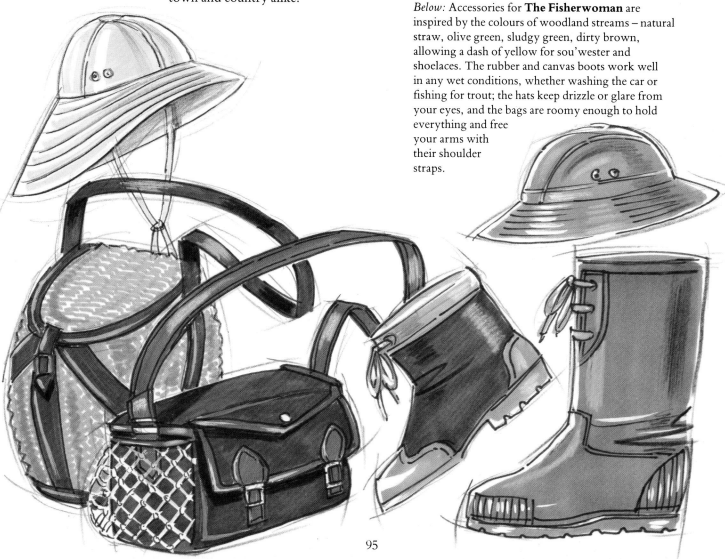

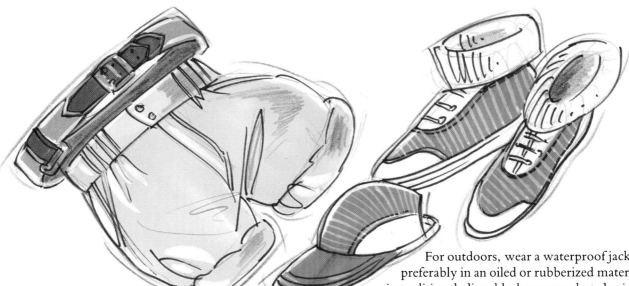

Above: In hotter weather, **The Fisherwoman** exchanges her overalls for shorts which can be rolled up, and her rubber boots for tennis shoes and socks which can be rolled down. Keep the cap though – there's a lot of glare off the water.

wools and rubberized materials are the fabrics to look for while the garments themselves should be roomy and comfortable. If the basic components of your outfit are loose-fitting, you will be able to adapt your look to all seasons of the year by the addition or removal of layers of thick jerseys, quilted or down waistcoats and heavy-knit socks.

THE FISHERWOMAN's colours are the slubby greens, olives and khaki of the river bank plus the beiges, browns and rich golden sands of the shore. Most of the colour combinations and styles recommended for this version of the look can also be worn by THE HORSEWOMAN, LANDOWNER, FAIR ISLANDER and even THE OUTDOOR GIRL and SCOTSWOMAN.

Trousers are an essential component of the look; they should be comfortable, protective and practical. Look for loosely fitting, baggy styles in sand, khaki or olive green; those with side pockets half way down the leg are perfect. (You could borrow the sand- or olive-coloured fatigues from THE SOLDIER). Be sure to tuck trousers into socks, whether you are sporting plain rubber boots, waterproof lace-ups or canvas deck shoes on your feet (see *Accessories*). Then plunder the cupboards of THE HORSEWOMAN and THE LANDOWNER for checked shirts and lambswool sweaters or that of THE SCOTSWOMAN for off-white Arans in oiled wool. Finish by topping the sweater with wide webbing belt, complete with clips and leather buckles.

For outdoors, wear a waterproof jacket, preferably in an oiled or rubberized material, in traditional olive, black or navy, but also in bright blue and yellow. You want a casually cut, loose shape, with ample pockets and zip or stud fastenings, which falls to mid-thigh – THE LANDOWNER has suggestions.

If an extra layer is required between sweater and jacket, add a sand- or khaki-coloured down waistcoat. In milder weather, discard the waistcoat and sweater and roll back the sleeves of your shirt over your jacket sleeves; or dispense with the jacket and keep the waistcoat.

For balmy, sunny days choose the same garments but in lighter fabrics; abandon trousers in favour of shorts – a pair of khaki- or sand-coloured ones with pleats at the waist (like those sold in army surplus stores) look great with co-ordinating T-shirt or shirt. Roll back cuffs on shorts and shirt, add a webbing belt and fishing bag.

For a more rough and ready version sported by real fishermen, go for an authentic fisherman's oiled wool jersey, worn for generations with good reason. Traditionally in navy blue or a natural creamy colour, with a crew neck and in a heavy ribbed knit, it is a great protection against water, spray and wind, since its oiled wool resists permeation. Over the last few years it has become a fashion classic and it is now easily available in a wide range of colours which co-ordinate well with THE FISHERWOMAN look.

ACCESSORIES
As with the other outdoor looks, there are a few accessories which make THE FISHERWOMAN instantly recognizable, such as a traditional fishing bag. This tough and spacious carry-all was first borrowed by photographers, who found it the ideal container for their equipment; it has now been universally adopted and co-ordinates well

with all the country looks. The bag should be large and roomy and made of strong, waterproof canvas, with several large outside pockets, a wide webbing shoulder strap and leather trim; soft sandy shades or olive green with brown trim are best. If, however, you prefer the idea of something a little different, look for an old-fashioned osier basket, beloved by anglers. Made from woven willow in an oval shape with a flat, slanting lid, this sturdy capacious container will withstand a lot of wear. Alternatively, you could use a fishing tackle box; all of these styles can be found in professional anglers' stores.

Waterproof footwear is, of course, essential. On wet days wear olive or black wellington boots, or waterproofed canvas lace-ups to ankle height. In summer, wear any canvas shape with a rubber sole. Bend the rules and consider navy, royal blue, scarlet or yellow, too. But always tuck your trousers into your socks so they don't flap around, and your ankles are kept dry.

Visit a river bank that is the favourite haunt of anglers on a Sunday afternoon and you will see the traditional fishing hat in abundance; in olive green and made of tough waterproof cotton or canvas with rows of stitching round the brim, it is the ideal hat to wear with fishing gear. However, you could also wear a canvas cap, trilby, sou'wester or wool hat. And don't forget webbing belt, fingerless gloves (which keep the hands warm but enable the fingers to grasp that rod tightly), and a large fishing umbrella.

FACE AND HAIR
All the fresh air should give you a truly healthy complexion and allow you to get away with as little make-up as you dare. But if you can't exist without it, make sure that what you do use is subtle. Choose waterproof mascara, around eyes shadowed in sludgy greens or blues. Add roses to your cheeks with a tawny blusher and protect your complexion from drying winds and sprays with an application of a clear gel, as used by skiiers and other outdoor girls – petroleum jelly will do the job cheaply.

Hair will for the most part be hidden under your hat, which will also help to keep it out of your eyes. You can also tie it back with leather or cotton shoelaces or use a wool scarf as a headband.

IDEAS
● Use a fishing tackle box as a handbag-cum-briefcase.

● Having emptied the fly box of its flies, use the latter as authentic finishing touches to your fishing outfits. Tuck one or two of the more brightly coloured ones into the band of your traditional fishing hat, or pin one in the buttonhole of your jacket.

● Make fingerless fishing gloves by cutting off the finger tops of old worn-through gloves (see THE FAIR ISLANDER for instructions).

● If you are a dab hand with knitting needles or a knitting machine and can follow a fairly complicated pattern, knit your own original Guernsey jersey. There are lots of beautiful traditional designs to choose from. Like the Fair Isle patterns, most of the Guernsey motif patterns are symbolic.

Below: Tackle boxes made terrific handbags, whether you're going fishing or not!

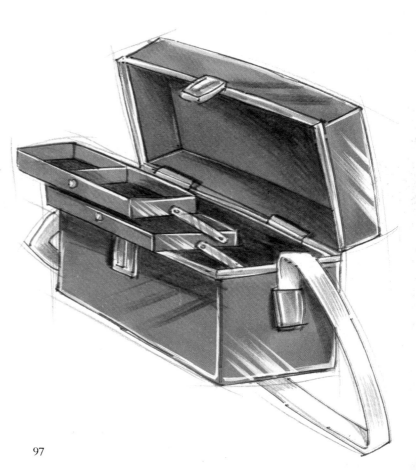

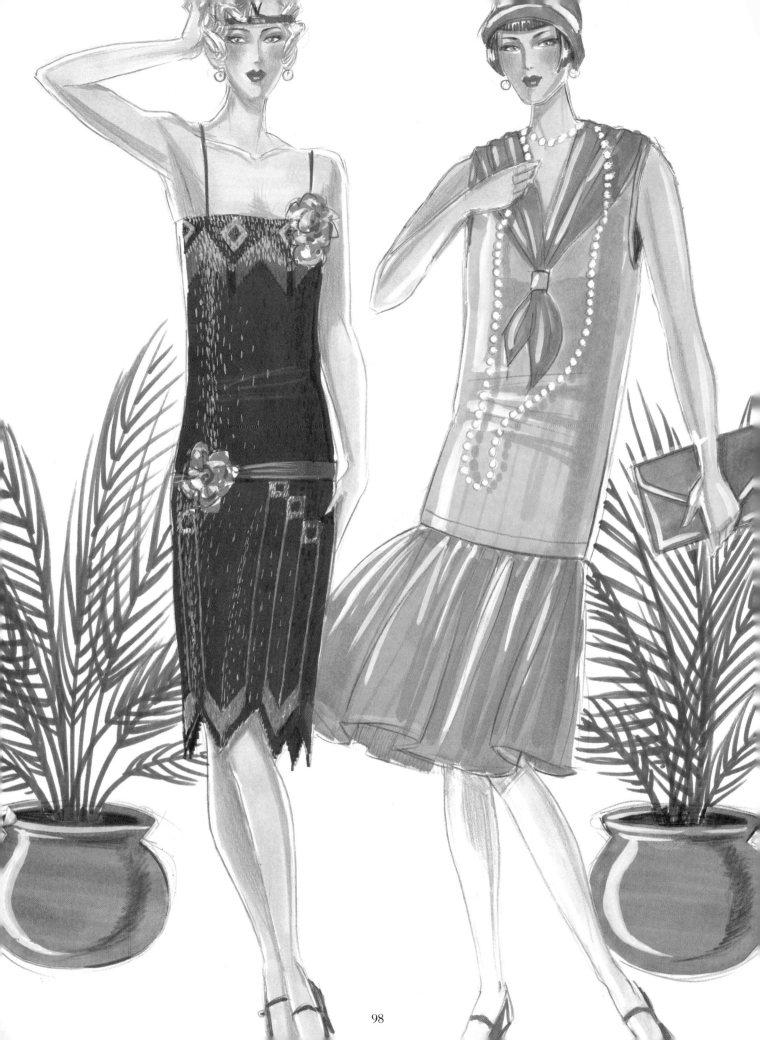

THE FLAPPER

BACKGROUND

The wardrobe of THE FLAPPER epitomized the zany atmosphere of the Roaring Twenties, a decade dedicated to frivolity. The hectic lifestyle of Scott and Zelda Fitzgerald and their glamorous circle was immortalized in Scott's novels: *The Great Gatsby, The Beautiful and the Damned, This Side of Paradise* and many more. While fortunes were being made on Wall Street, young fashionables bought the new gramophone records of Gershwin's 'sweet' jazz and Armstrong's 'hot' jazz and danced the Charleston, the black bottom and the shimmy till the small hours. The wave of prosperity spread like a fever through the USA, rising in a crescendo before the Wall Street crash in 1929.

The spirit of the Jazz Age crossed the Atlantic to Europe and for almost the first time America dictated fashion while Europe followed enthusiastically, women responding immediately to the emancipated style of their bare-legged and bobbed sisters across the sea. Off came the Edwardian corsets, into the bin went the tight laces, boned bodices and the stiff upholstered costumes. On went the loose-fitting, unrestricted, bustless, baggy and virtually shapeless garments of the free-thinking Twenties. And horror of horrors, hitherto hidden legs were now exposed! Even worse, off too came beautiful long locks, now all chopped to chin length. This bobbed fashion, cropped, kiss-curled and permanent waved, symbolized a new age for women.

Never before had women sported short hair, never before had women bared their legs, worn trousers or smoked cigarettes in public. Never before had women looked and behaved like men! It wasn't just coincidence that the New Woman took with alacrity to the boyish look in the Twenties – THE FLAPPER's new clothes summed up her new attitudes.

THE LOOK

THE FLAPPER lives mostly by night so this look comes into its own in the evening. For parties, dances and any other special evening occasion, the Flapper style appears year after year. A svelte figure is not an essential pre-requisite of this look, as your dress will be low-waisted and loose. The low-slung bodice is usually held up by thin shoulder straps or sheer short cap sleeves and the skirt will fall to knee-length. Sequinned, beaded, jet or rhinestone embroidery adds extra sparkle.

Below: **The Flapper** of today will choose the same accessories as her sister did sixty years ago: the clutch bag, the almond-toed shoes with the essential strap detail, the long, long strand of pearls or beads, the cloche hat for day, the feathered cap for evening and, of course, the ostrich feather boa.

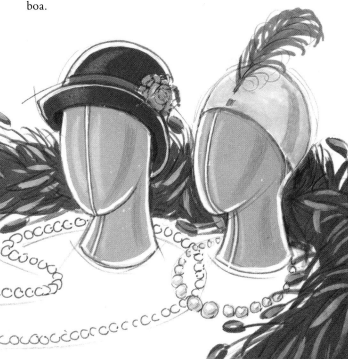

Many original examples of Twenties evening dresses can still be unearthed in antique markets or shops which specialize in period clothes; if you're lucky, you can pick up the genuine thing. If not, choose a straight-cut dress from your wardrobe, tie a wide satin or velvet sash around the hips finishing with a bow or double knot; hitch up the dress top to spill over the sash. Hemlines will accentuate those once forbidden legs – flounces, tiers, handkerchief points, a single frill, ostrich feather band or broad edge of fabric, contrasting with the main dress material, are all in keeping with this style.

Colours can be as loud as you like. Forget discreet and demure tones and choose the zappiest, zingiest Charleston-hopping shades you can imagine: bright pinks, fuschias, purples, gold and silver and lots of black. And remember that your chosen 'creation' will require similarly appropriate cover: a brocade or velvet three-quarters or knee-length coat with high fur collar and deep cuffs are perfect; fur stoles, feather boas, capes and short jackets in luxury fabrics trimmed with feathers or fur are also in keeping.

THE FLAPPER's day wear is based on the same loose outline; legs still show but the upper half of the body is more covered. For cooler days a loose-fitting but well-cut suit should be teamed with a small-collared silk or cotton blouse. Or try a broadly-pleated skirt with cardigan or pullover sweater falling to well below the hips, such as those worn by THE OCEAN VOYAGER, a style that also draws its inspiration from the Twenties.

If you get carried away by THE FLAPPER image remember that emancipation also meant the release from the restrictive underwear of previous decades. Liberation brought with it loose and comfortable camisoles, camiknickers, French knickers and the like. Slide into satin, silk and chiffon, or synthetic equivalents. Vintage underwear can also be found in secondhand clothing shops.

ACCESSORIES

Distinctive accessories give THE FLAPPER her particular style. For the toe-tapping, dance-till-you-drop look you must have a long rope of pearls, a band around your forehead, toning shoes with almond toes and buttoned straps, a feather boa and an exceedingly elegant cigarette holder. These are the trademarks of THE FLAPPER, so twirl the pearls, drape the boa and slouch when you're not dancing.

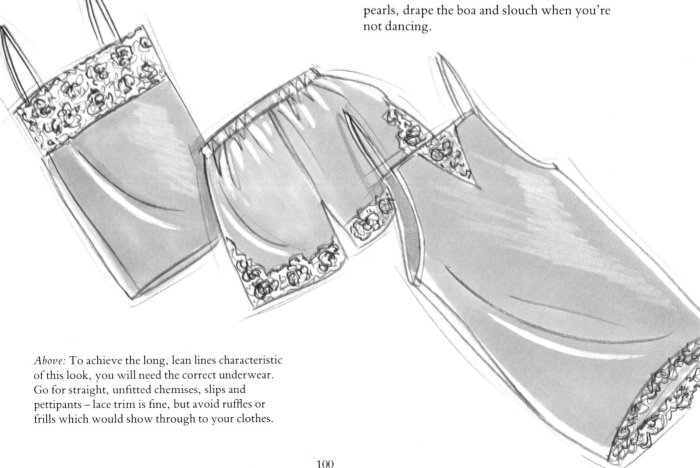

Above: To achieve the long, lean lines characteristic of this look, you will need the correct underwear. Go for straight, unfitted chemises, slips and pettipants – lace trim is fine, but avoid ruffles or frills which would show through to your clothes.

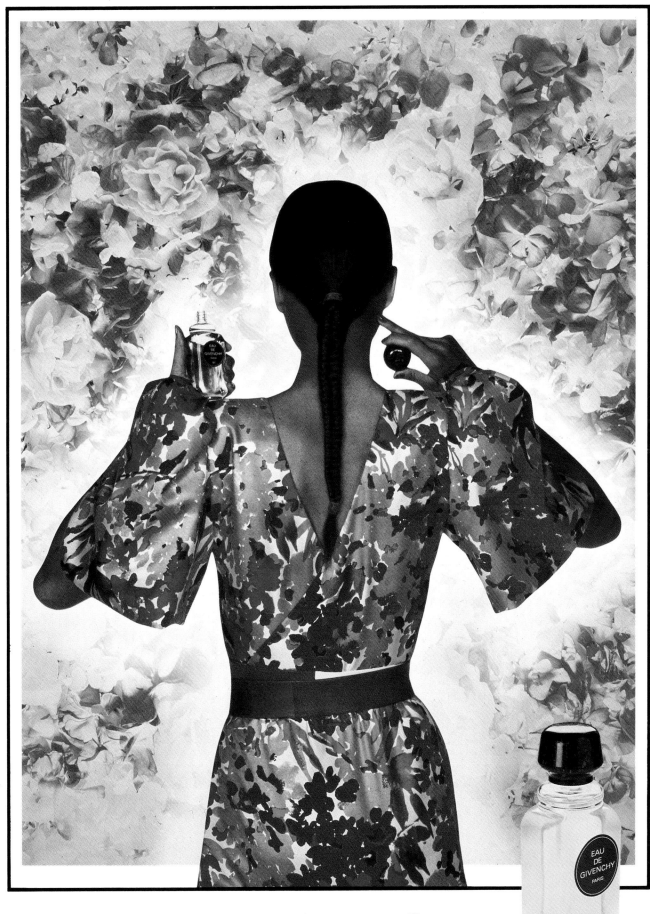

EAU DE GIVENCHY PARIS

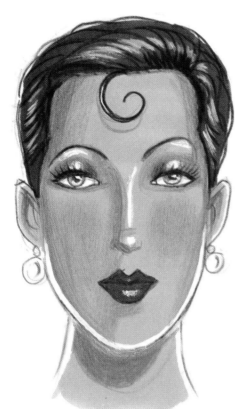

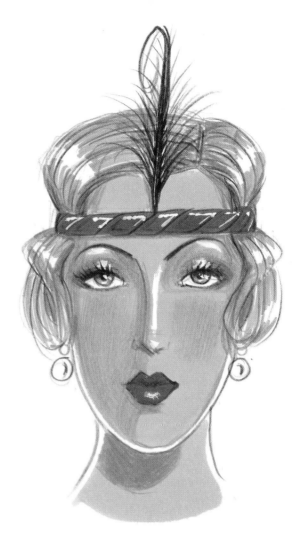

During the day a cloche hat is *the* characteristic accessory; in soft slouchy felt, or cotton for summer, wear it low over the brow. Trim it with grosgrain band, brooch or pheasant feather at a rakish angle. Leather shoes with a Louis heel and buttoned strap or two, silky beige stockings, lapel brooch, neat clutch bag and the essential pearls or beads put the finishing touches to THE FLAPPER's daytime look.

FACE AND HAIR

Whether fair or dark, you really ought to follow the example of Scott Fitzgerald's Bernice and have your hair bobbed! For a less drastic alternative, improvise. A loose but evenly permed style can be straightened by a careful blow dry or hair can be slicked with gel or setting lotion and one perfect kiss curl kept in place on the forehead in the same way.

As this is primarily a party look, THE FLAPPER can go to town with her make-up. Begin with a very pale foundation, dusted with a matching loose powder. Give the appearance of total boredom at another glass of champagne by making eyelids heavy with an application of dark grey eye shadow, accented with a line of grey eyeliner just inside the rim of the eye. Cheeks must be dotted with a clear red, applied towards the front of the face. Outline lips with a sharp red pencil, making points of the bow, then filling in with a clear red lipstick. If you dare, pluck eyebrows to a thin arched line.

Above: Two quick tricks with heads: try a kiss curl in the middle of your forehead and maybe at your nape, kept perfect with a dab of gel; on the right, an instant evening effect achieved with a stretchy headband or strip of ribbon tied tight to hold a small feather in place.

IDEAS

• Experiment with different ways of wearing a long rope necklace of pearls and beads: hanging loose, so that you can twiddle the ends in your fingers; tied in a single long knot; doubled up in two equal length loops; or doubled with one loop tight at the neck, the other hanging low.

• Forehead bands are easily made from velvet or satin ribbon; decorate with strips of glittery embroidery to match that on your dress; alternatively add a brooch to one side or wear a brooch on your hip sash. For real razzmatazz pin a couple of tall curled ostrich feathers to the back of the headband.

• Construct a simple turban for an authentic evening look; see THE COSSACK for instructions; finish by sticking a feather or a brooch in the folds or knot at the back.

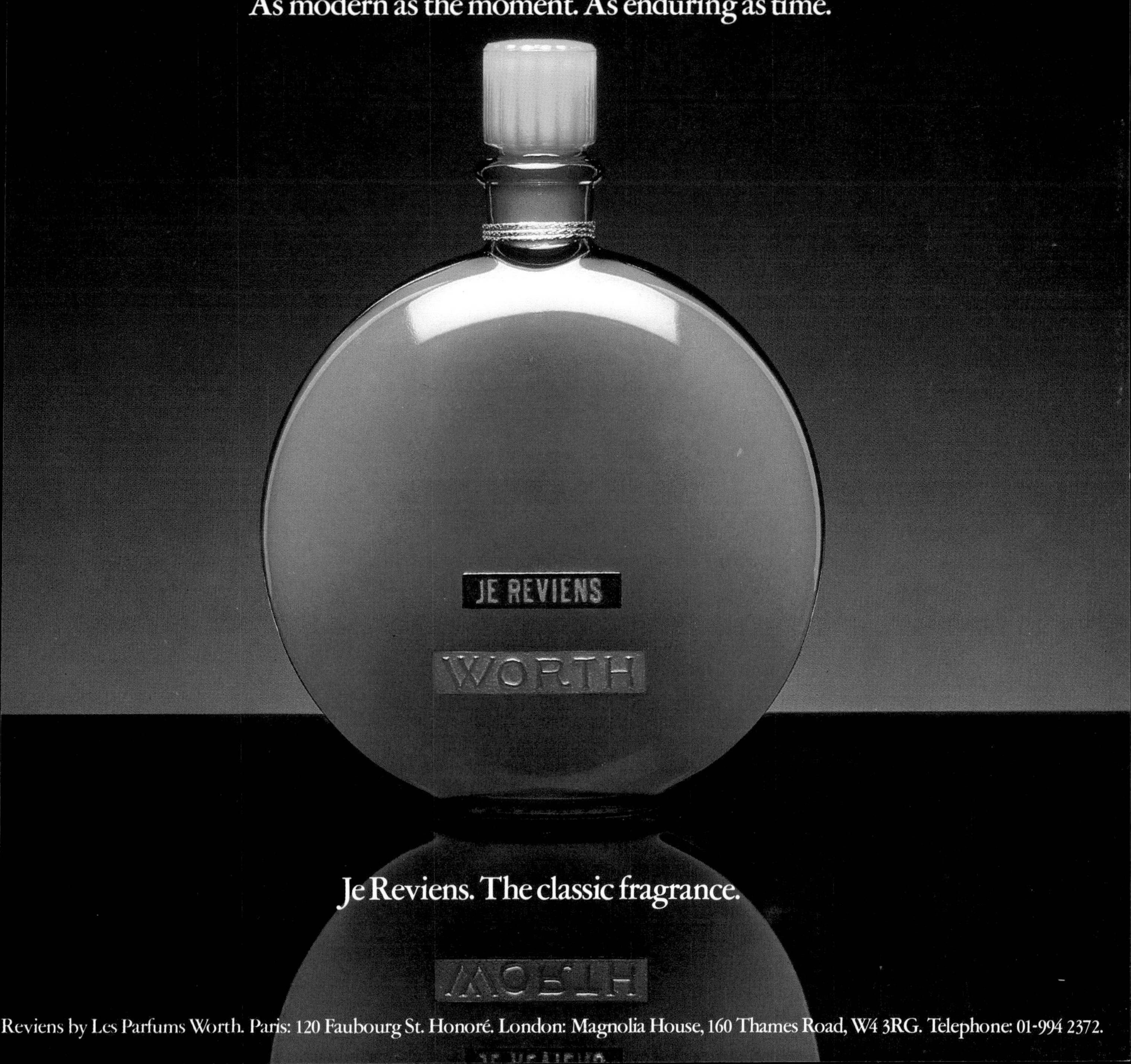

As modern as the moment. As enduring as time.

JE REVIENS

WORTH

Je Reviens. The classic fragrance.

Reviens by Les Parfums Worth. Paris: 120 Faubourg St. Honoré. London: Magnolia House, 160 Thames Road, W4 3RG. Telephone: 01-994 2372.

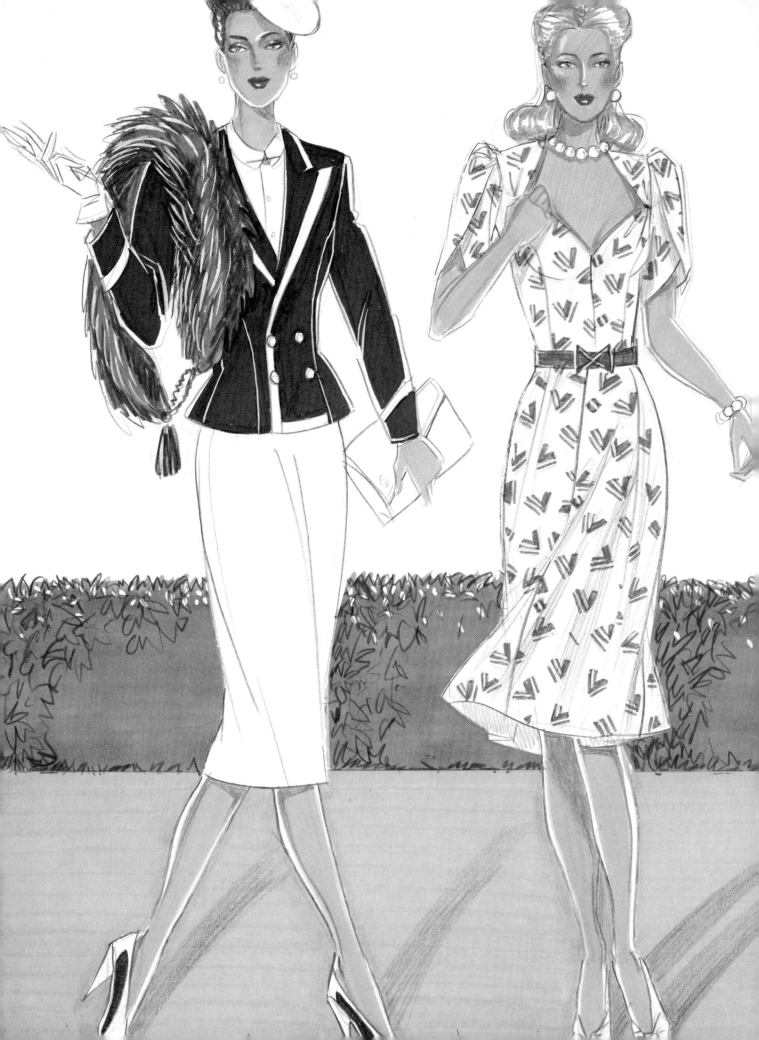

THE FORTIES FASHIONABLE

BACKGROUND

THE FORTIES FASHIONABLE comes to us from the decade of fashion between 1937 and 1947, beginning after the Great Depression, lasting through World War II and ending with Dior's 'New Look' launched in 1947. Cast your mind back to the glamourous side of the Thirties and Forties as glorified in all the Hollywood movies. As a look, it is the wealth of detailing in the clothing produced just before, and just after, the war that is striking. Fabric was pleated, tucked, frilled, ruched, draped, over-printed, furred and fitted.

Women were sculpted and made up (probably as a reaction to the extreme boyishness of the Twenties), and by the end of the Thirties had developed into curvaceous sirens: wrapped in bias cut dresses and gowns, cocooned in large coats and furs with heavily padded shoulders, made statuesque with hair piled on heads. Skirts were below the knee, gloves and hats were vital, colours were exquisite and pale – bois de rose, eau de nil and ecru were popular. Trousers were worn on the beach and for special occasions in the form of evening pyjamas. Schiaparelli paraded her 'shocking pink' and Balenciaga dressed women in stark contrasts of black and white.

Unfortunately, this great fluttering of style was interrupted by the outbreak of World War II. Although most of the Parisian couture houses managed to remain open during the Occupation, German authorities made repeated attempts to move these to Berlin.

After the austerities of the war, Paris began to work its fashion magic again in early 1945: everything was cut to fit and flatter the female form, nothing was left untrimmed or unadorned, there was braiding on collars; pleating on pockets; fringes on shawls; fruit clusters on hats and lapels; feathers on hats; fur everywhere; jet embroidery on evening clothes and hats were back with a vengeance.

Suffice to say that if you want to look like THE FORTIES FASHIONABLE, there are two basic approaches: firstly, the tailored suit complete with padded shoulders immortalized by the Hollywood stars of the Forties such as Bette Davies, Katherine Hepburn, and Joan Crawford, and more recently by Bianca Jagger and Bette Midler, and secondly, the

Below: When adding the finishing touches to this look, go for frankly forties accessories such as outrageous hats, seamed stockings, boxy or clutch-style handbags, ruched gloves, and platform shoes and sandals.

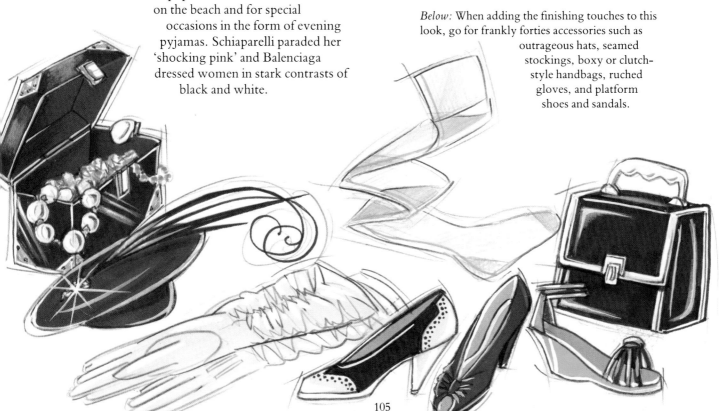

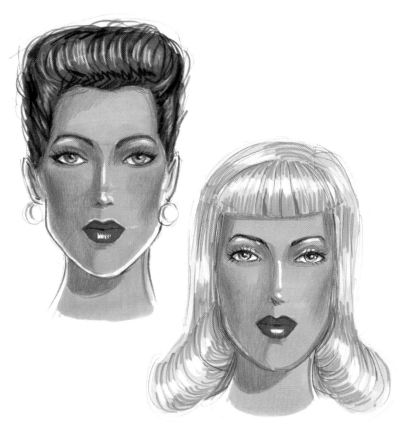

Above: Fashionables of the period wore their hair in one of two styles: swept up and caught in the back in a twist in a modified pompadour as on the left, or in a page-boy style shown on the right.

little-girl look epitomized by Judy Garland, who wore bias-cut, puffed-sleeved, knee-length dresses as she danced and sang her way over the rainbow and into everyone's heart (see also THE INNOCENT).

THE LOOK
Look for the gorgeously-tailored, impeccably-detailed suits of great designers like Georgio Armani, Piero de Monzi, Anne Klein. Better still, search for a secondhand Forties original for a fraction of the price of these modern imitations. If you're on a strict budget, get the jacket first, because the important detailing is here: it will also look ideal with trousers.

Look for cardigan jackets with roll back *revers*, cowl-necked belted shapes, and very fitted dressier ones with waist and pocket emphasis. Skirts should be in straight styles with deep kick pleats, angled patch pockets, or the fuller styles that heralded the late forties and early fifties. As a rule of thumb, the boxier the jacket, the straighter the skirt, while tighter nipped-in styles allow fuller skirts.

When hunting for originals, watch for chalky plain shades from the thirties – taupes and beiges; then speckly tweeds and houndstooths from the forties, resplendent with velvet collars, back belts, intricate pockets and beautiful buttons.

Wear the suit with plain-necked or tie-collar sweaters or beautifully made blouses in silk, cotton, crepe or man-made imitations with collars to peek out under the jacket.

In your hunt for this definitive suit, be on the lookout also for another authentic item from the same period – the princess-line, prettily-printed dress. This is the foundation of the second version of the look and will usually have puffed, dolman, or raglan sleeves, often ending just above the elbow. It should be adorned with front detailing like rows of round buttons, tucks or bias cut panels, and may have ties which knot at the back. These dresses look great for work or semi-formal occasions.

They are usually found in early imitation silk fabrics or cottons, printed with spots, squiggles, tiny flowers, even Art Deco motifs. Moreover, they are cut to flatter everyone – the unbelted princess line hides a too thick waist or hips; big sizes when belted add shape to too-thin figures, the bias cut bodice adds the illusion of a full bust. Wear them summer and winter, they always look great.

On top, wear a coat with fold back *revers* (lapels) or a stole in a fine wool such as a vicuna or a fur (fake or not). Stoles were very popular and are the perfect foil for tailored clothing.

ACCESSORIES
Oddly enough, THE FORTIES FASHIONABLE seems almost as accessory-obsessed as her older sister THE GIBSON GIRL. She, too, had to wear a hat and carry gloves. Certainly, hats reached the pinnacle of expressiveness during this period with Surrealist-influenced Schiaparelli shaping them like upside down shoes! Obviously, should you come across an inexpensive original in good condition, get it. If not, don a straw or suede cloche, a floppy beret, or big-brimmed hat and go to town with the trim. Use feathers, rhinestones, sequins, flowers, fruit, ribboning, netting. If you like changing a hat's ornament, use brooches to hold ribbons and ornaments in place rather than tacking them on.

Gloves should be elbow-length ruched cotton, or leather, maybe even nylon. Day and night, gloves are essential.

Search for early pieces of plastic jewellery, and imitations of semi-precious materials – this was the era of fabulous fakes. Costume jewellery was the brainchild of Coco Chanel, who realized in the late Twenties that the ever-expanding middle classes would not have easy access to real jewels. Thus fake baubles were born and worn to excess throughout the Thirties and Forties. Earrings, necklaces and bracelets in bold plain shades can match, or can be faceted chunky styles, sometimes teamed with metals or metal finishes.

During the war, silk stockings were painted on with leg make-up, sometimes even with a back seam. You don't need to go that far – stockings (called nylons during the war) should have ankle ribs and back seams. Shoes tend to be high, raised either on platform soles or with wedge heels, perhaps with peep toes and a riot of straps in summer. To be absolutely correct, your bag should match your shoes and ought to have a short handle, rather than a shoulder-strap.

FACE AND HAIR
Hair can be worn in a variety of styles: with demure suits and dresses, go for tight waves or curls, or else a smooth pageboy style, ending somewhere between chin and shoulder length, maybe with a curled fringe (bangs). More sophisticated molls might try the period variation on the pompadour – back-combing

the top, smoothing it over a roller, and hairpinning it in place as the illustration shows.

Make-up was heavy, so begin with a concealing foundation, dusted with matching powder. Apply medium brown or dusky blue over the lower eyelid, and a bit of ivory under the brow. Brows will be plucked very thin, and pencilled in, if too pale. Outline lips first in a very deep red pencil, filling with a very brilliant red lipstick. Paint nails to match lips.

IDEAS
● Use remnants from alterations to make bands for hats. Wrap a length at the base of the hat's crown, then tuck in any of the trimming suggested above.

● Should your blouse, suit jacket or dress be missing a button or two, replace them all with originals from junk shops or with modern imitations.

● Replace damaged shoulder pads (blouses and dresses often had padded shoulders) in original clothing with new foam ones – this is imperative to preserve the shape, though it may entail unpicking the lining.

● Give the effect of a blouse under a sweater by using insert collars (see illustration) – usually in starched white cotton and sometimes with a lacy edging – they save lots of ironing.

Below: Little details that complete the period effect such as geometrically inspired buttons – use similar geometric shapes to replace less interesting ones on sweaters and blouses. To save on blouses, use detachable collars in white cotton or lace.

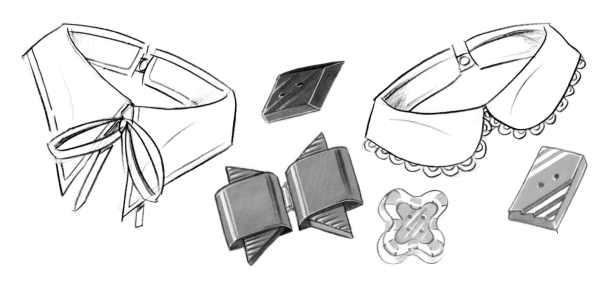

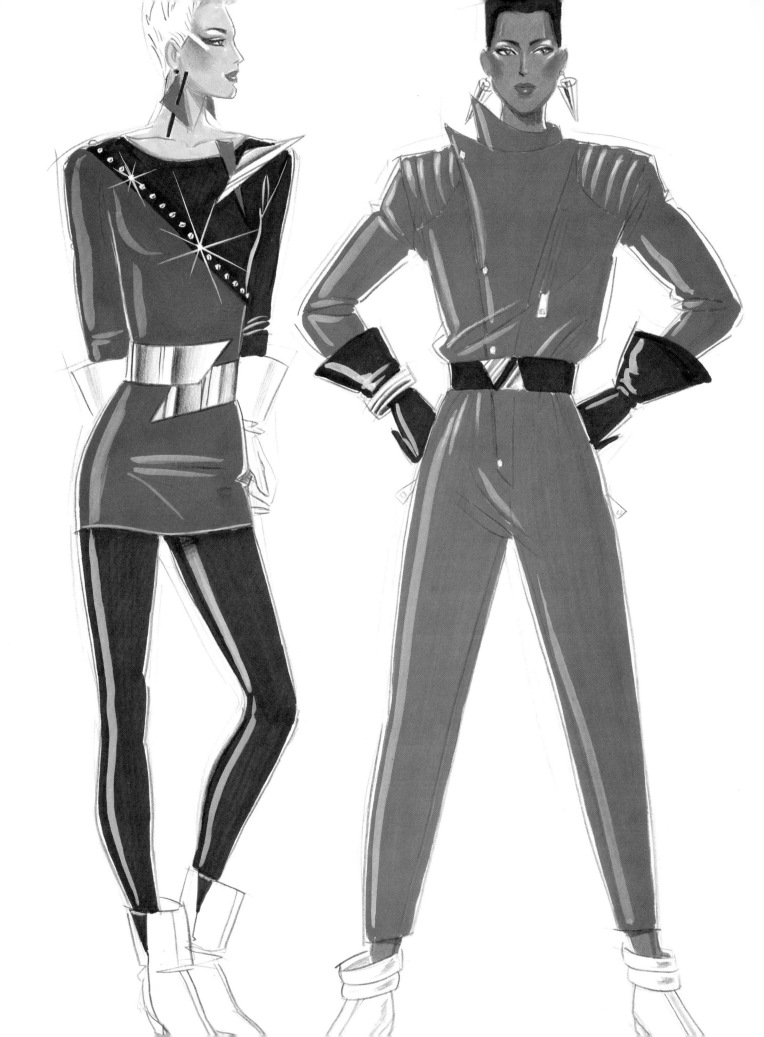

THE FUTURIST

BACKGROUND

Although nowadays you might associate it with the punk look, futuristic fashion has in fact been around at least as long as the twentieth century itself, and someday we may occupy the ultra-convenient worlds described by H.G. Wells and Asimov. You may, however, want to dress for them now. Heroines of science fiction comics and movies approach the problem of dressing in two different ways, although the components of each overlap. The first is a functional, fully-covered style, rather like THE WORKER, but more colourful and zappy.

The second variety of Futurist dressing is more way out, coming from the cult of sci-fi and hugely successful space odyssey films, such as *2001* and *Star Wars*, which have helped make this look into a popular and familiar style in recent years. Today THE FUTURIST parallels the high-tech movement of interior design which brings the elements of large-scale technology and factory design into the home just as Futurist fashion brings space age discoveries in materials and clothes design down to earth.

THE LOOK

Whichever version of the look you choose, this style is not for the timid or those short of imagination. Nor does it suit the overweight, unless the overalls are cut just right, and everyone except the super slim should forget microskirts. It can be worn everyday, but it is ideal for parties and nightspots.

Start with a bodystocking, or leotard, opaque tights and a high-necked T-shirt on top, all in electric colours. For the next layer, choose a jacket, tunic or mid-thigh-length dress, straight or A-line in shape. Ideally, it should be decorated with metallic details or geometric stitchery and have metal fastenings and either a large or small stand-up collar. Wear it over the body stocking and tights. Skirts are always short and made from plastic (clear, translucent or opaque depending on how much you want to conceal), and other rigid fabrics like felt, thick wools and quilted materials. They too can be either A-line, or cut on the bias like skating skirts.

Below: Sci-fi accessories suit **The Futurist.** For footwear choose calf-length boots, jewellery in plastic or metal, and close-fitting helmets and hoods, but to keep the starshine out of your eyes, add a brimless hat on top.

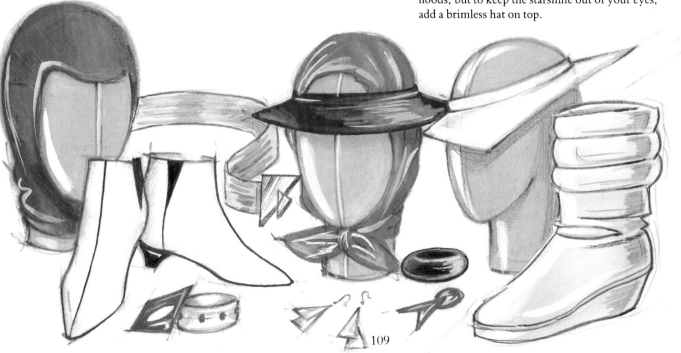

Tapered trousers, stretch pants (both from ski shops) or overalls are tucked into boots or, if they are tight at the ankle, worn with flat-heeled shoes (see below). Overalls, made of cire nylon or metallicized fabric, will have industrial fastenings, such as press studs, rivets, toggles, catches and velcro strips, but no buttons. They may be gathered at the waist and/or ankle, and be quilted and padded.

Both tunics and trousers should be made from softer fabrics than skirts; jerseys, silks, satins, or knits all work well, and are even better if they are shiny and in plain, shocking shades – avoid patterns and prints unless they are

simple and geometric. The final layer of the look can be a quilted duvet coat, a cape or a cheap, translucent, but colourful plastic raincoat.

ACCESSORIES

'Moon Boots' can be found in ski shops; look for crepe soles, wedge heels, quilted uppers and metallic accents, but avoid rustic-looking country-style ones – there is no mud in your space capsule. For cheap flat shoes, try ballet slippers – they come in a myriad of colours including gold and silver. There are, of course, more expensive flat-heeled alternatives in metallicized leathers.

Belts are big. Again look for metallicized leathers or bright plastics with stunning geometric clasps. Strips of metal sheeting will work too, but whatever your belt is made of, make sure it is bold. Wear it over a tunic or to define your waist where microskirt and T-shirt meet. Belts can also have several dog clips to hang keys, change purses, etc. from, so you don't have to carry a handbag. If you do, make it a shiny aluminium briefcase or a translucent or neon plastic satchel.

Jewellery is also very emphatic. Look for big pieces in anodized titanium or neon perspex, or choose battery-operated jewellery that glows in the dark. Try brooches, pendants, big earrings, and hair ornaments in geometric shapes. Alternatively, there is a lot of high-tech jewellery, based on plastics, wire grids and refractive foils – see *Ideas*.

To top off the look in cold weather, put on a balaclava, hood or knitted helmet with chin strap and/or visor. In warmer weather, wear a plastic hat brim like those illustrated.

FACE AND HAIR

THE FUTURIST, unlike most other looks in this book, can be conveyed by hair and make-up alone; both must be very extreme. Hair should be worn off the face and can be any colour including blue, green or pink – for the shy, streaks in these shades. Short hair can be greased with gel or setting lotion to make it stand up slightly, medium hair should be cut in geometric styles (very Sassoon, very sixties) long hair can be wrapped into a chignon worn

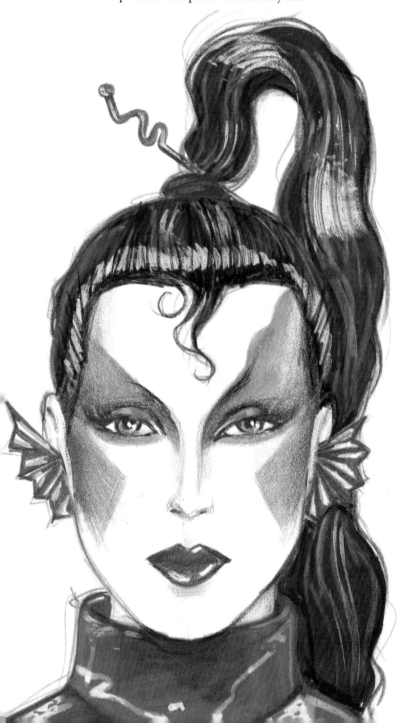

Left: A Futuristic look can be achieved with a Futuristic face. Follow the instructions given under *Face and Hair* on the opposite page, allowing the colouring to be as wild as you like.

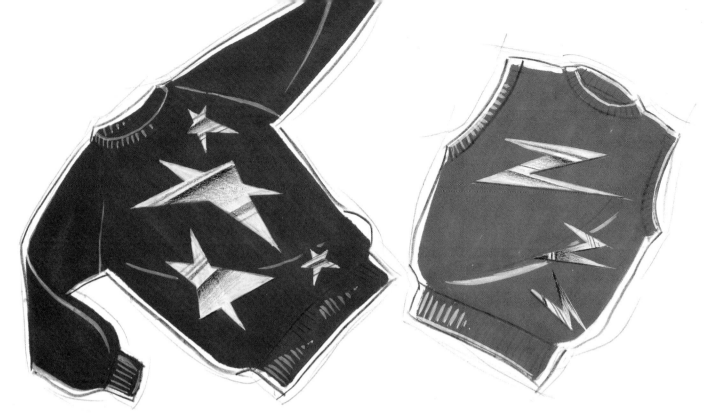

Above: Transform less-than-zappy sweatshirts and T-shirts with Futuristic appliqués cut from iron-on fabrics. Alternatively, stitch on your stars and lightning stripes.

over each ear or gathered in a ponytail at the top of the head as the illustration shows.

When making up, think of Grace Jones and Lene Lovich. Faces are decorated as if they were a blank canvas.

Step-by-Step Make-up Instructions

1. Apply a very pale, even whitish, or a very bronzed shade of foundation over the entire face, including eyelids.
2. Using an eyebrow pencil, draw a fine line from the outer corner of the eye to the end of the eyebrow *and* from the inner corner to the start of the eyebrow.
3. Start shading with an application of orangish or pinkish shade on the lid near the lashes, up to the crease.
4. Next apply a contrasting colour such as lime green or bright blue just under the eyebrow, working it towards the crease. (You can follow the line of your natural brow, or if your brows are pale enough, ignore them and draw new ones up to your hairline as in the illustration.)
5. Apply a third contour colour such as red, purple or navy in the crease line extending it to the inner corner of the eyelid so it completely encircles the eye.
6. Using a soft kohl pencil in navy, black or brown, according to your colour scheme, draw a wedge shape around the entire eye, just inside the eyelashes.
7. To emphasize cheeks, take a thick sheet of paper and hold it against your cheekbones up to your hairline. Apply frosted blusher below the cheekbones, keeping the paper in place to give the cheeks hard definition.
8. Finally, outline lips in tan or mauve, making the bow at the top like two mountain peaks and the bottom lip into an inverted triangle. Fill in with a sharp red, pink or fuschia lipstick. If you like, also use the outlining pencil for drawing small designs on your face – stars, crescent moons and zigzags.

IDEAS

● Decorate hair with a stylish hair-pin. It can be similar to your jewellery or an unusual substitute such as cocktail swizzle sticks, which are inexpensive and ideal.

● Add detail to outerwear using iron-on or quilted metallic fabrics. Reinforce elbows, knees and pockets with fabric patches or add geometric shapes as in the illustration.

● Do-it-yourself jewellery is easily achieved. Collect small electronic components or more mundane bits of hardware – washers, bolts, screws. Arrange on metal templates such as those used for making patchwork quilts, or simply hang from earring hooks or glue to pin backings from jewellery supply stores.

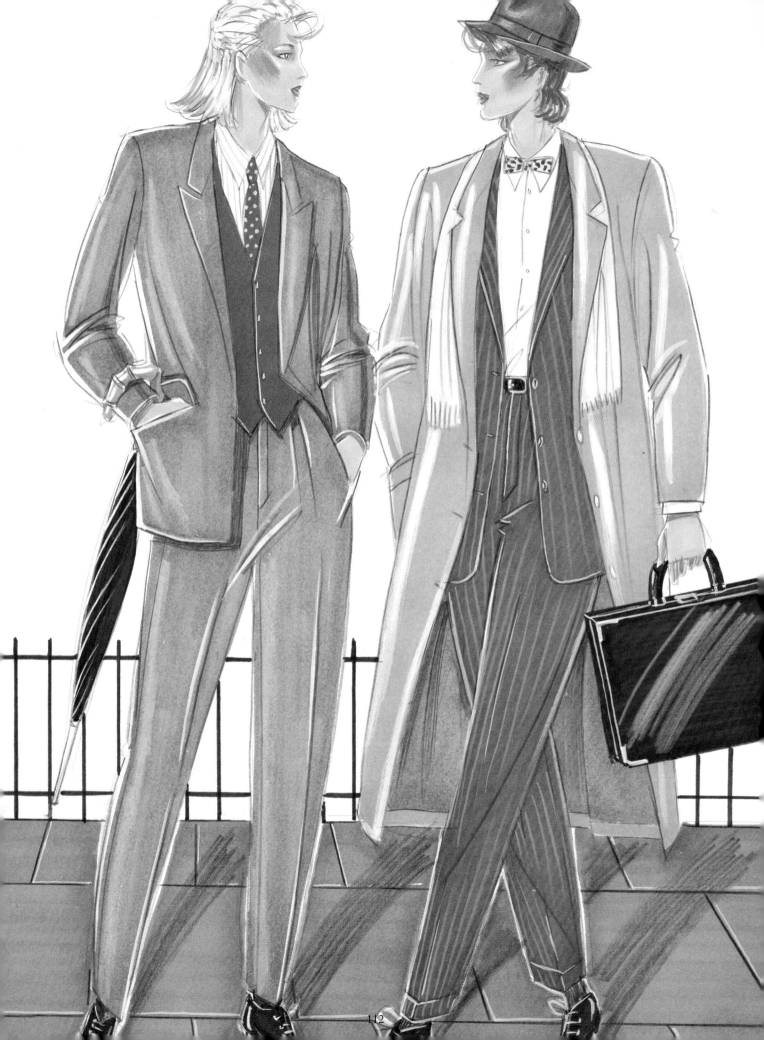

THE GENTLEMAN

BACKGROUND

There may be nothing like a dame, but there's nothing like a gent either. The gentleman is always perfectly mannered and perfectly dressed – never untidy or foppish. This look was born in the great tailoring establishments of London and New York and is still worn daily by executives throughout the world. It has stood the test of time because it is an easy look to achieve and is comfortable to wear, and has consequently become a perennial theme with both the French and Italian designers. It's currently favoured by Cerrutti, Armani and Piero di Monzi. The basis of the look, the tailored suit, is now sported by men and women alike, in virtually every colour and texture. For our purposes, we'll stick to traditional masculine attire; see the BUSINESSWOMAN for the modified feminine version.

Below: Choose mannish accessories for **The Gentleman,** such as low-heeled lace-up shoes or loafers worn with Argyle plaid socks, neckties with traditional spots or stripes, and plain belts in classic colours.

THE LOOK

Start with the two- or three-piece suit. It should be of plain wool flannel, in grey, black or navy, perhaps with a fine pin-stripe. The jacket should be perfectly tailored, with notched lapels, back vents, two or three front buttons and the trousers cut according to the current men's fashion. Get the suit from a man in your life (if he's the same size), a menswear shop, or a secondhand clothing store. If you find that you love this way of dressing, consider having a suit made by a tailor. Alternatively, get a secondhand suit that nearly fits and have it altered. Bear in mind that it is very important for the suit to fit correctly, or else THE GENTLEMAN starts looking like THE IMMIGRANT.

Under the suit, wear a classic white cotton shirt with collar and cuffs. Those gents who are less colour-shy might wear light or mid-blue pinstriped shirts, but in any event avoid wearing shirts with pintucks or ruffles. Reserve those for evening – see THE DANDY.

For outerwear, don a classic trenchcoat or a man's overcoat in a fine tweed or plain camel, navy or grey. According to the fashion dictates of the day, the overcoat may be above-knee or calf-length, cut large or close-fitting.

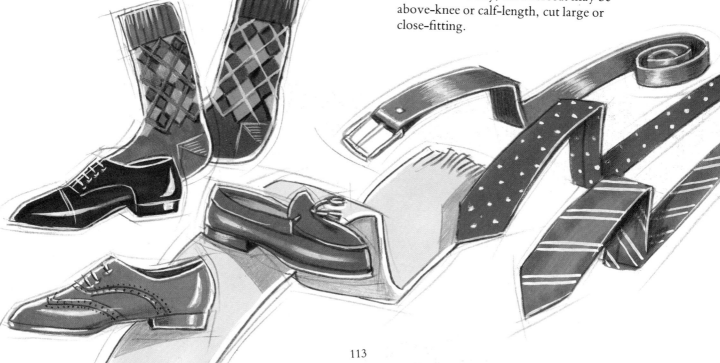

ACCESSORIES

THE GENTLEMAN's accessories can be found in any menswear store. If you love the look, buy the best – if you're wearing it with tongue-in-cheek, go for the inexpensive. Begin with a subtly striped or white-dotted necktie (slightly nattier gentlemen may opt for a bow tie in the same traditional patterns). Choose sober shades of blue, burgundy, green, occasionally allowing a splash of pale yellow, blue or pink. Knot the tie as the illustration shows, securing it with a tie clip, stick pin or stud pin if you like, but beware of anything flashy.

On your feet, wear brogues, loafers or Oxfords in black, wine brown or navy with matching or contrasting socks. If you're attracted to patterned socks, make sure they are in tasteful neutral shades. Your belt can be plain leather to match your shoes or might be webbing in the classic combinations of burgundy/navy or black/grey stripes. Alternatively, hold up your trousers with braces – these delightful anachronisms are especially appropriate under a waistcoat, when a belt buckle might make an ugly bulge.

Carry a briefcase to hold your papers and make-up (the inside pockets are marvellous organizers). If a briefcase seems too large and bulky for your needs, get a slim leather envelope with a zip fastening on three sides. For money and credit cards, get a wallet to match.

Handkerchiefs, like bow ties, can be used to add a dash of colour – tuck a cotton or silk one, plain, paisley, or dotted, into the outside breast pocket of your jacket. Alternatively, carry the white starched variety in a trouser pocket. A monogrammed handkerchief is a nice touch, too.

As for jewellery, we must ultimately leave that to your discretion – and discretion is the word. If you feel in need of adding a 'feminine touch' to the strict lines of your outfit then a fine gold chain at neck or wrist, simple classic gold bands, flat or twisted, and neat ear-studs in gold, pearl or coral work best. This look does not lend itself to the home-made, the glittery, ethnic or outrageous, so jewellery should be chosen with restraint – a classic watch with kid or lizard-skin strap may well be your best and only investment. Cuffs can be secured with tasteful cufflinks.

By way of hats, again, go for the understated. A well-fitting trilby or fedora is just right.

Below and opposite: Plain, white or pastel-tinted Oxford cloth shirts are basic to this look, but you might vary these a little by allowing a contrasting white collar against a coloured shirt, a few pintucks down the front, or a bib-front style with detachable collar. Real gents would approve and think nothing of changing their shirt and collar twice a day!

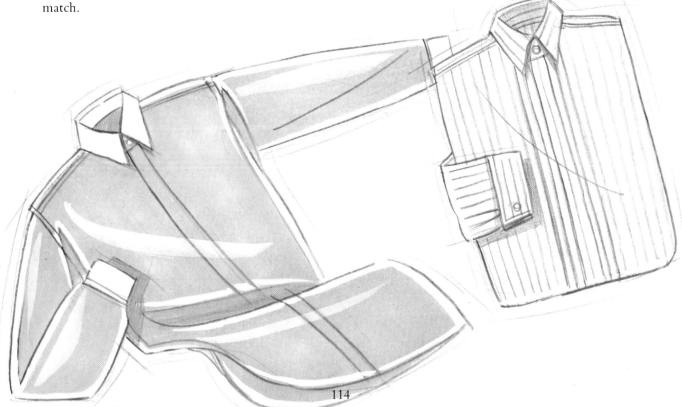

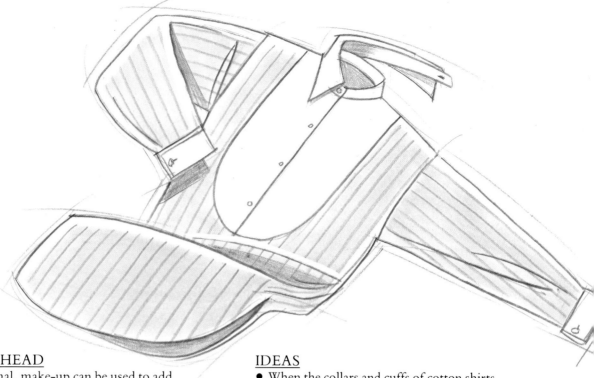

FACE AND HEAD

Though minimal, make-up can be used to add much-needed colour to this look. Use neutral shades like grey and cream for eyes, pale apricots and pinks for lips. Eyebrows must be thick, either naturally, or pencilled in. Hair should be sleek and neat, preferably above shoulder length, though short, cropped styles are ideal. If short, slick back with gel. The final emphasis is on the jaw bone. To widen, apply ivory highlighter at the corner of the jaw, then apply a taupe-coloured powder under the jaw bone for a squares effect.

IDEAS

● When the collars and cuffs of cotton shirts wear thin, replace them with plain white ones. A gentleman's shirtmaker will do this for you, or you may be able to purchase replacements from a haberdashery shop. The new white collar and cuffs will look fine with coloured or pinstriped shirts, but may not match an older white shirt very well. In that case, remove the collar completely, turn up the cuffs, and wear the collarless shirt with THE IMMIGRANT.

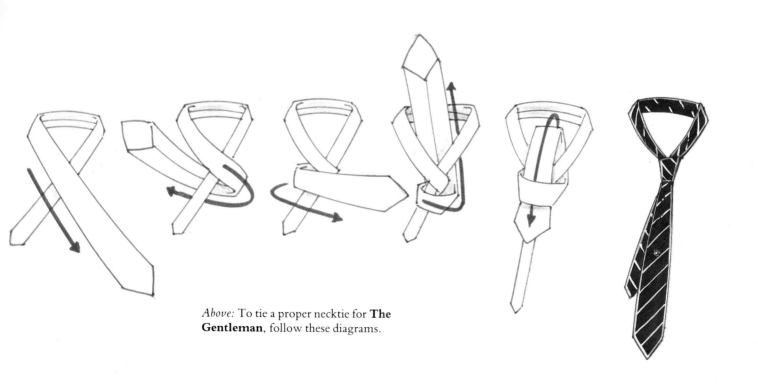

Above: To tie a proper necktie for **The Gentleman,** follow these diagrams.

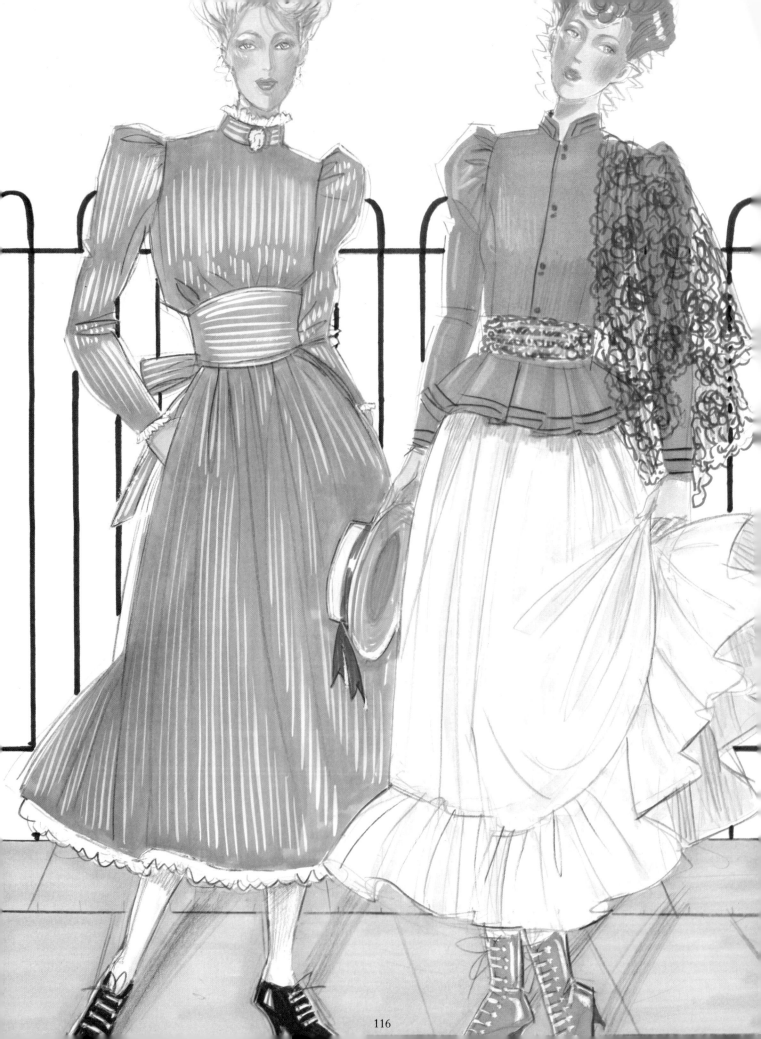

THE GIBSON GIRL

BACKGROUND

THE GIBSON GIRL comes to us straight from the turn of the century when the middle classes in Europe and America were enjoying ever-increasing prosperity, oblivious to the gathering war clouds.

The Gibson Girl gets her name from the captivating drawings of Charles Dana Gibson, the American illustrator. He was married to Nancy Astor's elder sister, a renowned beauty, and it was her delicate aristocratic features, long neck, and elegant, slender figure that he immortalized.

It was a period of emancipation for women. The suffragette movement was at its height, the bicycle had arrived, and clothing was rapidly becoming less restrictive. Although corsets were still worn, some of the multiple layers of underclothes were thrown aside. Voluminous skirts which swept the ground were replaced by flared or gored ones of lighter, less cumbersome fabrics. These developments facilitated the newly popular sporting activities and for bicycling it soon became acceptable for women to sport knickerbockers. Freedom of movement was the essence and it led to a new romantic style of dress.

As with all romantic movements the original inspiration was soon lost as the look became more and more accentuated. The gently flowing curves of the Edwardian line evolved into the outrageous, serpentine decadence and hot-house motifs of Art Nouveau.

THE LOOK

Variations on THE GIBSON GIRL look have been popular ever since and have been re-established during the last decade by the designer Laura Ashley, with her high necklines, soft ruffles and gently sprigged fabrics. Designers of evening wear, such as John Bates, Gina Fratini, Zandra Rhodes and Oscar de la Renta have used the full skirt and sleeve for years, but it was Laura Ashley, more than anyone else, who established the look as acceptable day wear.

Below: **The Gibson Girl** has a heyday with accessories: shoes can be simple black pumps or the period-correct laced or buttoned ankle boot with Louis-shaped heel; gloves will be lacy or leather, preferably with a frill at the wrist; jewellery is antique or imitations thereof; bags are soft drawstring styles; belts are wide and stockings are always coloured, either dark or pale.

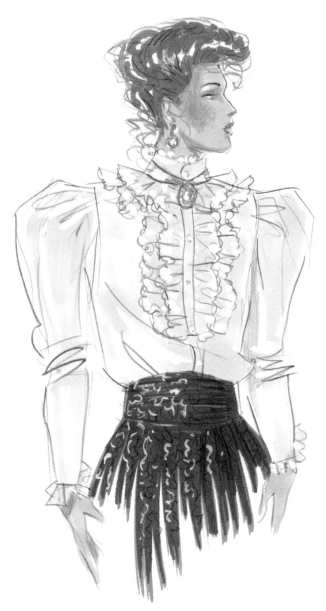

Left: For evening, nothing beats **The Gibson Girl** for making a feminine impression. Choose a white or cream-coloured, high-necked, ruffle-fronted blouse. Add a knee- or calf-length skirt in any fabric from suede to brocade, sweep up your hair, add a cameo or similar pin to your neck, and while the late hours away.

Under the jacket wear a high-necked blouse. Traditionally, the blouse was white with a ruffle or lace at the neckline, cuffs, and down the front panel, but today the choice is wide.

Original colours were subdued for winter – browns, navy, bottle greens and dark reds – and paler, creamy shades for summer. Stripes were also very popular, from the pin-line to the very bold. Nowadays, your choice is much less rigid: decide on your own combinations but don't mix two contrasting types of stripe or too many different colours.

For authenticity – and the prettiest effect – the peplum top should be teamed with a full, mid-calf-length skirt in lightweight wool, corduroy, challis, for winter day wear, and seersucker or similar weight cottons for summer.

For winter outerwear, if your peplum jacket is not warm enough, choose a coat with a fitted waist and, preferably, full sleeves. It can be any length from three-quarters to ankle length. A voluminous three-quarter-length untailored coat works well with this look, too. For a lighter outer layer, consider shawls – lacy wool or spider's web mohair give the final romantic touch to your outfit.

Begin with your feet. Boots should be worn with the daytime, winter version of the look. They can be classic, to-the-knee style; better still, buy calf-length fitted boots with lace-up or button-up fronts. Heels are at least two inches high and might be shaped. For summer and evening wear, ankle-strapped shoes or any mid-heeled style in soft kid. Patent leather, lace or velveteen are best for evening. With footwear, wear stockings if you want to go all the way. (Even your underwear can be from the correct period – use the camisole and petticoat from THE SHEPHERDESS). Look for stockings in silky, sheer textures, or choose thicker, cottony ones like the original cotton lisle. Wear white or cream with pastel shades, summer clothes and evening fabrics; darker ones for winter days and darker clothing. A flash of coloured leg is also in keeping – maybe bright red or emerald green.

You can dress like a Gibson Girl whether it's day or evening, summer or winter. The components (given below) remain the same, only the fabrics change. It is a wonderfully flattering way of dressing, suiting both the thin, because of the fullness of sleeve and skirt, and those who wish to disguise their hips and thighs. It also makes for spectacular evening wear in rich fabrics.

A jacket (or blouse for summer) with a peplum waist (that is, with a fitted bodice and short flared piece at the waistline) is the distinctive garment for this look. The garment has slightly puffed or leg-o'-mutton sleeves and it can button, snap up or fasten with frogs – the important thing is the characteristic shape. A similar effect can be achieved by simply belting a short jacket or sweater which comes two to four inches below your waistline, but the properly styled jacket gives the best effect.

Emphasize the waist on your skirt or jacket with a thick belt (up to six inches wide), in leather, suede webbing or any of the fabrics recommended for evening wear. Belts can buckle, lace up or wrap to fasten, but the main thing is to cinch, cinch, cinch your waist.

Jewellery should be old-fashioned-looking or better still, antique. You can get away with quite a lot of it – the Edwardians thought nothing of wearing earrings, bracelets, a necklace and a brooch all together. If you have no antique jewellery, see *Ideas* for a simple choker.

On your hands, wear gloves or at least carry them. They can be short white ones in cotton ecru, or kid for summer; longer push-up or gauntlet styles for winter; lacy fingerless mitts for dressy occasions.

And to top it all off, a huge brimmed hat, ideally bedecked with flowers and feathers. Look for them in secondhand clothing stores, steam into shape over a bowl in a bathtub and retrim as the illustration shows.

FACE AND HAIR
Upswept locks were *de rigueur* at the turn of the century. Ringlets and waves are also right (see THE IMMIGRANT for instructions on making rag curls). A bunch of artificial flowers or ribbons looks very charming at the back or to tie up strands of hair from the front and sides. However, make sure that they go with your outfit. Also consider patterned ribbons with stripes, plaids and floral designs.

Make-up is equally subtle. Foundation should be natural, dusted with a thorough application of loose powder. Begin eye make-up by applying a pinkish shadow over the entire lid, blending it into a grey or brownish tone applied in the crease. Bring this same colour around under the lower lashes to give a dewy-eyed effect, but make sure this line is soft and smudged. Finish with a pinkish blusher and a very natural shade of lipstick.

IDEAS
• Make a choker by tying an 18-inch (46 cms) ribbon around the neck of your blouse or jacket, knotting it into a single or double bow in front. Or, use a 1 – 1½ inch (3 cms) wide ribbon and pin a brooch in the centre of the length, tying the ribbon at the back of your neck.

• Use thin satiny ribbons for lacing through lace on summer whites like petticoats, blouses, camisoles, and wear the same colour ribbon in your hair and/or on your hat.

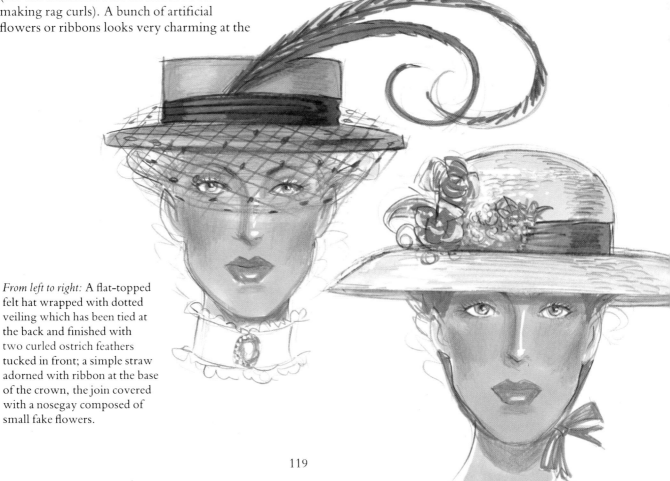

From left to right: A flat-topped felt hat wrapped with dotted veiling which has been tied at the back and finished with two curled ostrich feathers tucked in front; a simple straw adorned with ribbon at the base of the crown, the join covered with a nosegay composed of small fake flowers.

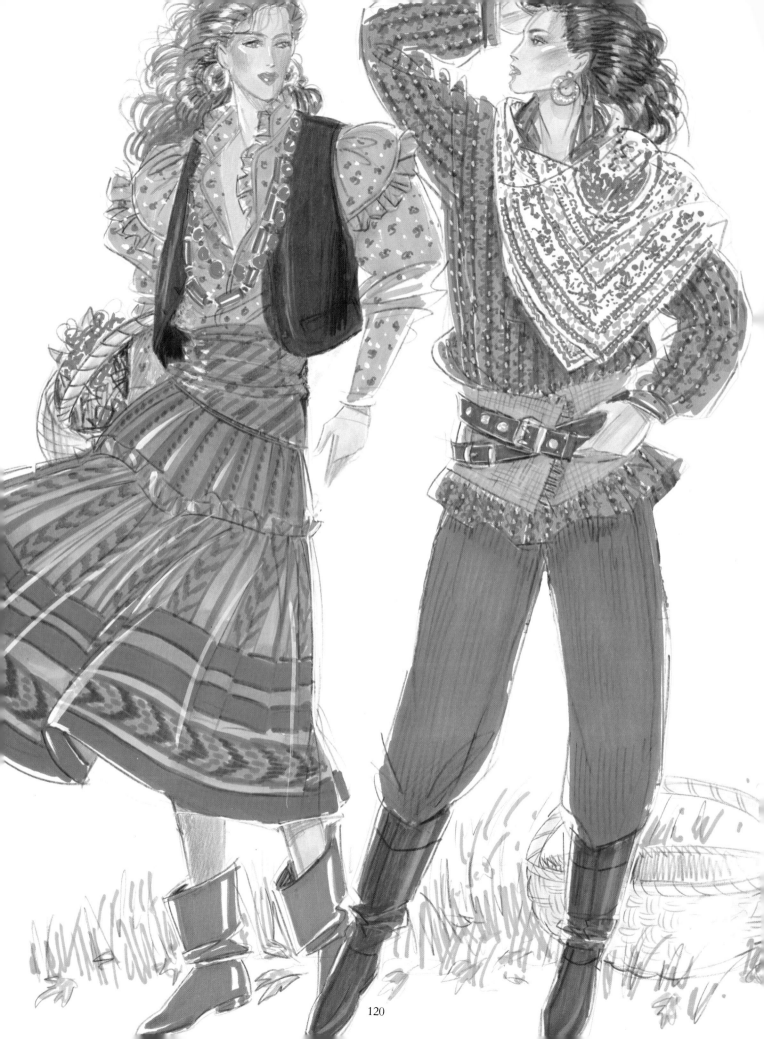

THE GYPSY

BACKGROUND

The advent of the flower children of the Sixties and their pointed attempts to ignore mainstream fashion in favour of colourful ethnic clothing, brought about a re-birth of the Gypsy style. However, the origins of the look are much older. Originally a Romany-speaking people scattered throughout Europe and North America, gypsies, even today, maintain a nomadic and independent way of life in the midst of industrialized societies. They migrated from north-west India during the twelfth to fifteenth centuries, and were thought to have come from Egypt – hence Gypsies. Like all travellers, they collected customs and articles as they went, evolving an exotic and eclectic appearance.

Of course, like all looks born in the wild, THE GYPSY was tamed and refined by fashion designers such as Yves St Laurent and Oscar de la Renta and re-presented in a more amenable and luxurious package. THE GYPSY

look is both practical for everyday wear and exotic enough for special occasions. It can be worn by every figure type and looks best on those women whose complexions allow them to wear a medley of the very bright characteristic colours. So wear vibrant tones like red, orange, gold and yellow set off by tan, black, brown and white, and accented by dashes of bright blue, turquoise and green.

In addition, THE GYPSY is the perfect look for playing with pattern, and with the influx of traditionally-printed separates from India and China, there is no shortage of such clothing. The small prints from the Provençal region of France are also ideal, though usually far more expensive. Traditional American calico prints will also do, as will any of the brighter Laura Ashley motifs.

THE LOOK

Like many of the looks in this book, THE GYPSY has a trousered and a skirted version. The trousers can be made of anything from

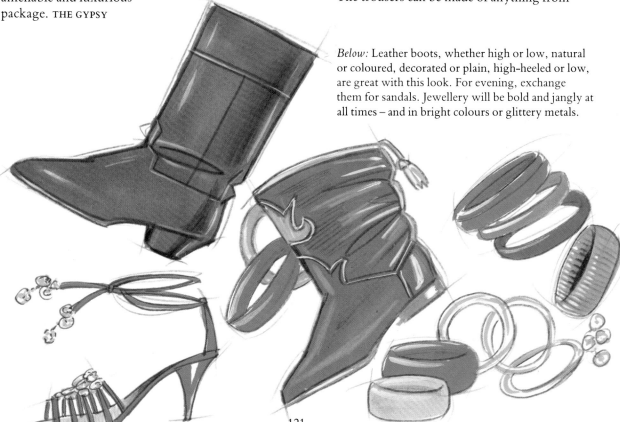

Below: Leather boots, whether high or low, natural or coloured, decorated or plain, high-heeled or low, are great with this look. For evening, exchange them for sandals. Jewellery will be bold and jangly at all times – and in bright colours or glittery metals.

gauzy inexpensive cottons for summer to heavier velvets and wools for winter; a rich Gypsy might even wear leather or suede. However, trousers should be harem or zouave-style (as in THE ARABIAN). For an instant effect, tuck baggy trousers into calf- or knee-length dark leather boots and let the excess fabric fall luxuriously over the tops.

Next, a big blouse on top – traditionally white with very full blowsy sleeves, slash neckline and pointed collar, but any loose-fitting style will do. Tuck it in, or wear it over the pants with a belt if it comes down to your hips. On top of this, add a short bolero or buttonless waistcoat.

If you prefer a more authentic gypsy style, choose full, tiered skirts. These come in every fabric imaginable from cotton voile to satin, but stick to plain bright shades or small prints. For a really full and romantic effect, wear several gathered skirts in bold co-ordinating colours as layers, with white Victorian lace-trimmed petticoats underneath. On top, wear a white blouse and embroidered or printed bolero jacket.

Whether wrapping up on cool summer nights or keeping warm around the caravan's campfire, choose a poncho cape or large shawl. (These squares of fabric are immensely versatile – wear them with THE IMMIGRANT, THE COSSACK, THE LATIN, THE ARABIAN, and THE YOUNG ROMANTIC depending on the fabric and texture.) For THE GYPSY, they can either be of plain bright colours, embroidered or floral-printed – the gaily-patterned ones look marvellous with unpatterned clothing, or if you're confident about your colour sense, wear two and add pattern to pattern. In summer, the wrap could be thin silk or cotton; in winter, embroidered wool or even a blanket wrap.

From left to right: Four ways of wearing either a large square scarf which has been folded on the diagonal or a triangular-shaped shawl: over both shoulders and crossed in front with the ends knotted in back of the waist; over your head with both ends thrown over your shoulders; over both shoulders with the knot in front, secured with a brooch; and over one shoulder with both ends knotted on the opposite hip.

Shawls can be worn a number of ways as the illustration shows – over both shoulders, fastened in front with a brooch or knot, over one shoulder and tied at the opposite hip, or bunched up like a serape and wrapped round and round.

ACCESSORIES

Indulgers in excess will love THE GYPSY. It is a very ornamented look; nothing is too much. Wear bracelets by the dozens, belts in threes, scarves everywhere.

For the cold weather version of this look, a pair of boots is essential. They can be flat or high-heeled, and should be of plain colours such as red, brown, burgundy or black. Embroidered or embossed boots, such as those described in THE COWBOY are also in keeping. Tuck the cuffs of pants into the boot top (as described earlier), or wear them with full skirts in cold weather – they are essential. In summer, exchange them for sandals – low-heeled with laces and coins, or high-heeled with your full summery skirts. Metallic accents be they coins, jewels, or

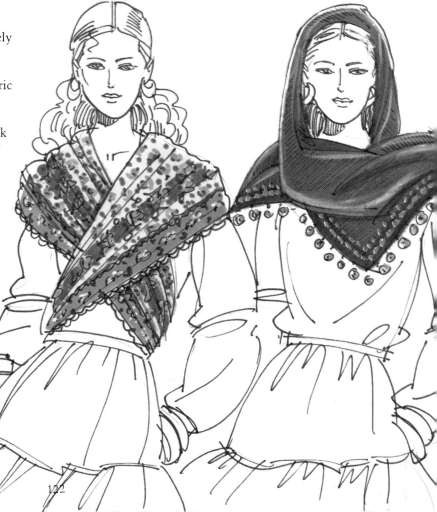

bronzed leathers on any footwear will lend an appropriately exotic look.

Another requisite is a well-wrapped waist. Scarves, fabric remnants or pieces of leather or suede will all make wide cummerbunds. Use the same waist-wrapping technique as outlined in THE ARABIAN – first a wide swathe of cummerbund, secured with a thinner rope, be it a thin belt, a satin curtain cord, a strip of cotton or a scarf rolled into a belt. Alternatively tie a shawl round your waist so that it hangs like an overskirt, diagonally over the hip.

Scarves are also essential for making headwear appropriate to THE GYPSY. The tradition-minded vagabond will knot a gaily-printed floral one behind her head at the nape of her neck, but you can knot it to one side, or at your chin if you choose. The important thing is that the scarf should be decorated with rich floral patterns or spots and even fringed. Tie a paisley-printed or polka-dotted neckerchief round your neck for a more casual use of THE GYPSY's scarf. You might then add another scarf on top of the first one, rolled into a rouleaux, as the introductory illustration shows. See THE COSSACK for another treatment.

Jewellery knows no limits. Begin with hooped earrings, but don't stop with one pair – if you have pierced ears wear several of different sizes. Alternatively, wear only one, peeping out from behind a scarf-wrapped head. For necklaces, wear chunky gold, silver, brass or bronze chains with huge pieces of stone such as agate, amber or coral dangling from them – the more the merrier. Bracelets, too, are best in numbers – stack them up your arm, mixing metals and styles. Wear them further up your arm as armbands with tanned arms in the summer and wear anklets with sandals. Finally, wear as many rings as you have. There is nothing discreet about the wealth of THE GYPSY.

FACE AND HAIR

Start with an application of warm honey-coloured foundation and matching powder unless you have a naturally tawny complexion. Use sandy shadow over the entire lid and a darker brown blended into the crease line. Give yourself deep, mysterious eyes by drawing a fine line next to the lashes and inside the inner rim with a black kohl pencil. Blush cheeks with a rusty shade, using approximately the same colour on lips.

Wear your hair as wavy and wild as possible, either by brushing out the ringlets achieved with rag curls (see THE IMMIGRANT) or by using conventional curlers and setting lotion.

IDEAS
● Use large squares of chintz, loosely-woven, flower-printed fabric to make shawls. Unravel each edge to make self fringe or attach ready-made fringing or tasselling.

● Seek out those shops that sell ethnic clothing such as those devoted to the goods of nations such as Russia, Hungary, Greece, for more authentic and unusual patterns and items: soft wool floral headsquares from Slavic countries, raw, warm-striped cotton from Greece are examples.

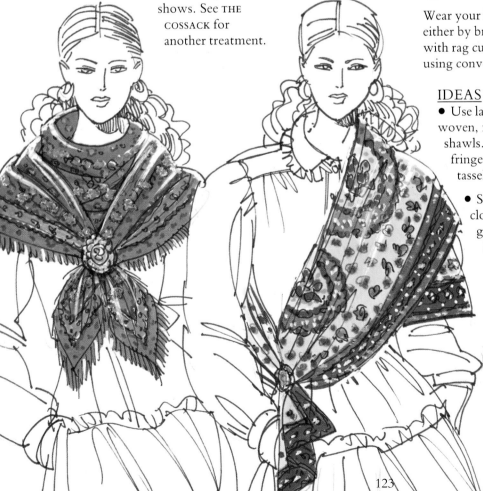

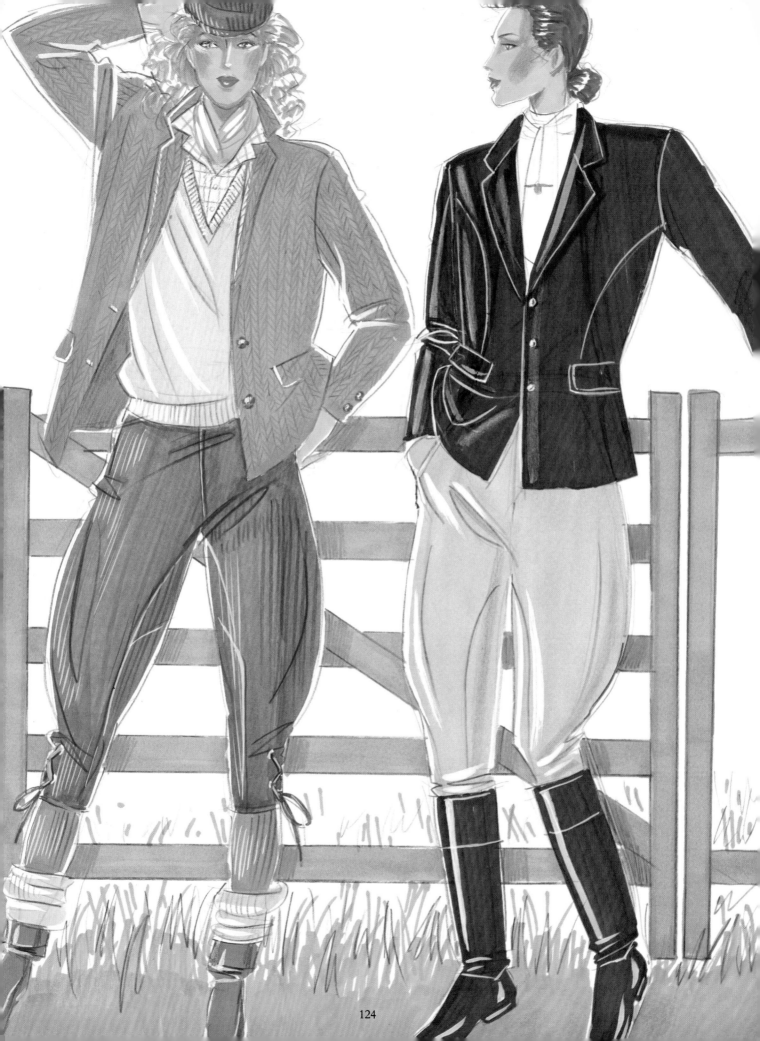

THE HORSEWOMAN

BACKGROUND

Misty mornings, frosty fields, tack over arm and out to the stable yard to saddle up, in good time to make the Meet at the manor house; groomed and prancing hunters, gentlemen in 'pink' coats and black hats, ladies in habits or smart black jackets and immaculate white stocks, all ready for the Master's call. Hounds underfoot, fox in the distance, 'Tally-ho!' and They're off!

If this scenario sounds to you like an archaic tradition pursued only by the last of the 'landed gentry', you may be turned off completely. But before you demolish the motives and manners of those who ride to hounds with the smart hunts, stop to think what we owe them, sartorially speaking. Those horsey ladies have provided one of the most comfortable and practical looks in your wardrobe, not to mention a range of versatile components (such as the hacking jacket and the riding boot) which have become fashion staples for all of us.

THE LOOK

THE HORSEWOMAN can choose from two different styles of dress, though the outline and basic components are similar. Aficionados of the smart hunt or dressage event make a point of being 'well turned out' while clothes for a relaxed cross-country gallop are naturally more informal.

Hacking jacket and riding boots are the crucial ingredients of both versions of the look. Nowadays, they are readily available from sources other than traditional riding outfitters; jackets come in a mass of different colours and patterns, and boots in many variations, so there will be no problem in finding something to suit every taste.

Below: Not to be confused with **The Cowgirl**, this is a much more refined look, and chic enough to take you to town. Make sure your boots are clean and polished, your cravat and string gloves immaculate. The correct riding hat is shown, but less equestrian-minded fans of this look can choose a cap in corduroy or tweed.

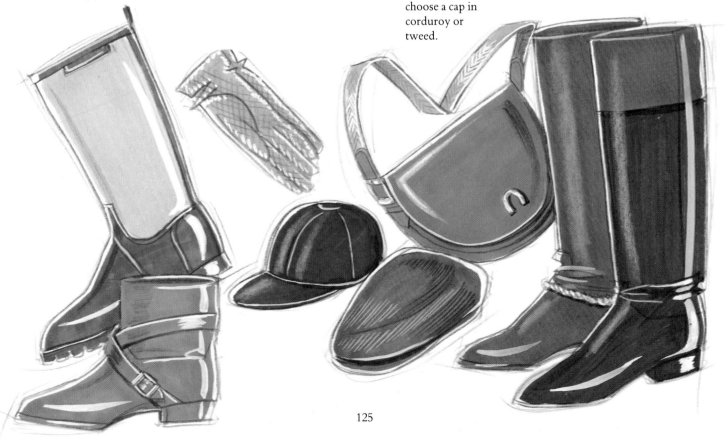

As far as colours go, you are on rather a tight rein with the more formal look and you should really opt for black, white and beige or stone. Your hacking jacket should be of black worsted: well-fitting, single breasted, with small *revers* and collar, and slanted side pockets (probably containing sugar lumps for Dobbin). It has characteristic back or side vents to allow it to fall correctly over the horse's rump. A spotless white shirt and stock go under the jacket. The elegant stock, a length of silk or cotton about three inches wide, is tied high round the neck, its ends falling at the front and kept in position with a stock pin (see *Ideas*). Beige twill jodhpurs (one of the legacies of the British Raj) are baggy and comfortable over the hip and thigh but tight and fitted from knee to ankle.

The alternative relaxed, informal style is the easier of the riding looks to adopt. Choose comfortable, natural fabrics: tweeds, corduroys, wools, and brushed cottons, choosing the fabric weights according to the season. Take nature's subtler colours: moss, olive and leafy green, rust, chestnut, sand and earthy browns in plain, flecked, herringbone, houndstooth or other patterns for your tweed hacking jacket and beige, stone, sand or olive for corduroy or twill jodhpurs.

The tweedy hacking jacket of this version of THE HORSEWOMAN look is cut on the same lines as the smarter black alternative. And the classic jodhpurs feature here, too, though you can exchange them for less strictly styled examples: soft corduroy jodhpurs with laces up the outsides of the calves, breeches buttoned under the knee, or even country farmers' baggy cords are suitable, but tuck the latter into boots to prevent hems from flapping. If you have an aversion to jodhpurs and the like, but are attracted by the rest of this equestrian look, try instead a soft tweedy skirt or pair of tweed or corduroy culottes.

Viyella or cotton shirts with small pointed collars, in plain colours or traditional tattersall checks, are just right under cosy V-necked Shetland or lambswool jerseys, sleeveless pullovers, knitted waistcoats or even THE CLANSWOMAN's Aran. Use the sweater to give the colour scheme of your outfit a lift; a burgundy jersey under an olive jacket, or a yellow pullover with a rust or moss coat.

Because this is a hardworking outdoor look (horses kick up a lot of mud) you are allowed

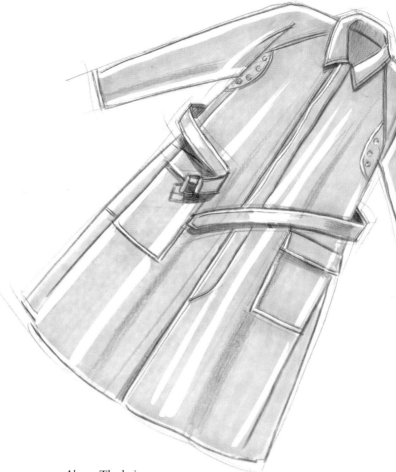

Above: The beige or light loden green rubberized raincoat is indispensable, whether you're a bona fide **Horsewoman** or not. Tie the belt in a self knot rather than threading it through the buckle for a more casual look.

one extra layer with which to insulate yourself against cold and wet: a classic stone-coloured riding mac. This stiff rubberized garment was specifically designed to be worn on horseback; the deep vent at the back allows the wearer to sit easily on the saddle and the studded air holes under the arms prevent any discomfort.

However comfortable you feel in your riding gear, don't forget how the true horsewoman holds herself. Posture – ramrod-straight back and head held high – is all important. The fitted cut of the riding clothes will only emphasize round shoulders, so emulate the ladies of the saddle and carry yourself well.

ACCESSORIES

Many contemporary styles of boots are based on the traditional British riding boot, so there should be no problem in acquiring a pair. This classic low-heeled knee-high leather boot is simple in shape and beautifully made. Choose black to go with the formal black hacking jacket and white stock, and make sure the boots are well polished. For the more casual style of dress, try either full-length dark brown or chestnut-coloured leather boots, brown leather lace-ups or jodhpur boots (these are ankle height with inside zips, elasticated side panels or criss-cross leather straps and buckles). The full-length type with a wide contrasting fawn-coloured band at the top is beautiful and, because of its mix of black and brown, can be worn with either of the horsewoman looks. Alternatively, there's the perfect partner for the riding mac – the recently revived canvas riding boot; a strong rubber foot may have replaced the leather one, but the leg is still in stone-coloured canvas.

Hats are also crucial to THE HORSEWOMAN. With the smarter outfit wear a black velvet hard hat; this is the traditional riding hat. For the more informal look opt for a flat tweed cap which looks great with all kinds of informal country clothes. Or, as a last resort, try a headscarf (after all the Queen of England often wears one).

You will also need warm socks, riding gloves (beige or yellow string for preference) and a tie. The stock counts as your tie for the black coat look, but for the casual style select a knitted or rough woven wool full-length tie, a soft bow-tie or a paisley cravat tucked into your shirt. A horsewoman rarely carries a bag (where does she put all her gear?) but one of the canvas shooting or fishing kinds would be suitable (see THE COUNTRY LANDOWNER and THE FISHERWOMAN).

FACE AND HAIR
THE HORSEWOMAN spends virtually all her time outdoors. As a result, faces are healthy and natural looking with the characteristic rosy cheeks much in evidence. Apply a light foundation for a more even skin tone, followed by golden shadow all over the eyelid with a rust colour in the crease and maybe a forest green in the outer corner, smudged into the rust. Blush cheeks if they're not ruddy already with a toffee shade and finally apply a rusty-apricot lipstick.

Despite the wind, or because of it, every sensible horsewoman knows that hair must be kept out of the eyes. Ladies with short hair have few problems here, but those with long hair should experiment with some of the traditional styles shown in the illustrations below.

IDEAS
• Use woven wool fabric scraps to make full-length or bow ties; or knit up a simple square-ended length (2 × 18 inches – 5 × 46 cms) in olive or rust-coloured rough textured yarn.

• Treat your leather accessories as if they were your tack and give them frequent applications of good old-fashioned saddle soap. Over the years you'll build up a marvellous patina, and boots and bags will acquire that wonderful leather aroma of the best-kept tack rooms.

Below: Four ideas for keeping your hair out of your eyes as you canter along: the ever-classic chignon, or bun, worn at the nape of the neck; a fuller bun or long ponytail tucked in and covered with a woven snood, as worn by 19th-century horsewomen; the ever-popular ponytail, with a fringe or not, plus ribbon if you like; and plaits with ribbon tied at both ends.

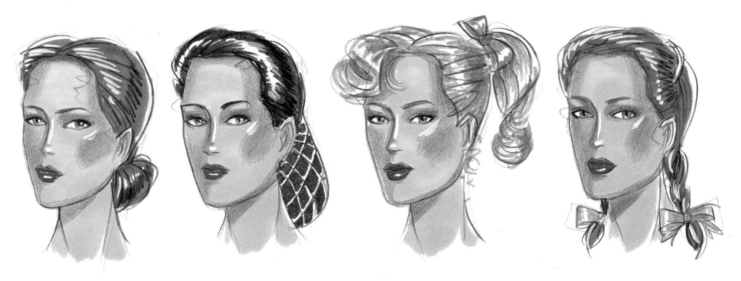

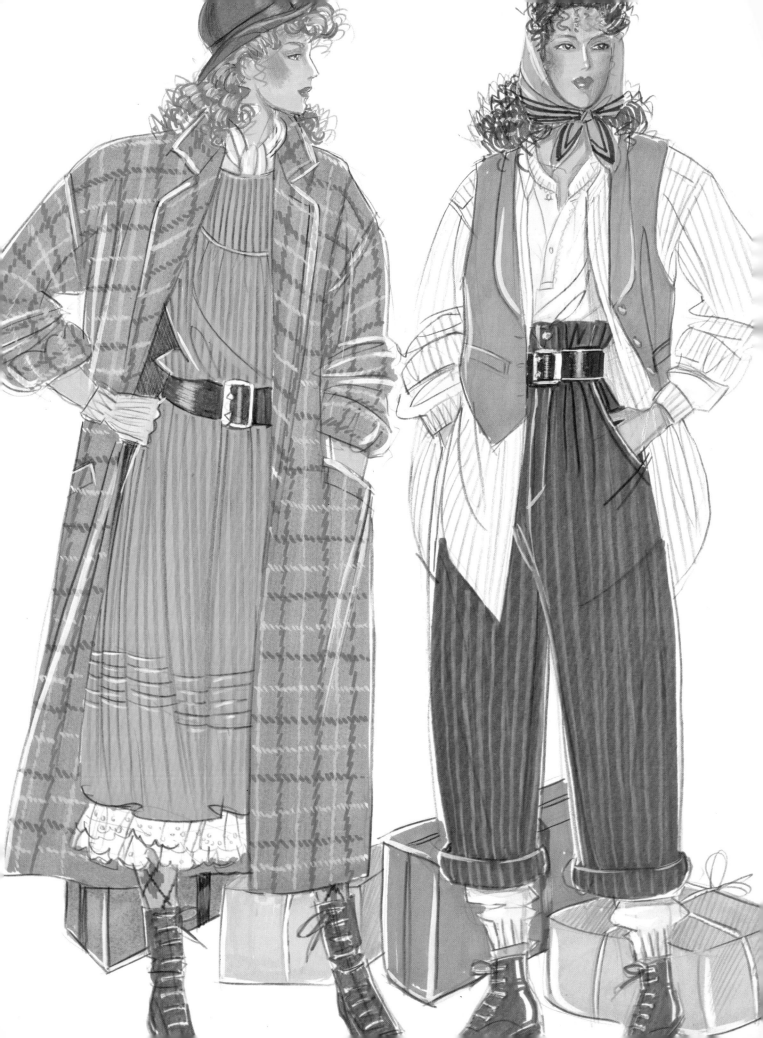

THE IMMIGRANT
THE ANNIE HALL LOOK

BACKGROUND
Imagine that you have to leave home tonight, taking only the clothes that you can put on your back with you, and you'll have a good idea of how to dress like THE IMMIGRANT. In dressing for your imaginary departure, you'd find that you put smaller, more fitted clothes on first, the roomier ones next, maybe ending in a final layer from your father or older brother's cupboard. THE IMMIGRANT is the ultimate layered look.

Without question, the person who popularized this way of dressing was Diane Keaton, in Woody Allen's film *Annie Hall* (1977). Her fetching and eccentric style contrasting tom-boy props with mischievous femininity left its mark on the fashion scene for the next two years; indeed several designers still use it as a basis for their collections.

THE LOOK
Although complicated, dressing like THE IMMIGRANT is very adaptable, and, because of its many layers, is an ideal cold-weather look, yet it can be adapted for warmer weather by changing the fabrics and removing a few of the layers. Additionally, there is both a feminine and more masculine version within the look, though the accessories and proportions remain the same whichever you choose.

Begin by thinking big. Look for outsize clothes in secondhand clothing shops. Search out collarless shirts, hand-knitted sweaters, large waistcoats, single-breasted jackets and overcoats in traditional fabrics such as cottons, worsteds, tweeds and corduroy. Men's trousers will also be useful, even if they don't fit perfectly. Don't worry if your garments are a little threadbare – this look really is a bargain-hunter's delight. You can pay a small fortune for these clothes from famous designers, but you can spend a few pennies by browsing through a few flea markets, auctions and secondhand shops.

Begin dressing with a long-sleeved T-shirt, or off-white wool vest if the weather is cold. Next add a blouse or shirt (the mannish version is pinstriped, collarless, perhaps tucked or bib-fronted; the feminine one has

Below: The more decorative men's clothing such as Argyle plaids and paisley patterns work well with this look. Chunky, laced boots with thick soles, roomy carpet bags and a slightly too big man's hat complete the ragbag effect of dressing like **The Immigrant.**

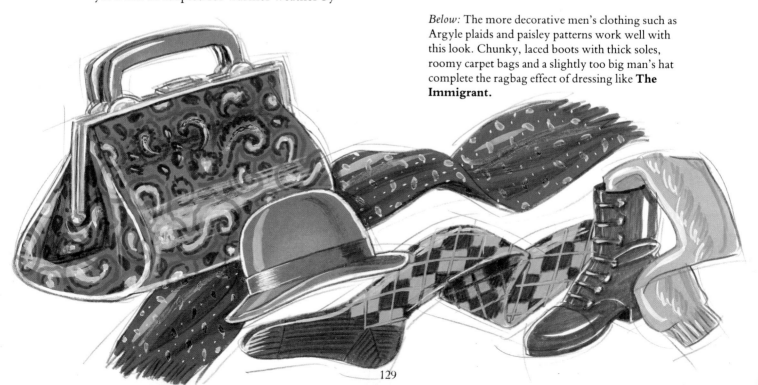

slightly puffed sleeves and can be daintily floral printed). If the blouse is fairly fitted, tuck it into trousers or a full skirt; if it's largish or longer than hip-length, consider wearing it over the trousers or skirt and belting it.

If you are wearing a skirt, make sure it is fairly full and let an assortment of garments peep out underneath – petticoats, long underwear, leg-warmers, even trousers. If you choose the trousered version, remember that trousers don't have to fit. If too large at the waist, cinch with a belt (see *Ideas* and *Accessories* below); if above the ankle, roll up the cuffs a little more and let your socks show.

Over top and bottoms, wear a roomy waistcoat, or if the weather allows, a sweater first, then a waistcoat. On top of all this, add a biggish jacket, then an overcoat, shawl or scarf. Immigrants keep *really* warm! For summer wear, eliminate the overcoat and choose lighter-weight fabrics such as linens, challis, cottons, corduroy. Your skirt may also be shorter, even above the knee and your blouse might have short sleeves. However, the waistcoat and scarf details remain.

There are no rigid colour schemes; the choice is yours. You can stick to the traditional colours used in menswear like navy, brown and black, accenting with their paler cousins, pale blue, beige and grey. Or you can introduce more colourful accents. For example, you may have a blue and white pinstriped jacket with a navy waistcoat, over a pink sweater and blue plaid trousers. This is the perfect look for unmatched but colour-co-ordinated textures too. Think nothing of mixing stripes, prints, tweed and plaids, provided that the colours don't clash.

ACCESSORIES

When looking for secondhand clothes, also watch for secondhand accessories such as men's hats, belts, braces, scarves, shoes and boots. With your layers of immigrant clothing, wear a man's fedora or Mark Twain style straw hat, but make sure it looks a little too big and falls slightly over your eyes. If it's really too big for you, but otherwise perfect, make your head fit the hat by wrapping it with a scarf or headband first.

Almost any type of belt will tie in with this look, be it large and masculine or fine and feminine. Wrap long ones twice around your waist, or tuck in the extra inches by wrapping them round and round the belt itself. Twisted lengths of fabrics or scarves will double as belts – even a length of rope or cording will look right. Alternatively, you can hold up your skirt or trousers with braces.

Boots should be ankle-length lace-up styles, with crepe or leather soles, and as chunky as you like. Edwardian bootlets or spat styles will also look effective, but you're entering the realm of the rich immigrant with these on your feet. Under a skirt, wear textured or patterned thick tights with the boots – if you don't like too much pattern, ribbing is the classic, but predominant textures like Argyll plaids and cable knits look even better. If it's very cold, wear another pair of socks over

Below: **The Immigrant** is a perfect look for long hair. Wear it twisted and wrapped into buns over or above each ear; in two plaits joined at the centre back with a single ribbon; or plaited at each side and then crossed over the top of your head, with ribbons at the begining of each plait. Alternatively, create rag curls as instructed opposite.

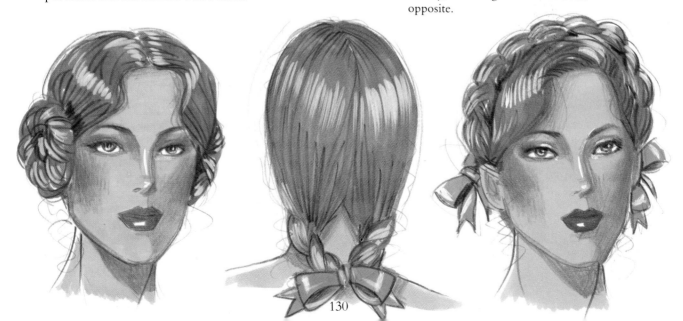

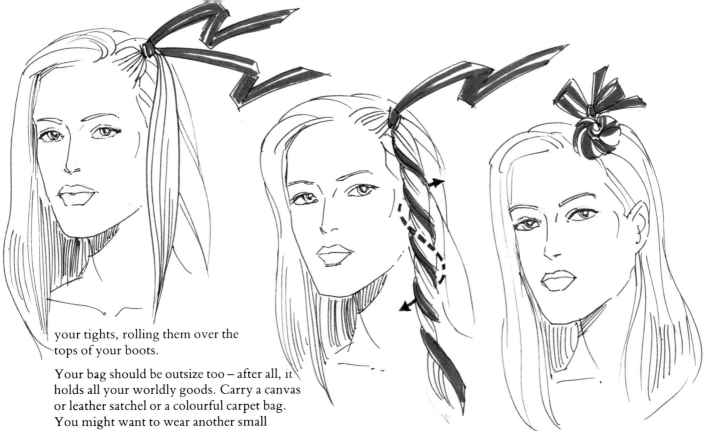

your tights, rolling them over the tops of your boots.

Your bag should be outsize too – after all, it holds all your worldly goods. Carry a canvas or leather satchel or a colourful carpet bag. You might want to wear another small shoulder bag on top of your outer layer to hold small change and lipstick. This shoulder bag is also useful for holding scarves and shawls in place. Wear these in paisley patterns, brightly-flowered prints or blanket checks. (See THE GYPSY for ways to drape them.)

Avoid flashy, elaborate jewellery. You might have a simple ring or two, a pair of fine earrings, or an antique brooch to pin on your jacket, but that's sufficient.

FACE AND HAIR

THE IMMIGRANT is essentially a healthy look, and so restrain make-up, save blusher on your cheeks and a little lip colour. You might also apply eyeliner inside the bottom rim, perhaps in blue or green, for a more wide-eyed look.

Finish by plaiting your hair if it is long enough; the pictures show different ways. Or simply wear them down your back tied with unmatching ribbons. If your hair is too fine or too short for any of these treatments, plait a strand or two and decorate the end with a thin ribbon tied in a bow.

However, for real authenticity, curl your hair with rags. Depending on the thickness and length of your hair, use pieces of thickish cotton fabric 6–12 inches long and about 4-inches wide. Fold the fabric in half, and wrap the bottom of a lock of hair around the rag, dampening hair beforehand if it is fine or flyaway. Using the rag as a roller, wind the hair up to the scalp, then secure the rag curl

Above: Rag curls are the ideal accompaniment for many ethnically based looks in this book such as **The Gypsy**, **The Cossack** and, of course, **The Immigrant.** To make rag curls, follow the instructions under *Face and Hair*.

with a loose knot. The thinner the length of hair, the tighter the curl; if you have very long hair, use the entire length of the rag to spiral the hair round, then roll it up and secure with a knot. This age-old trick has several modern advantages – you can sleep in the soft 'curlers', they look quite stylish while they are in, and you can have ringlets if you leave the curls unbrushed, or gorgeous waves if brushed. If you're daring, you might even appear on the street in rags co-ordinated with what you're wearing – certainly less offensive than rollers.

IDEAS

● Twist a length of fabric, or a scarf, at least 24 inches (61 cms) long into a roll. Use as a belt or headband, as the illustration shows. See THE COSSACK for suggestions for positioning the headband.

● Off-white one-piece long-johns look terrific under a full gathered skirt. Just add a waistcoat and go.

● The ultimate skirt would be made from old bits of quilting à la Ralph Lauren. Make yours from scraps for a fraction of the price.

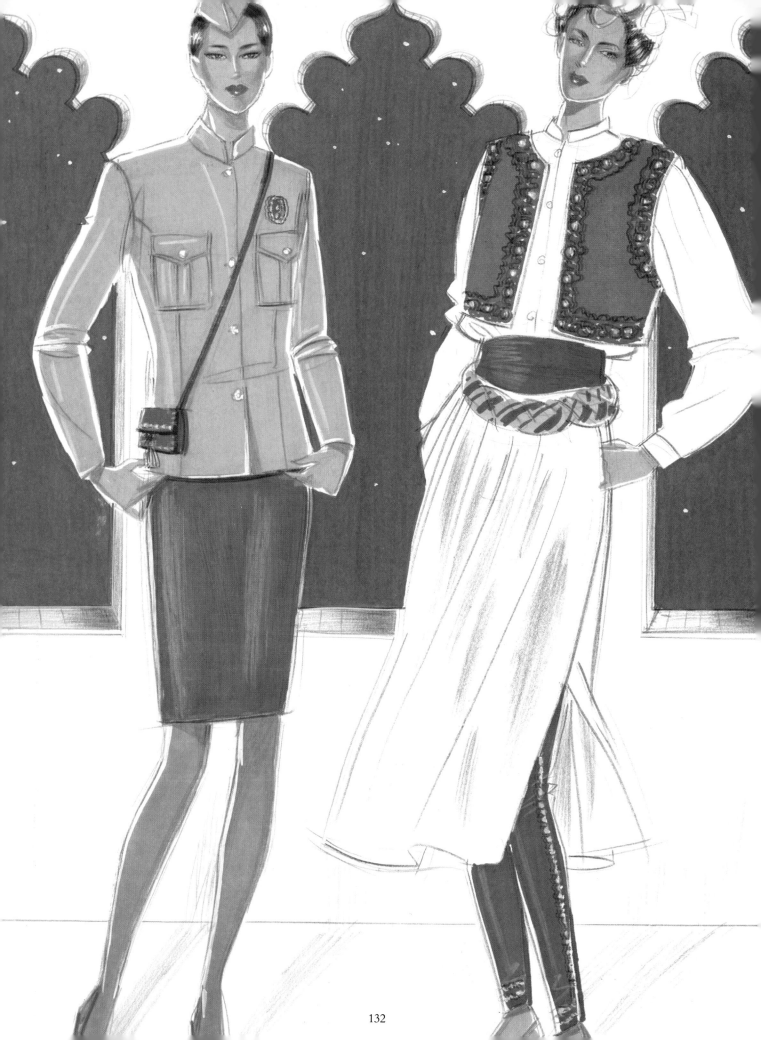

THE INDIAN

BACKGROUND

Steaming, teeming cities, cool hill stations and lofty mountain ranges, barren deserts, sleepy coastal villages, fertile farms and tea plantations; temples, shrines and holy rivers with burning pyres and pilgrims; the glittering magnificence of Maharajahs, their marble palaces and bejewelled elephants; Moghul emperors' wondrous monuments, the ethereal Taj Mahal; the British Raj, the Dutch, the Portuguese; Kipling's *Plain Tales from the Hills*, Scott's *Raj Quartet*, Rushdie's *Midnight's Children* and most recently Attenborough's *Gandhi:* this is India.

From one of the world's great continents comes the inspiration for a fashion look which reflects the conundrum of its country of origin, for India is a patchwork of diverse influences, a melting-pot of religions, civilizations and cultures. Invaded, liberated and re-conquered since time immemorial, dynasties and empires flourished and declined until unification and independence in 1947.

The fascination of India did not end with the last days of the Raj. It drew the flower children of the Sixties when they began their search for enlightenment and an alternative to the bankrupt values of the West. They returned not just with gurus, meditation methods and yoga techniques; in addition they brought back with them the trappings of Indian life.

THE LOOK

Few Westerners have the poise to carry off the supremely elegant sari; but other styles have found a place in the wardrobe of many a Western woman and in many a designer collection. These included the *salwars* and *kameez* of Northern India and the sikhs – trousers, tight at the waist and ankle but loose elsewhere, worn with a long, loose tunic; the *churidhar* and *kurta* version – trousers, baggy over the thigh but ultra tight from knee to ankle, worn under a fitted tunic with side slits, mandarin collar and a soft matching cotton shawl; the country 'pyjama' (from the Urdu and Hindu words for 'leg' and 'clothing') – trousers with drawstring waist and loose half-mast legs.

With so many traditional components to choose from THE INDIAN is a comparatively

Below: **The Indian** can be as ornamented as she likes: hats can be turbans, Nehru-style or skullcaps, shoes can be embroidered, scarves and bags can shimmer with metallic threads and little mirrors and jewellery knows no limits.

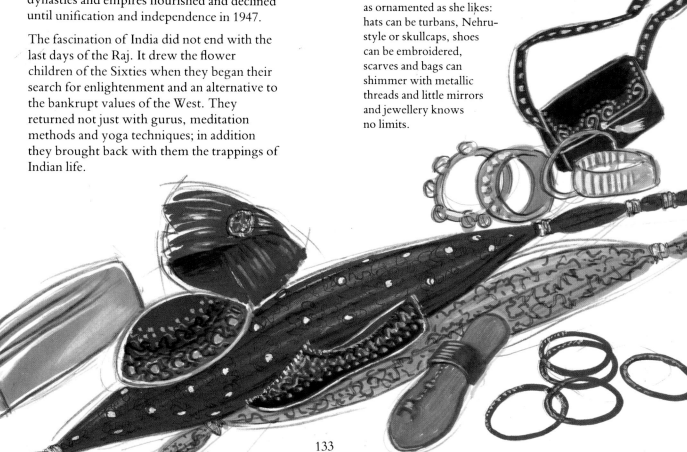

easy look to put together. And, what's more, you can decide between two rather different alternatives: a cool and elegant clean-cut style for day, a billowingly glamorous and gold-encrusted version for night. The former, which could be termed the 'Nehru style' (after Jawaharal Nehru, the first Prime Minister of the Republic of India, 1889–1964), is based on the apparel adopted by the educated business people of India. The latter is an amalgam of traditional Rajesthani 'Maharajah' attire.

To dress for the steaming streets follow the example of the Indians themselves. Go for well-cut layered separates in crisp and cool natural fabrics: cotton, linens, calicos and raw silks. Begin with one of the following: a longish jacket, a side-slit tunic, a straight-cut three-quarters coat, a coat-dress or a long man's shirt. As a general rule 'Mandarin' or 'Nehru' collars are best. Underneath your chosen top add a straight skirt (to knee or mid-calf) or a pair of the tapered trousers already described, but avoid the tightest styles unless you are ultra-skinny. Wear the top belted or hanging loose; it can fall to hip length, mid thigh or, if a tunic, to the knee. If you do select a knee-length tunic or coat-dress, try a waistcoat on top for cooler days.

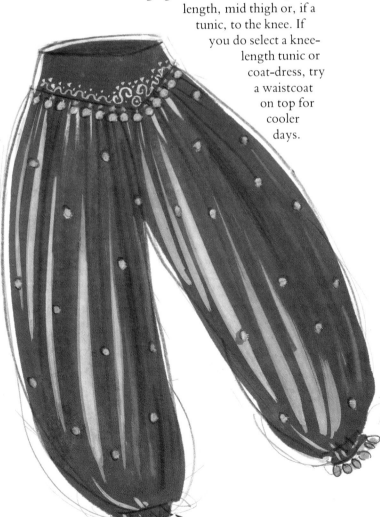

Always opt for plain rather than patterned fabrics for this daytime look; leave the florals and geometrics to come into their own in the evening. For colours, choose from the oriental spice shades: paprika red, nutmeg brown, cinnamon tan, curry gold, saffron yellow and black and white pepper.

The most surprising sources for 'Nehru' jackets are restaurant supply firms: the waiter's thick white cotton classic jacket with stand-up collar, patch pockets and a single row of white buttons down the front is a good facsimile of the Indian jacket.

When the sun goes down, shine in place of the sun, glitter like a princess in a Moghul miniature or glimmer like the timeless moonlight reflected in palace lakes.

Most importantly, head for the shimmery fabrics; there is a wealth of relatively inexpensive Indian materials available today with gold or silver thread woven through them. Don't hesitate to mix fabrics, patterns and colours: comfortable cotton with satin, slubbed silk with chiffon, prints with stripes, spots with florals.

Lines and proportions need not now be so strictly observed, so let blouses billow, trousers balloon and skirts swirl. Decoration *is* the order of the evening, see *Ideas*. Embroidered waistcoats sprinkled with little mirrors and trouser ankle bands hemmed with tiny tinkling bells.

ACCESSORIES

THE INDIAN is a look which can be evoked by the clever use of a few appropriate accessories. The archetypal headgear for day is the now-classic, double-peaked 'Nehru' hat, traditionally in white canvas. Wear the peaks front and back, with your hair long and free or wound up into a neat and elegant chignon.

For a less tailored look, try a soft thin shawl draped round the head, with one end swung over the shoulder or draped from front to back, so that both ends hang down over your shoulders, with a soft, low cowl shape at the front; or try it as a *lunghi*, folded on the diagonal and tied in a knot at the side hip.

For more extravagant occasions an opulent brocade, satin or silk draped turban will look

Left: Voluminous evening trousers studded with golden dots and jingling with little coins.

magnificent with a matching or toning brocade tunic jacket and tapered trousers. Add a large flashy jewel at the front of the turban. For more subdued night-time events, try a neat skull cap decorated with tiny mirrors.

For footwear, choose sandals for preference; lavish styles with a medium-high heel look most elegant for evening, though single-thonged, flat styles look right for daytime. Belts, too, will be ornamental: look for lacings of fine chains, wrappings of cottons and metallic threads, tasselled satin strands and woven and embroidered fabrics. Your bag could be a tiny embroidered pouch, or a large envelope, but wear it diagonally.

Discretion by day, daring by night is the rule to follow for jewellery. In the evening you can cover arms with bangles and bracelets, necks with chains and semi-precious stones, fingers with rings and ears with studs and dangling hoops. Add a couple of anklets, a toe ring or two or even a nose stud if you are feeling very exotic. During the day a single silver and coral bracelet, for example, or a pair of stunning amber earrings will suffice.

FACE AND HAIR
To achieve the face that matches THE INDIAN look up start with as dark a foundation as you can without appearing artificial, and blend it right down into the neck unless you have naturally dark-skinned looks. Follow with a matching loose face powder. Use a kohl pencil for the eyes; smudge this around the lower lid and lashes and line the inside of the lids with it too. Then add black mascara to both top and bottom lashes. Apply a warm burgundy blusher to the cheekbones and create a sultry Eastern mouth by lining the lips with a burgundy/plum-coloured outline pencil and filling in with a claret-coloured matt lipstick. For a final touch use a little of the lipstick to make the traditional mark in the centre of the forehead, or use a little red food dye to colour the hair parting.

If you are naturally endowed with long and straight dark brown or black glossy hair let it hang loose. If you are not so lucky, tuck your hair up in a bun in the traditional style.

IDEAS
• On summer nights try wearing one of the cool, short-sleeved, midrif-baring garments which Indian women wear under their saris.

• Make your evening accessories more decorative by sewing tiny brass or silver bells and faceted baubles onto the ends of scarves and onto belts and slippers; and use similar items instead of buttons.

• Too baggy trouser bottoms can be gathered by inserting a strip of elastic as long as the circumference of your ankle into the hem; join the ends of the elastic with a few stitches and sew up the gap in each hem. Finish with ankle bands from strips of embroidered ribbon.

Below: plain trousers and scarf being transformed with the addition of golden bells and by inserting elastic through the hem to gather the legs.

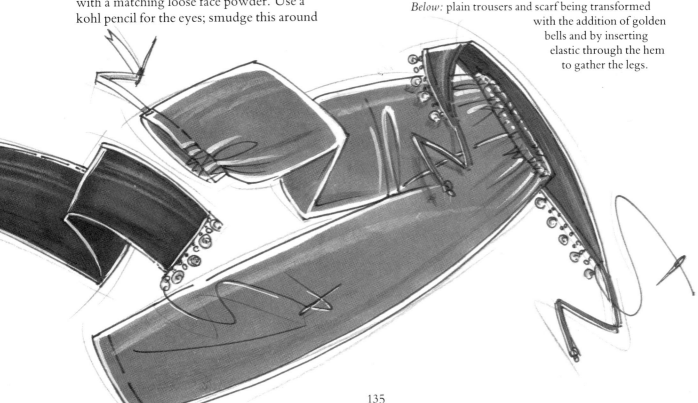

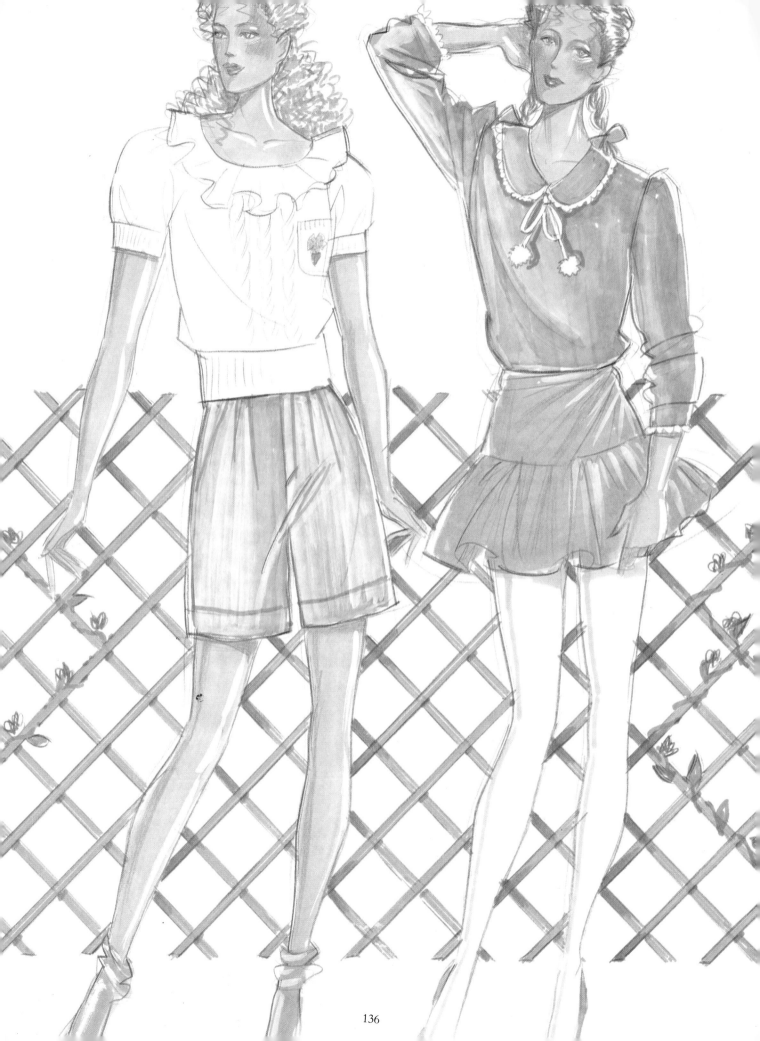

THE INNOCENT

BACKGROUND

Sugar and spice and all things nice, that's what little girls are made of. THE INNOCENT is appealingly vulnerable. Sweet, delicate and totally lacking in guile or edge, she is the princess in the fairy tale who was so sensitive that she could feel a single pea under dozens of mattresses. She is Shirley Temple in *Bright Eyes* (1934) and *Rebecca of Sunny Brook Farm* (1938); even Marilyn Monroe in *Some Like It Hot*, all soft naïvety and wide-eyed sex appeal.

The image actually goes right back to the late eighteenth century when for the first time children were no longer considered merely as miniature adults, but encouraged to be themselves and dressed in simple, loose clothes that gave them the freedom to play and reflected their childish innocence.

THE LOOK

Innocence is the prerogative of the young, or at least the young at heart. The essence of the look is naïve purity, so clothing is either entirely white, or in pastel shades. Begin with a white blouse, trimmed with a banding of lace or ruffles. The blouse may have short puff sleeves or fuller three-quarter-length ones; for summer it might be a camisole style, but white it must be. Small Peter Pan collars and tiny round pearl buttons add a nice touch. Ideally, the blouse will be in a fine natural fabric such as pure cotton, linen or silk. Wear this demure little garment with a short white skirt or culottes. The skirt can be rara style, bias cut or soft and full; it can be edged with a frill or have a drop waist, but should be above the knee, unless you're an older innocent in which case the skirt or culottes should be just below the knee.

Although an ideal summer look, it can be adapted for winter. Quite simply change to more wintery textures, but retain the same colour scheme, with the addition perhaps of a touch of dove grey, chinchilla beige, soft pigeon blue and bunny rabbit brown, but only in the form of overcoats and jackets or footwear.

Almost everyone has some white separates in their wardrobe, but what distinguishes this

Below: **The Innocent** must keep her accessories sweet and simple: purses and shoes will always be white or pastel, heels will be flattish, jewellery will be flowery and, above all, demure.

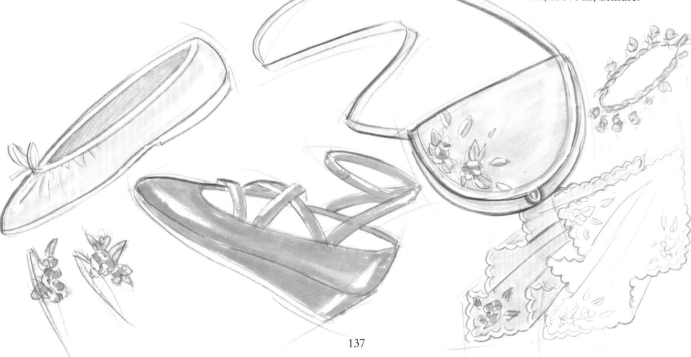

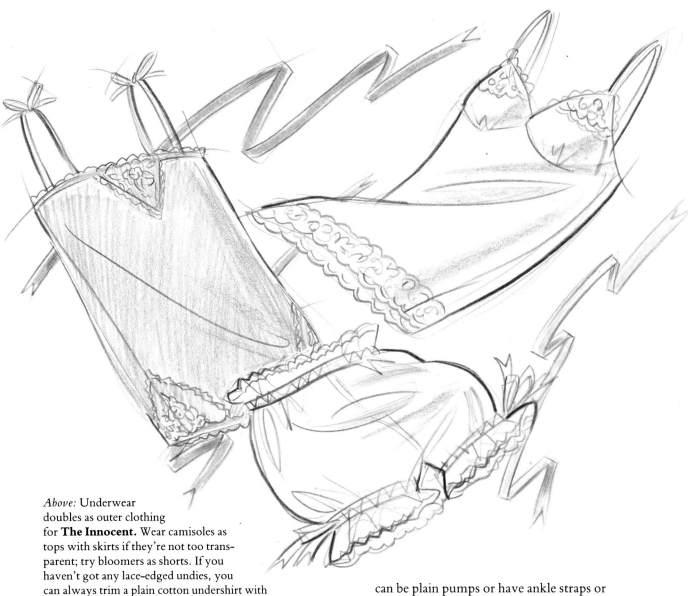

Above: Underwear doubles as outer clothing for **The Innocent.** Wear camisoles as tops with skirts if they're not too transparent; try bloomers as shorts. If you haven't got any lace-edged undies, you can always trim a plain cotton undershirt with broderie anglaise edging.

look as specifically innocent is a frilly or fluffy sweater worn with it. This should either end at the waist or have a small peplum; it can be a cardigan or pullover but it must be white, sugar pink, baby blue, creamy yellow or pale minty green. It might be decorated with tiny bunches of embroidered flowers, have a lacy collar, or be in the softest of stripes; it might be cobweb knit, or plain lambswool, but whatever it is it will be the ultimate in feminine girlishness (see also THE DANCER). Make it as sweet as you can. In winter, the sweater could be thick angora or soft mohair; in summer, choose a finely-knit mixture of linen and silk.

ACCESSORIES
Of course, the youthful impression must extend to your feet. Choose white or pastel shades for slipper styles with flat heels. These can be plain pumps or have ankle straps or thin gossamer laces for tying around your delicate ankles. Wear these light little shoes with bare, tanned legs, fine, cotton anklet socks or the sheerest, palest tights, depending on the dressiness of the occasion and your outfit.

For jewellery, opt for anything with hearts and flowers. A golden locket for your neck, brooches with bunches of flowers, hair ornaments with butterflies or other childish motifs. If you have pierced ears, try simple pearl studs or enamelled hearts on small hoops; above all avoid anything chunky or brash. Wear a single silver or gold chain at your wrist or neck, and only one delicate ring at a time. Bracelets are of the charm variety – linked chains rather than bangles which would lend an undesirably hard quality to this tender look. Carry a lace-edged hankie in a pocket of your sweater or in a pretty pastel shoulder bag.

Underwear can double as clothing with this

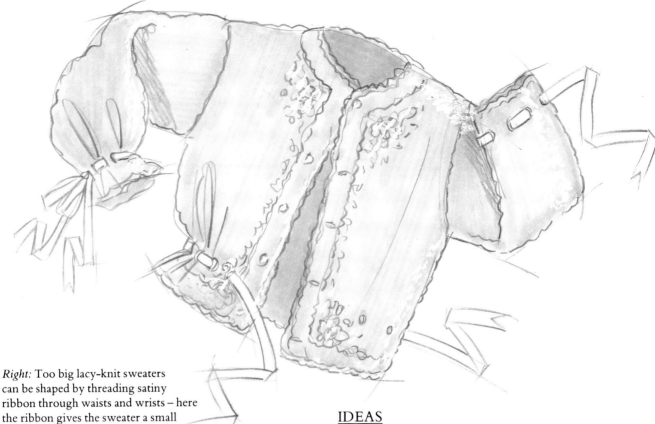

Right: Too big lacy-knit sweaters can be shaped by threading satiny ribbon through waists and wrists – here the ribbon gives the sweater a small peplum too.

look – camisole tops, bloomers, petticoats, all modern imitations or authentic antiques will work provided they are purest white and ironed to perfection.

FACE AND HAIR

Give yourself a pale, vulnerable face with an application of lighter than normal foundation in an ivory shade. Shadow eyes in pearlized colours such as palest pink, grey, taupe or barely blue. Use navy mascara on lashes and create big baby eyes with a fine line drawn inside the rim of the eyes very close to the lashes using a blue or grey pencil. Blush cheeks with a mist of pink; shine lips with a pearly pink or just a hint of lipgloss.

Hair should be caught back off the face by thin headbands or gathered into a ponytail or bunches, decorated with little-girl hair clips complete with small furry animals, tiny bunches of flowers or ribbons. If your hair's not long enough for these treatments, wear it slightly wavy or in loose ringlets.

IDEAS

• Thread lace-edged clothing and undergarments with satin ribbons. Weave white or pastel satin ribboning, no wider than one-half inch. The same ribbons can also be used to give shape to a lacy sweater which has become baggy or stretched at the waist or sleeves. Again, simply thread the ribbon through at equal intervals to form gathers, pull to fit and tie opposite ends in a tiny bow.

• Make an inexpensive locket by using an inexpensive heart-shaped charm threaded onto a length of satin ribbon. Wear it choker tight or dangling down.

• If you're handy with a needle and thread, embroider single stems or bunches of flowers on a spare, shrunken sweater – perfect for this little-girl look.

• Sew fine ruffled lace or broderie anglaise to the edges of ankle socks, underwear and petticoats using small running stitches.

Right: Lockets become necklaces or bracelets depending on the length of ribbon they hang from – see *Ideas.*

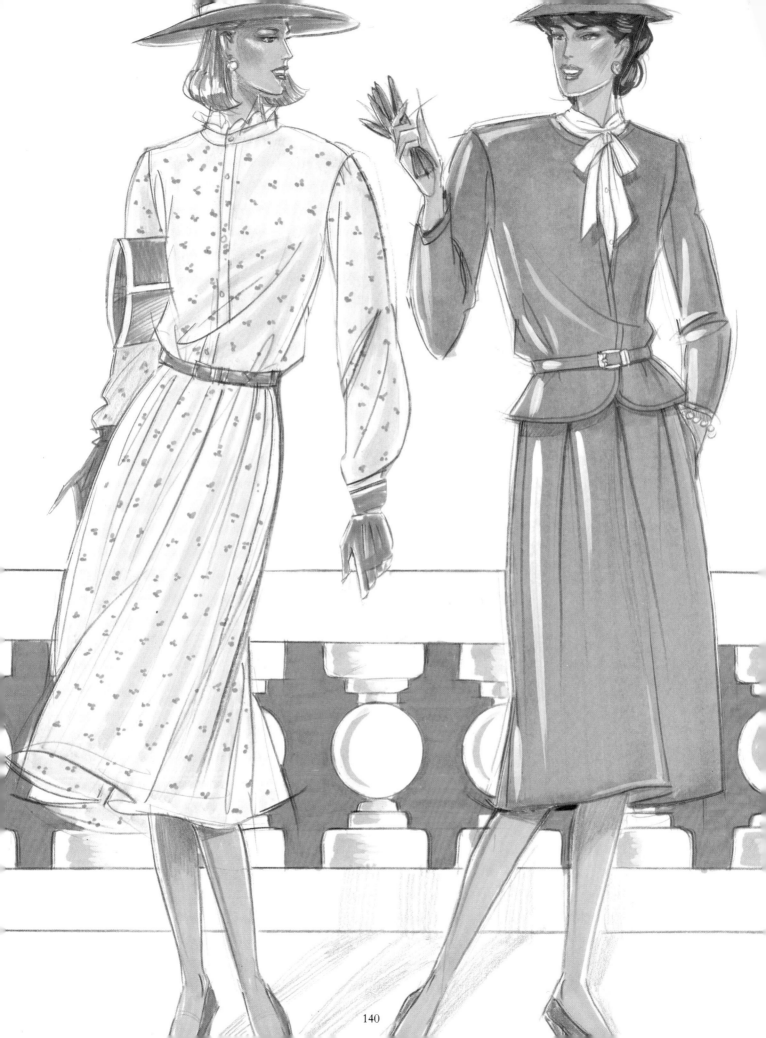

THE LADY

BACKGROUND

Princess Diana and Catherine Deneuve exude the breeding and charm which distinguishes THE LADY. They have, and Princess Grace had, the dignified femininity which is the essence of this look.

She may have vaults of jewels but will never speak of her wealth, she may have a title but will rarely mention her background, she may have inherited acres of land but will never brag – in short she possesses a quiet consistent grace and impeccable manners.

But you don't have to possess great riches, beauty or breeding to be a lady. You can certainly behave like a lady and you can easily dress like one.

THE LOOK

For special occasions like state balls, THE LADY will dress as THE DEBUTANTE; on informal occasions as THE CLASSICIST; on transatlantic journeys as THE OCEAN VOYAGER and in the country as THE LANDOWNER. But there is a distinctive style adopted by THE LADY for semi-formal daytime events such as teas, luncheons and bridge parties. For these occasions THE LADY wears lots of cream, teaming it with raspberry red, sky blue, apricot, eau de nil green, and sometimes navy or pewter grey.

Although propriety is the order of the day and the components of the look are fashion classics, the look can still be worn with imagination and style. In fact, virtually every

movie star of the Forties and Fifties posed for the camera in one version or another of the shirtwaister dress – a fashion perennial of THE LADY. Traditionally, the top is styled like a blouse or shirt with collar and a buttoned front, while the skirt is straight, A-line or neatly pleated into the waist. For winter, the shirtwaister can be made from lightweight wool, fine plaids or corduroy; for summer a lightweight cotton, linen, silk or man-made equivalent. Whichever season, it must be plain coloured or printed with the most discreet of patterns – thin strips, tiny flowers, subtle checks, tasteful abstract motifs. Let nothing flashy or garish distract from the calm self-possession of the wearer. For more formal occasions, the shirtwaister might have a ruffle at the neckline, a lace-trimmed collar, or be

Below: Make a real **Lady** of yourself by choosing the right accessories: low-heeled shoes, strands of pearls, pure white wrist-length gloves with pearly button fastenings, unobtrusive jewellery, sleek handbags, and hats as glamorous as you like, whether adorned with fake flowers or veiling.

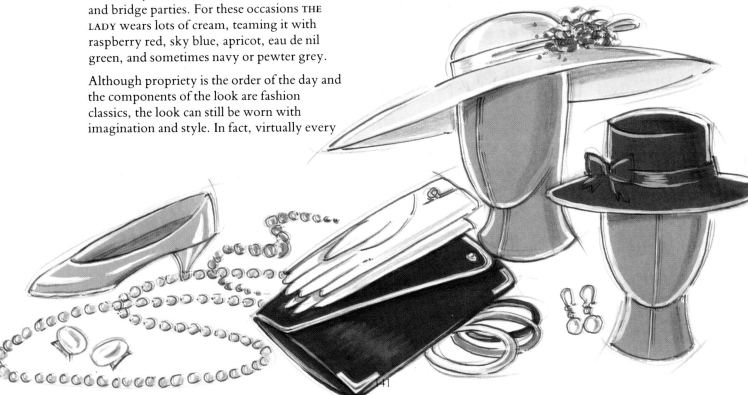

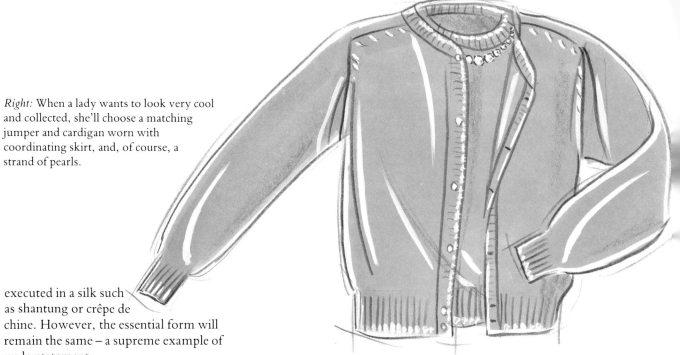

Right: When a lady wants to look very cool and collected, she'll choose a matching jumper and cardigan worn with coordinating skirt, and, of course, a strand of pearls.

executed in a silk such as shantung or crêpe de chine. However, the essential form will remain the same – a supreme example of understatement.

On cooler days wear a cardigan over your shirtwaister dress. Again style and fabric depend on season and occasion – in winter, it might be of fine lambswool or cashmere with a V-neck; in summer a botany wool or cotton/wool mixture with mother-of-pearl buttons. On less formal occasions, wear the same cardigan over a matching short-sleeved sweater. Team it up with a matching or co-ordinating skirt for the true 'twin-set and pearls' look, but for a less dated appearance, wear a silk blouse in place of the short-sleeved jumper.

Alternatively, THE LADY might choose a suit, especially if the weather is a little chilly. In that case, search for a classic, simple style, with a single-breasted jacket and A-line, straight or pleated skirt. (Nothing mannish.) The skirt will be a modest length, just below the knee, and the jacket will be large enough to add a sweater underneath. In the Twenties, Chanel popularized the buttonless boxy jacket trimmed with contrast braiding, worn by all great ladies since. This suit usually has a relatively straight skirt, and because of the braiding needs very little accessorizing – just add a hat, gloves and a strand of pearls.

Wear these suits over a neat blouse in silk, fine cotton or linen. In colder weather, a high-necked lambswool, angora or cashmere jumper will give an extra layer of warmth.

For outerwear, choose a beautifully made wool or cashmere coat with an A-line shape – either single- or double-breasted. It should swirl slightly as you walk, completing your totally graceful appearance.

ACCESSORIES

THE LADY is incomplete without a hat. In summer, wear a large-brimmed straw style to match your shoes (see right); in winter one of a similar style in felt.

A lady also must have gloves. Carry them in one hand if you like, or lay them across your handbag, but they must be in evidence. Wrist-length white cotton or kid for summer, the same length in leather for winter. Handbags are very sedate – no shoulder styles, huge clasps or wild colours. The bag will have a small handle or might be a modest clutch style, and it should match your shoes.

Can you imagine a lady without her string of pearls? My dear, she would feel absolutely naked! Wear single short or choker lengths by day at the neck of shirtwaister, or sweater, longer lengths or double strands and chokers for night. In fact, pearls appear everywhere – on ear lobes, on fingers, at wrists. They should always be small and delicate though, never the oversized specimens that no oyster could ever produce. Other kinds of jewellery might be gold or silver chains, or plain bangle bracelets, brooches, cameos, but on no account wear anything obviously fake or flashy.

Footwear must be sensible – lowish heels no more than two inches for day, maybe up to three inches for special occasions. They should be very plain, and should match your bag and hat. No lady would appear without stockings, even in the height of summer, so choose the sheerest ones you can find in cream or taupe shades depending on your outfit.

Belts, too, will be fine and of excellent quality. No fancy buckles, no designer signatures, no manufacturer's patterns – just thin strips of leather with discreet gold or silver buckles to accentuate the waist of your shirtwaister or cardigan.

FACE AND HAIR

Give your skin a flawless finish by applying a covering creamy-toned foundation, followed by a dusting of matching loose powder. Shadow eyes with a soft stone colour over the lower lid, a soft shell or ivory shade under the brow and a dab of grey, taupe or sludgy blue in the outer corner. Bring this around into the crease, around the eye, with just a smudge under the lower lashes. Define eyes a little more with a bit of pencil liner along the lower lashes, keeping the line as soft as possible. Define your gloriously high cheekbones with a dusty pink blusher and finish with a rosy shade of lipstick.

Keep hairstyles simple. A classic blunt cut from any length from page boy to shoulder length or the more traditional treatments such as the chignon, worn in this case at the nape of the neck or at the back of the head, are all appropriate. Use velveteen headbands for winter and simple gold or silvery clasps anytime to secure longer hair, but remember, the whole effect should be stylish, neat and calm.

IDEAS

● Fake a shirtwaister dress by wearing matching or toning skirt and blouse, but be sure to define your waist with a narrow leather or fabric belt in a complementary shade.

● Replace plastic or matching buttons on cardigans, coats and dresses with pearly ones – anything from the flat, abalone, four-holed kind to the round-topped tiny ones, depending on the size required. Ladies simply love rows of little pearl buttons!

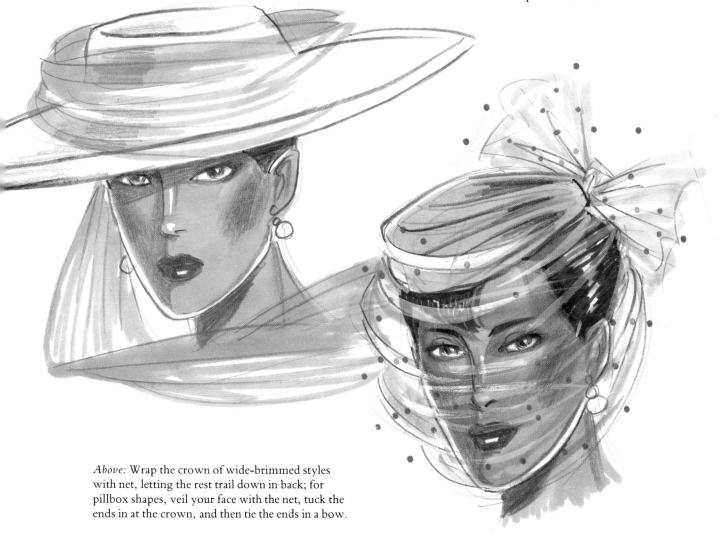

Above: Wrap the crown of wide-brimmed styles with net, letting the rest trail down in back; for pillbox shapes, veil your face with the net, tuck the ends in at the crown, and then tie the ends in a bow.

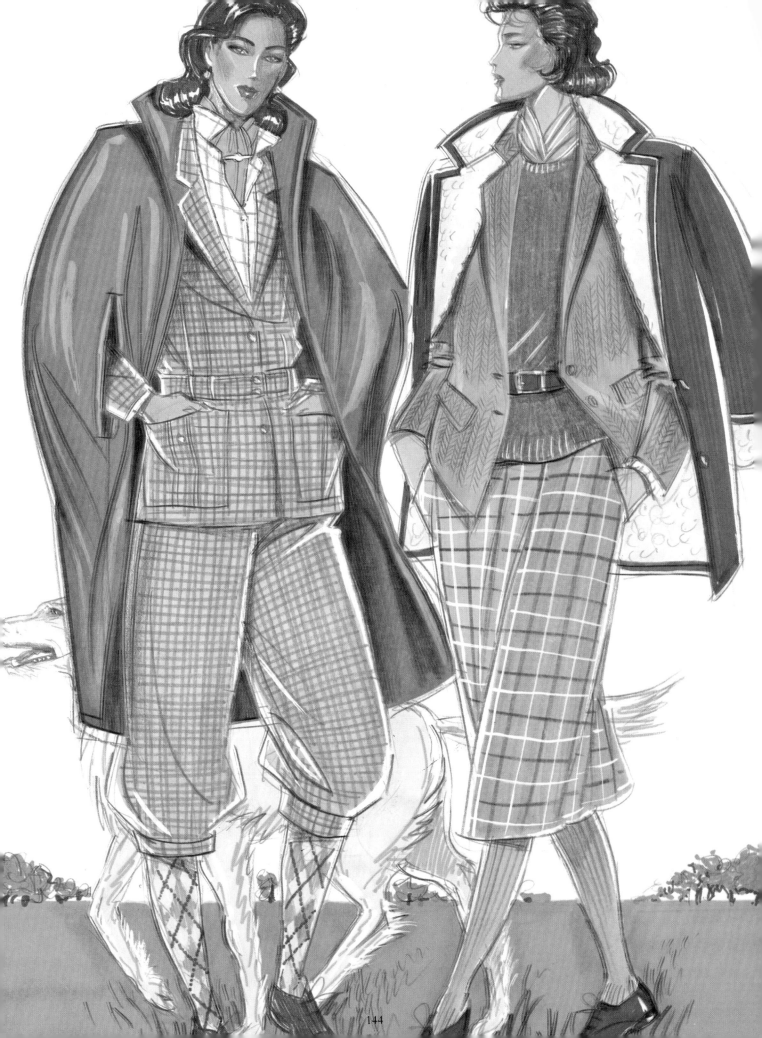

THE LANDOWNER

BACKGROUND

In traditional 'county' circles, one generation follows in the footsteps of another, and today's Sloanes and Preppies are no exception; they too emulate their parents' lifestyle. Off they trot to the same shooting parties, the point-to-points, the Sunday morning service and the estate and village events. And what do they wear for all these hale and hearty highlights of their country life? A timeless collection of pretty much what Mummy wore on such occasions.

Hardly a recipe for a fashionable look, one might think; but several factors ensure that the style of THE LANDOWNER does move with the times without losing its traditional character. Put together correctly there is no need for this look to appear frumpy or old-fashioned.

THE LANDOWNER is basically THE CLASSICIST in the country. Both styles have found favour with fashion designers, especially in France, Italy and America. 'Le style anglais' is rightly considered a classic look and fashion houses have improved the basic elements so the style can be worn by anyone.

Below: Sensible walking shoes and bags roomy enough for binoculars form the backbone of **The Landowner**'s accessories. Go for outside pockets and stitched detailing on canvas or leather handbags.

The look's popularity with designers such as Jaeger, Kenzo and Margaret Howell mean that its elements are not difficult to obtain, though you may prefer the traditional outfitters such as the Preppy 'mecca' L.L. Bean in Maine, or Brooks Brothers, in New York; Burberry's or The Scotch House in London.

THE LOOK

Like THE OUTDOOR GIRL, the LANDOWNER seeks out shades which echo those of her environment; hues of brown and green are appropriate, but bump up this basic palette by adding the heathery shades of moorland and heathland: soft purples and blues, tinges of pink and deeper rosy reds, shades of gold and pewter.

Fabrics are warm and comfortable, durable and practical; they need to be for such a brisk and bracing outdoor life. Layer yourself up with flannel and Viyella, Shetland and lambswool, tweeds and corduroys, and masses of heavily waterproofed and quilted materials. Take inspiration from THE HORSEWOMAN and THE SCOTSWOMAN too.

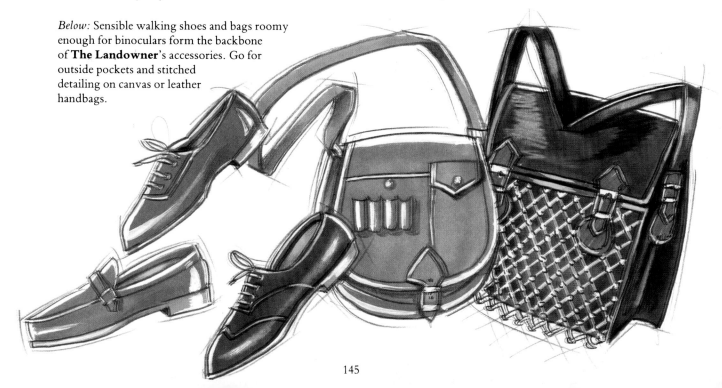

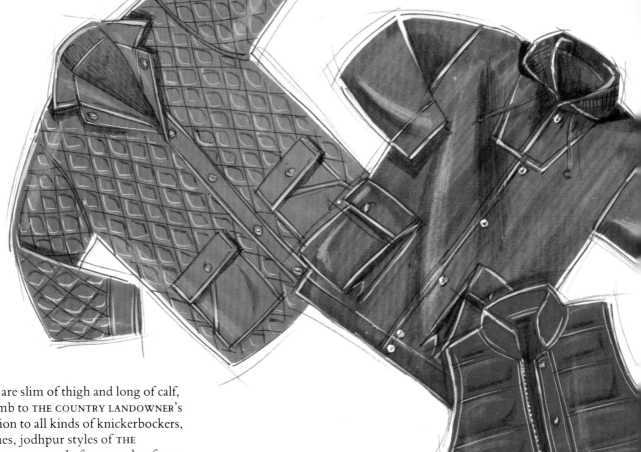

If you are slim of thigh and long of calf, succumb to THE COUNTRY LANDOWNER's addiction to all kinds of knickerbockers, breeches, jodhpur styles of THE HORSEWOMAN, and of course plus-fours. The latter were originally the preserve of the male country landowner, but they look marvellous on a lady, too. Ultra-baggy over the knee, they fasten slightly lower under the knee than average knickerbockers (see *Ideas*). Wear them with a traditional Norfolk jacket of matching tweed, characterized by tailored box pleats at front and back and a nipped in, belted waist. For this outfit don't hesitate to mix interesting tweeds; checked, patterned, flecked and other variations are all appropriate. Argyll knee socks, brogues, and matching tweed deerstalker (or Sherlock Holmes type hat) complete this very traditional look, always worn by grouse shooters on the Scottish moors.

Knickerbockers in wool or tweed mixes or in corduroy can be worn in the same way, with a matching or contrasting waistcoat, hacking jacket, or thick wool cardigan such as an Aran. Alternatively, exchange the breeches for warm trousers in the same fabrics, with turn-ups and pleats at the waist, if you are less adventurous.

Soft tweed suits or tweedy skirts with toning overcoats are the basic components of a more formal version of the look. A subtle plaid or patterned tweed skirt can be worn with a matching or plain jacket. Follow THE LANDOWNER's code and keep cut and proportions classic.

Above: Ideal outerwear for **The Landowner** comprises jackets which are big and well-pocketed. From the left, a quilted jacket, a rubberized olive parka and, of course, the essential down vest.

For everyday wear, THE LANDOWNER wears tattersall checked Viyella shirts and lambswool or heavy-knit, self-colour sweaters. For Sunday lunch or drinks with the Vicar, keep the tweeds the same but add a simple toning silk shirt with a round or V-necked cardigan on top. Alternatively, try a twinset, with pearls at the neck (see THE LADY); choose a colour which goes with your gently gathered or pleated wool skirt.

Outdoor wear of THE LANDOWNER is very distinctive and offers many possibilities. A good tweed overcoat, that will last a lifetime, is essential; single- or double-breasted, it is best with a vent or pleat at the back. A Sherlock Holmes-type cape, a loden jacket or coat, or a sheepskin jacket would also be suitable.

More importantly, for the thoroughly-active LANDOWNER who participates in all the country pursuits, the traditional shooting jacket made by Barbour is the waterproof garment beloved by Sloane and Preppy alike. Made in olive-green waxed cotton with a corduroy collar, it is loose fitting with large pockets and a hood, falling to mid-thigh. Alternatively you can sport the classic country jacket of today, the Husky – a warmly criss-cross quilted jacket or waistcoat in olive green or navy. Another favourite (the Puffa) is horizontally quilted in wide bands like a duvet; this too, comes in jacket or waistcoat form in olive or navy.

ACCESSORIES

Sturdy bags, boots and shoes are essential for this look; buy from such stores as Hunting World (New York) or Moss Bros (London) or any traditional country outfitters. Shooting bags are definitely suitable. There are several styles to choose from: cartridge bags in soft brown or sandy-coloured leather, similar styles in mid- or bottle green canvas with brown leather strap and trim; satchel shapes in olive canvas with net mesh outer pockets – all with long adjustable straps to enable them to be worn diagonally across the body.

For feet, don brogues with laces, sturdy moccasins or loafers and other flat casual leather slip-ons. Borrow the riding boots of THE HORSEWOMAN and the archetypal 'green wellies' of THE FISHERWOMAN. Keep heels as flat as you can and always buy hard-wearing materials. Wool shooting stockings, knee socks or ribbed tights in earthy colours should be worn with knickerbockers or plus-fours on freezing outdoor days; wear toning tights (or natural ones) with skirts and suits.

Raid the hatters of the country gents: flat tweed caps, trilbies or variants, deerstalkers and Sherlock Holmes styles with earflaps, or the ubiquitous Hermès scarf all work well with this look. And whatever you do, don't forget the shooting stick!

FACE AND HAIR

Charming, well-bred faces indicate a landed gentry pedigree, so avoid the glamorous and exotic. Echo the palette of your wardrobe in your choice of eye colours, exchanging the

greens and browns for the heathery colours to give a less conventional look. An outdoor flush achieved by a dusting of rosy blusher on the cheeks and a slightly tinted lipstick will help to bring compliments your way. Well-groomed sleek and healthy hair in tidy styles should be as shiny as a sleek black labrador or a glowing golden retriever!

IDEAS

● Experiment with trimming country hats in different ways: use dog leads and collars or leather belts with buckles round the crowns of trilbies of deer-stalkers – they make interesting alternatives to the more ordinary braids and bands. Or twist a length of yarn around the crown to match a sweater or your gloves. Add a pheasant feather or two for extra panache.

● Revamp baggy trousers with wide bottoms as plus-fours; cut off the lower calves, allowing for an overhang over the cuff; gather raw edges into a neat band made from the piece you have cut off which fits around your leg under the knee and add a button; the plus-fours will then hang over the top. (See THE FAIR ISLANDER for instructions of how to transform knickerbockers similarly).

● Patch elbows of tweed or wool jackets, or even Henry Higgins cardigans, with leather or suede in true-impoverished-stately-home-owner style.

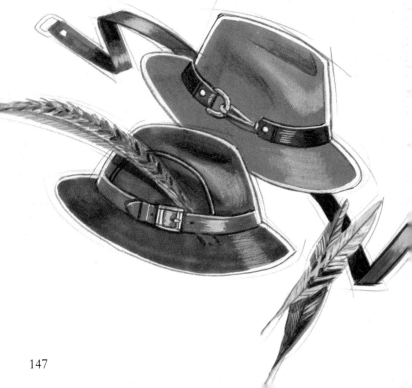

Right: Trim a plain hat with your finds from the fields such as pheasant feathers, or use short leather straps or dog collars. (see *Ideas*.)

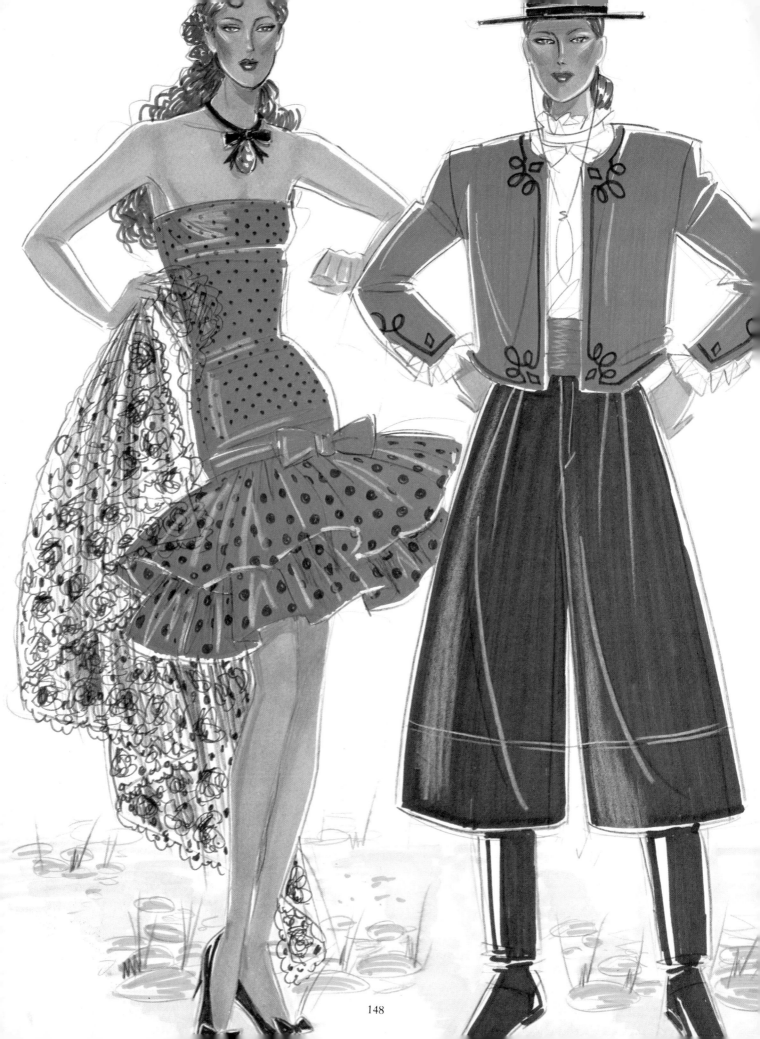

THE LATIN

BACKGROUND

The fierce pride of the Spaniard, handed down to us through the pages of history and legend, lies behind this look: Christopher Columbus, the Conquistadores, Don Quixote, Catherine of Aragon, Picasso, the great stars of the bullring – a motley crew, indeed, but all possessing the pride, the daring and the hot-blooded temperament of the Latin. The drama and passion of their history is reflected in the contrasts of this look, from the severity of the matador's outfit to the frilled flamboyance of the flamenco dancer's dress. Dark-haired, hot-blooded Latin lady or not, you can capture the dashing glamour of the gaucho, the matador or the flamenco dancer simply by choosing the right clothes.

THE LOOK

The party version of this look derives directly from the spectacular costumes of flamenco. Carmen Miranda, the Brazilian bombshell, took this colourful style to extremes. Decked out in excessively flounced and ruffled dresses, three-inch platform shoes and half an orchard on top of her head, she still stunned with the speed of her Samba! Nowadays, you would find it a little difficult to enjoy the average party in such an outfit – so save your Carmen

Miranda look for a costume party. The adapted and toned-down version of the flamenco dress does, however, make spectacular party wear.

The dress is based on a tight-fitting basque bodice, with a low-cut, boned decolleté; this can be in silk, satin, velvet or other fine fabrics, either strapless or with slender shoe-string shoulder straps. It can be cut straight across the back or scooped down to show a sensual length of brown back; in front, the decolleté is heart-shaped for preference, not straight across, the idea being to create a deliberately provocative look.

The skirt of the dress should be full and flounced from the waist, ending either just above or below the knee. Alternatively, the skirt could be tight-fitting à la flamenco dancer, flouncing from the knee down in a cascade of tiered and undulating ruffles, edged with lace or lined with contrasting silk.

Below: **The Latin** has some of the most distinctive accessories around: the lace mantilla, tasselled fan and sombrero hat come first. Finish the effect with wide belts, shiny black boots and gauntlet gloves in a bright colour.

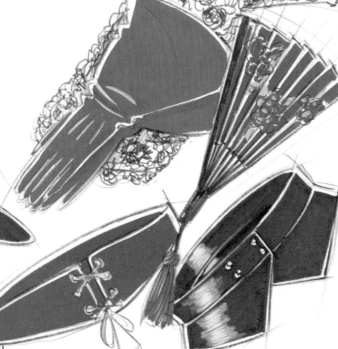

Choice of colour is vital in capturing the essence of the Latin look. The drama of black predominates and is offset with scarlet, bright yellow, cobalt blue and rich dark purple. So finish your party outfit off with huge imitation hot-house flowers, made from chintz and organza, in one or two of these violent hues; pin them in your hair, at your cleavage or at your hip (see also *Accessories*).

Luckily for those of a less flamboyant nature, there is a more street-worthy look for the Latin and many of the components of this version of the look are common to other ethnic looks such as THE COSSACK and THE GYPSY. Begin with baggy trousers or a full or tiered skirt. Choose black or dark brown, in fine wool or thick-textured cotton, but make sure the effect is generous. The skirt should be fairly long, and certainly cover the tops of your gleaming boots. Tuck trousers into boots or wrap them with leather laces around your ankles. Alternatively, search for genuine toreador pants for a perfect look. These are tight black pants ending above the ankle. Cotton or wool, or even leather are best for day; for evening, choose exotic black velveteen or satin. Wear these toreadors with flat shiny black patent pumps or black high heels and an embroidered or decorated jacket or cape unless the pants are leather, in which case one of the looser wraps described later will look best. Alternatively, for evenings, replace the toreador pants with a tiered skirt in lace, velveteen or satin and wear with the same beautifully decorated jacket and shoes. On top, wear a white blouse with billowing sleeves, notched neckline, pointed collar and maybe a ruffle at the wrist (see also THE GYPSY and THE PIRATE).

Black bottoms and contrasting white top are the basis of THE LATIN look, but to make it truly authentic, wear a characteristic outer garment in one of the strong Latin colours. If you favour tailored clothing, choose a bolero, with or without sleeves, cut well above the waist, or a waist-length, slightly boxy cardigan jacket with black passementerie (braiding worked into swirls as shown in the illustration). For informal occasions, a longer wool felt jacket embroidered with floral designs is ideal.

Right: The less formal Latin wears a bright blanket as serape and completes the matador effect with gaucho gloves and toreador pants trimmed with characteristic braiding.

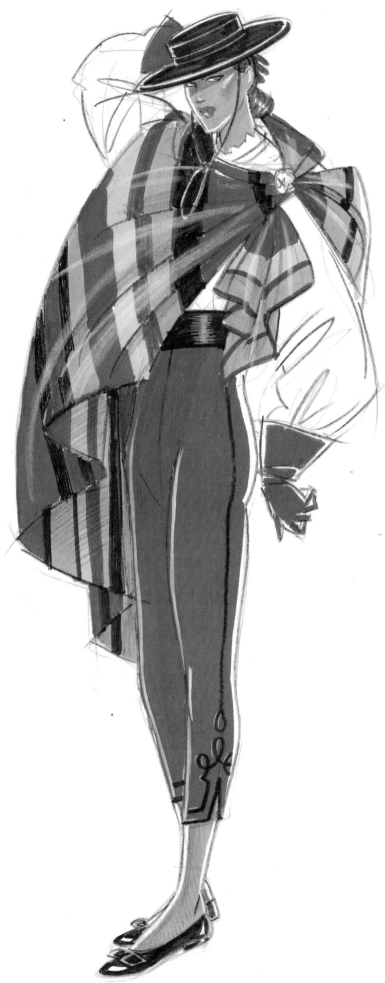

When riding on the huge grassy plains or just to keep warm on cold streets, wear one of the gaucho's perennials – the cape, poncho or serape. Capes can come just below the waist, or nearly to the ankles; ponchos can be fringed and with the same variation of length; the serape is anything from a hand-woven horse blanket to the finest piece of alpaca from the indigenous long-haired llama. To distinguish, the poncho is a square of fabric, usually worn with the points in front and behind with a hole for the head, while the serape is simply a length of fabric big enough to wrap around you. Wear these marvellous and versatile garments thrown loosely over your shoulders, secure them with a large blanket pin, or adorn them with a bold silvery brooch or thick leather belt.

For tips on working with wraps see THE GYPSY, but bear in mind that the serape is generally longer and more oblong than THE GYPSY's shawl, so you may have to wrap the serape around several times.

ACCESSORIES

For your party outfit, accessories distinguishing the Latin dancer are few but nonetheless essential. Unless the event requires fancy dress leave your castanets at home, but do make sure you wear a mantilla. This is a kind of veil worn off the face, for effect rather than practicality and can be either a large square of ornate black lace – the soft, heavy variety not the stiff nylon net sort – pinned to the back of the head with a splendid curved and cut tortoiseshell comb, or else a silk shawl of any size, but always beautifully fringed with long, silken threads and a frenzy of rich colour, preferably in traditional flower patterns.

Wear a black velvet or satin ribbon tied around your neck as a choker and carry a silken draw-string purse, embroidered, tasselled or plain. In summer you can heighten the Spanish flavour by also carrying a fan.

For footwear choose black high-heeled pumps in leather, suede or patent, pointed or almond-toed, or highish-heeled shiny black leather boots. Wear fishnet tights, scarlet stockings or black tights.

For your day version of this look don a charactcristic black flat-crowned and brimmed gaucho hat, now highly fashionable, and a pair of gauntlet gloves. Handbags should be small and elegant to suit the dressy

version – fine black kid is perfect, but for range-riding, anything squashy, hand-made, fringed, top-stitched and big is right.

Jewellery should be concentrated on ears and wrists. Earrings can be big dangles of gold, silver or similar semi-precious metals such as brass, or hung with brightly coloured stones such as coral and jet.

FACE AND HAIR

Begin with an application of foundation and powder slightly darker than normal, unless you have a slight tan or very good natural colour. Use very dark grey or brown shadow all over the lower lid up to the crease, smudging it around under the lower lashes. Apply ivory highlighter under the eyebrow, blending it into the lid colour. Use a black or dark brown kohl pencil to line just inside the rim of the eye and also to fill out eyebrows to make them appear as full as possible. Apply claret blusher just under the cheekbones and finish the look with an application of red liner on the lips filled in with a creamy red lipstick. Paint nails to match.

Wear hair pulled back into a chignon at the nape of the neck or emulate luxurious Latin waves by making rag curls (as directed in THE IMMIGRANT) and brushing them out until they fall in soft waves. Both hair treatments look right blowing in the wind or under the gaucho hat.

IDEAS

● Make a serape by fringing the end of a loosely woven length of thick cotton or wool using a large needle (see THE GYSPY). Alternatively, add ready-made wool or cotton fringing sold by the yard or metre.

● Similarly, a poncho can be easily made from a large square or rectangle of substantial wool fabric, by cutting a hole for the head and binding the edges with strips of leather or the classic blanket stitch.

● Decorate an existing plain, short-waisted jacket with braiding. Edge pockets, necklines and cuffs with a double row, making a large loop in the top row as the illustration shows.

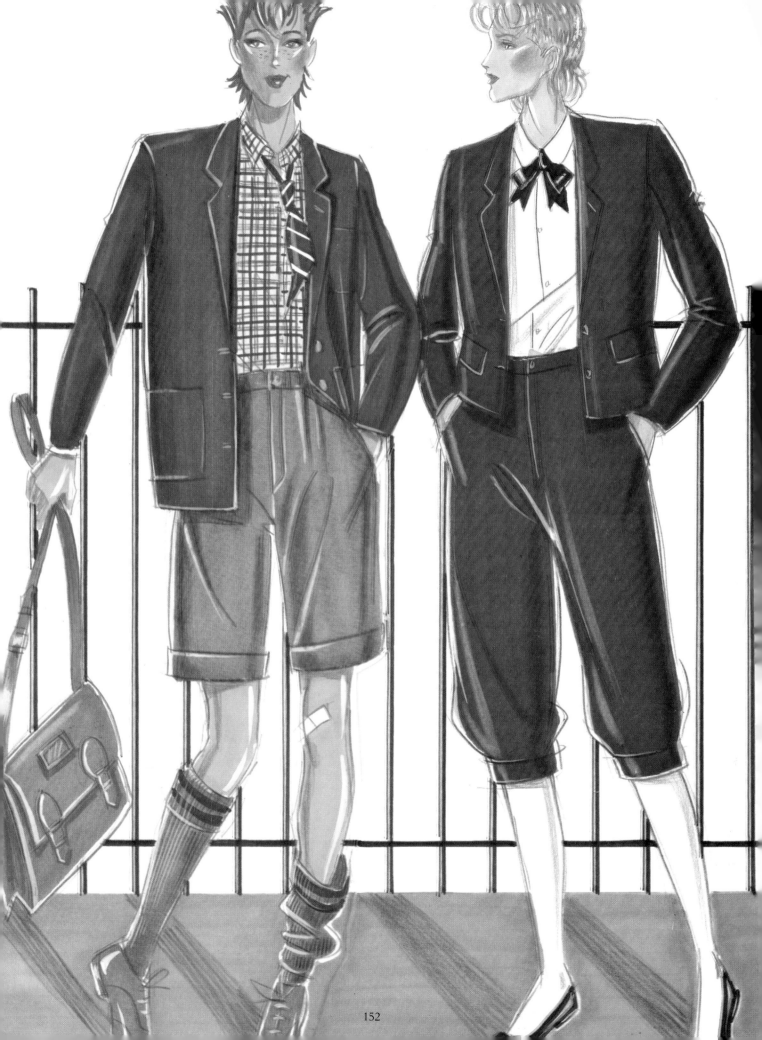

THE LITTLE BOY

BACKGROUND

Snails and satchels, freckles and blazers –
that's what little boys are made of. Think of
Just William; of Jean Seberg's urchin cut in
Jean-Luc Godard's *Au bout de Souffle* (1960); or
of young Tatum O'Neil's clothes in *Paper
Moon* (1973) or *Oliver*, to conjure up this
mischievous image.

The French word, *gamin* and its feminine form
gamine, are still regularly used to describe this
style. *Gamin* means urchin, kid or tearaway,
and the look took a hold with Jean Seberg's
fresh, boyish face and radical hair-cut in
Godard's film. It was a dominant style right
through that decade from Twiggy's
adolescent figure to the anything-goes, on-
the-streets, let's-have-fun ethics of Swinging
London and the Beatles.

The look is now a fashion staple. However,
it's a look that only works really well if you
are fairly slightly built, your face has an 'open'
appearance and you have a playful
temperament to match.

THE LOOK

Dressing like a little boy is easy. It's a versatile
look and will take you almost anywhere since
there are essentially three versions within the
look itself: the urchin, the schoolboy, and
Little Lord Fauntleroy. It is also an
international look and a great designer's
favourite – Dior, Valentino, Kenzo and Yves
St Laurent have used it again and again with
terrific success. It has a deep-rooted appeal
and always looks terrific.

The urchin is the most casual version, and a
marvellous summertime look. Amass plain or
boldly-striped T-shirts and baggy shorts in
any colours that suit you. Roll up the sleeves
of the T-shirt (and the cuffs of the shorts if
you like). For footwear wear tennis shoes or
any crepe-soled style and cotton ribbed socks.
For outerwear, don a sweatshirt or blouson
jacket – go for hardwearing fabrics like
denim, poplin or drill for the shorts and
jacket. Wear these knock-about clothes with a
slight tan and freckles (to fake the latter see
Face and Hair below).

The second version of this look relies on
schoolboy gear. For career wear, team a
blazer-style jacket with matching or
co-ordinating culottes or knickerbockers.

Below: **The Little Boy**'s requirements are few: a
simple watch, maybe with Mickey Mouse on the
face, lace-up shoes, canvas or brown leather school
satchel and a striped scarf.

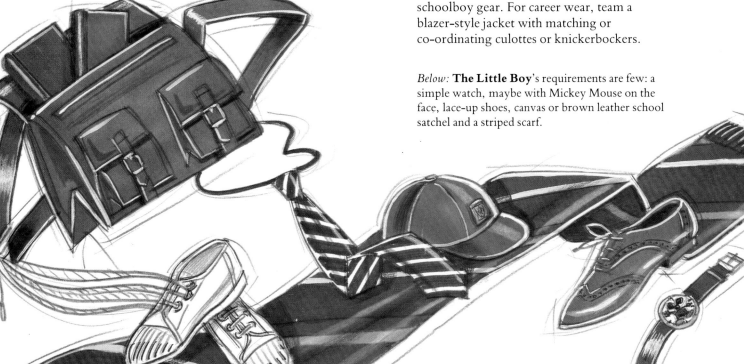

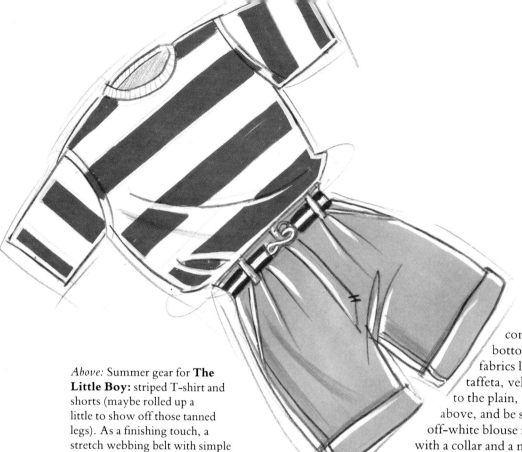

Above: Summer gear for **The Little Boy:** striped T-shirt and shorts (maybe rolled up a little to show off those tanned legs). As a finishing touch, a stretch webbing belt with simple clasp buckle, and you're set!

Knickerbockers can be just above the knee or just below; culottes can be from well above the knee to mid-calf, depending on the current fashion, occasion and the weather. Fabrics should be hardwearing – maybe seer sucker for summer, corduroy or flannel for winter. (If you're wearing THE LITTLE BOY for business occasions, avoid *really* short culottes and very bright colours. Adhere to traditional school shades like burgundy, navy, grey or dark green with accents of beige, yellow, white and pale blue.)

With this 'suit' wear cotton shirts with collars. Go for pinstriped, checked or plain colours – school outfitters and young men's shops will have them far cheaper than women's stores if you don't mind them buttoning up left to right. However, don't stop with the shirt. To be a well-dressed little boy, you must have a tie of some sort. Consider the traditional, short, schoolboy's striped necktie, a pre-tied, clip-on bow tie, or any of the alternatives given in *Ideas* below. If you're a tidy little boy, knot the tie neatly under the collar of your shirt. However, to look more roguish, tie it half way down, or wear it slightly askew.

The third and evening version of this look derives from the pageboy. Wear the same components of jacket and bottoms, but get them luxury fabrics like satin, brocade, taffeta, velvet or velveteen. Stick to the plain, traditional colours given above, and be sure to have a white or off-white blouse in fine cotton or silk with a collar and a minimum of frill. If you want to look like a rich kid, wear a bright satiny or plaid taffeta ribbon tied at the neck of the blouse, just under the collar, and maybe wear a matching ribbon in your hair.

Outerwear is predictable; choose anything a young boy would wear for Sunday best. In summer the blazer rules supreme. In winter a chesterfield or balmacaan style coat in plain shades such as navy or camel or in classic textures like tweed or tiny checks is the ideal garment. This overcoat can be any length from above knee to mid-calf, depending on the proportions of the rest of your clothing. Bear in mind that this perennial favourite will also work with other looks like THE BUSINESSWOMAN, THE CLASSICIST, THE FAIR ISLANDER, THE GENTLEMAN, THE IMMIGRANT and THE SCHOOLGIRL.

ACCESSORIES

For hats, choose caps. They can either match or contrast with your blazer or overcoat, with an emblem in front or without. The cap can be schoolboy style – small and neat, with a little visor; or urchin style – baggy with a large brim, perfect for tucking your hair into.

Socks and shoes should be highly functional and comfortable. Tennis shoes, brogues and lace-ups with ankle or knee-socks are perfect. Socks can be patterned or plain; ribbed white cotton ones for summer, Argyll or cable knits for winter. (Knee-socks are the most versatile since you can wear them pulled up or rolled down.) For evening, wear flat black pumps (best in patent or with a bow) and white stockings.

To add a dash of colour, wear a long scarf to wrap round the neck of your blazer or overcoat. Striped school scarves are ideal. If it's really cold, keep your hands warm in knitted gloves or mittens – as sombre or as colourful as you like. Look for them in children's departments and school outfitters if your hands aren't too big.

For a handbag, carry a satchel in leather or canvas trimmed in leather. Get one intended for schoolkids: you'll find it amazingly useful with its outside pocket and roomy interior.

Jewellery, as such, is minimal. You might wear a Micky Mouse or Superman watch by day, or cufflinks for evening, but his is really an unadorned look.

FACE AND HAIR

Use a tinted moisturizer to even out your complexion, but no face powder. Apply rosy blusher much further forward than normal to give a 'chubby cheeked' look. Imitate freckles with a very light tan eyebrow pencil sharpened to a fine point. Scatter them across the upper cheeks and bridge of the nose.

Hair should be short, or worn pageboy-style maybe even urchin-style spiked with a daub of hair gel. Alternatively, tuck long hair into a baggy cap, tomboy-style.

IDEAS

● Personalize your satchel, blazer or cap with badges – use traditional crests, or more zany ones like rainbows and cartoon characters.

● Brighten up lace-up shoes by changing shoelaces. Look for striped, polka-dotted and brightly-coloured ones.

● A necktie may be 24 to 36 inches (61– 95 cms) of velvet, grosgrain or satin ribbon. Ribbons in various lengths and textures will come in handy for accessorizing many other looks. For THE LITTLE BOY, wear a burgundy or navy, black or brown velvet one with your white evening shirt; by day, a length of thick grosgrain could become a necktie. For bow ties, tie single or double bows, wearing the knot at your neck or hanging slightly loose (see THE GENTLEMAN).

● Join mittens with a length of ribbon, string or thick yarn and thread them so they dangle from your coat sleeves.

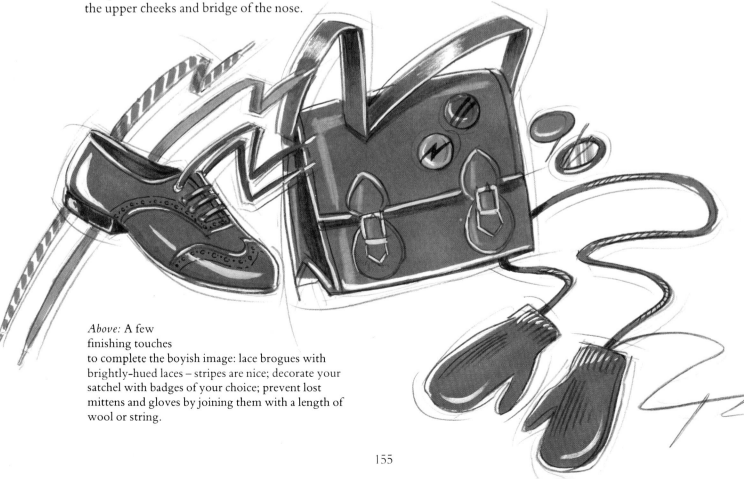

Above: A few finishing touches to complete the boyish image: lace brogues with brightly-hued laces – stripes are nice; decorate your satchel with badges of your choice; prevent lost mittens and gloves by joining them with a length of wool or string.

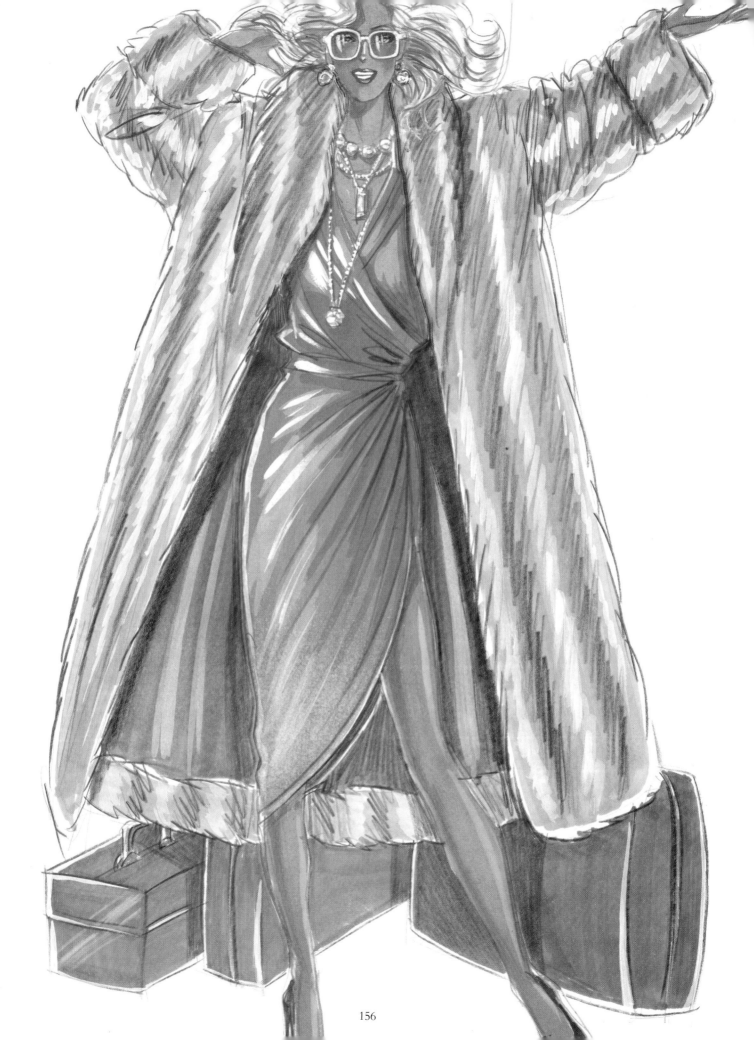

THE MOVIE STAR

BACKGROUND

'As the girl said, "A kiss on the wrist feels good, but a diamond bracelet lasts forever"'.★

And so it is with THE MOVIE STAR. Stars are attracted to all that glitters whether it's the bright lights, expensive jewellery or the star-studded sky shining over the centre of their universe, Hollywood.

Star appeal, or charisma, is that indefinable quality which makes heads instantly turn, shining out as special no matter what the occasion. THE MOVIE STAR, epitomized by such all-time greats as Rita Hayworth, Greta Garbo, Marlene Dietrich and Sophia Loren, more often than not has the kind of beauty which steals the breath away. But underlying the charisma and the glamour of a star there is a supreme, deep-rooted self-confidence that makes her out-shine everyone else.

Of course most of us are not stars – though we may yearn for their looks and self-confidence. While bone structure and long legs are God-given, THE MOVIE-STAR look in terms of clothes and style is surprisingly easy to achieve.

★Adlai Stevenson (1900–1965) in an address given to the Chicago Council on Foreign Relations, March 22, 1946.

THE LOOK

Just as a great MOVIE STAR becomes an all-time classic figure, so the trappings that distinguish her are not the kind of clothes that go out of fashion from one season to the next. The ideal clothes come in simple shapes but are executed in expensive fabrics. If you like the style, but don't have the diamonds to pay for it, don't despair – buy sparingly and selectively.

For THE MOVIE STAR, colours are above all tasteful. Wear white, ivory, bone, beige, tan, grey, gold, and silver deepening occasionally to charcoal, brown and black, if these dark shades are flattering on you. THE MOVIE STAR leads an international life so the clothes she wears are the stylish and costly classics that look right in Rome or New York, this year or next. The look begins with an essential calf-length fur coat. Ideally, it's of a long-haired fur in one of the neutral shades

Below: Ultimately luxurious accessories for this ultimately expensive look. Gilded leathers are the perfect refinement for shoes and bags, gloves are long and ruched and ideally kid or suede, jewellery is real or at least looks it. Scarves, big hats and sunglasses are all for travelling incognito.

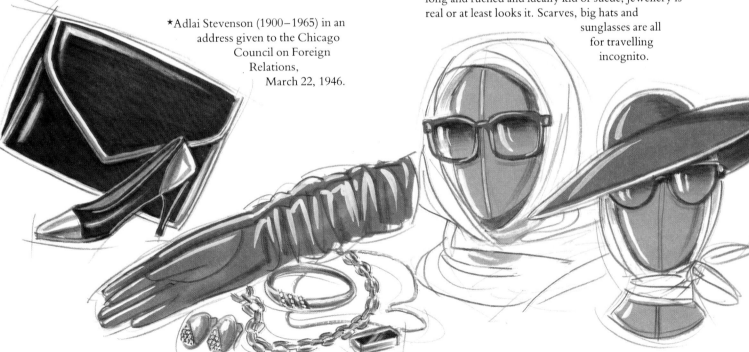

157

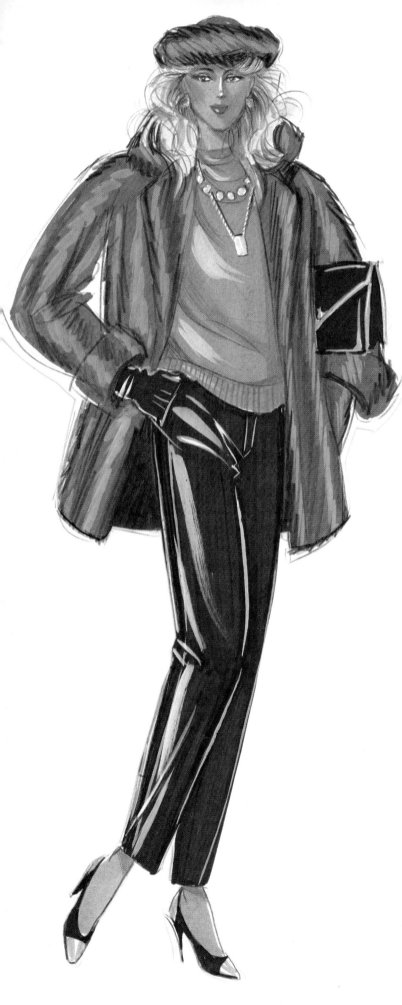

mentioned above. If you're opposed to wearing dead animals on your back, consider the marvellously convincing imitation furs now on the market. Fake fur is easier to keep clean, lighter in weight and is more easily restyled when shapes and/or hemlines change. A good imitation fur will set you back several hundred pounds, as opposed to several thousand for the real thing, and it will look and feel almost as nice. When choosing fur coats, go for an uncluttered design – at least for your first fur! Underneath your fur, the luxury continues. Wear beautifully-cut, draped dresses in real suede, silk, or fine wool jersey, or at least convincing imitations. For evening the same fabrics treated to a bit of sparkle such as sequins or diamante.

For more informal occasions (like lunch with your agent) wear a shorter fur coat, plain lambswool or cashmere sweater with suede, leather or silk trousers plus a few of your favourite jewels. In warmer weather, shed your fur and join THE OCEAN VOYAGER or THE LADY dressing in the palest shades.

Remember that quality clothing is the essence of this look. There is nothing cheap or vulgar about THE MOVIE STAR. She moves with quiet confidence, secure that she will always be the centre of attention.

ACCESSORIES
Without question, sunglasses are THE MOVIE STAR's distinguishing accessory. Weary of the adoring fans who greet her everywhere she goes, her one desire is to travel incognito. So she invests in several pairs. Choose them in a shape and colour to flatter, bearing in mind that the paler your looks, the paler your frames and lenses should be. For special occasions, you might like to gaze coolly through a Fifties wing-tipped or diamanté-studded pair. (See *Ideas* below.)

Stars hold their heads high so flattering headgear is *de rigueur*. Wrap your head in a long, silk, chiffon or cashmere scarf, and optionally add a wide-brimmed hat (as well as the obligatory sunglasses).

Left: A daytime look for **The Movie Star:** fur (or fake fur) hat and jacket, leather or suede pants and cashmere sweater. In summer, she'll wear silk or linen trousers with a silk shirt – wonderfully simple, isn't it?

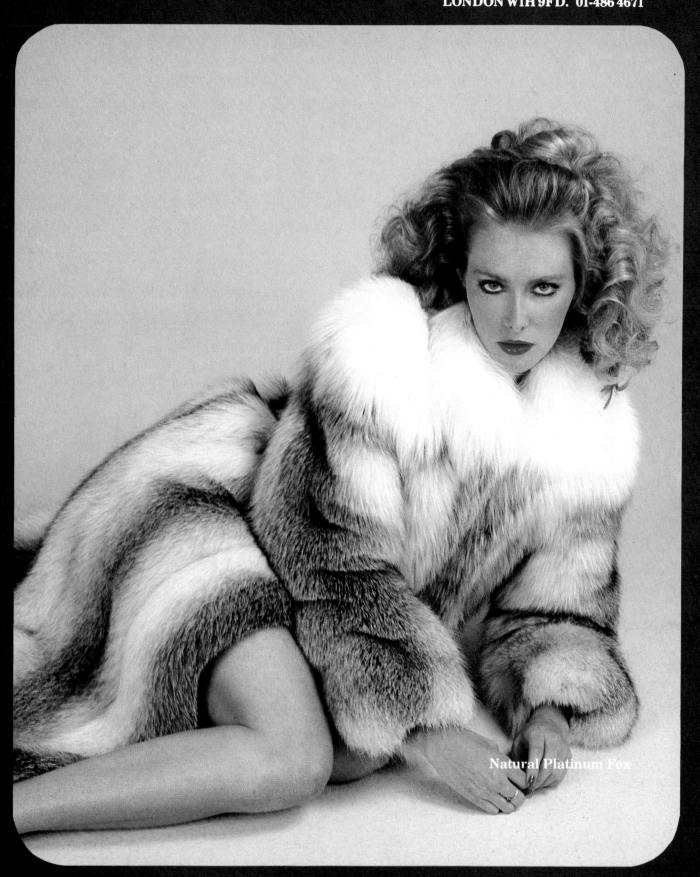

Stephen Glass
at Face Facts

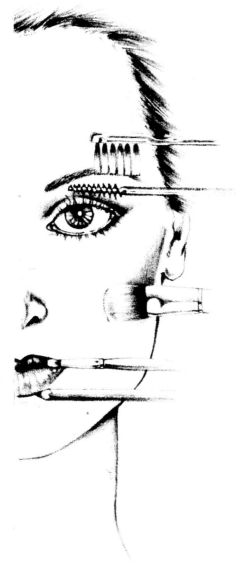

It's a woman's prerogative
to change her mind
why not her make-up?

75 GEORGE STREET
LONDON W1H 5PL
01-486 8287

Immaculate manicures can be protected by leather gloves – preferably long and ruched to go with the fur coat of the day or to match your hat or scarf. On colder days, wrap your head in fur, too. A Russian-style hat with a band of thick fur looks perfect.

To be chic, jewellery must be underplayed (to distinguish from THE VAMP again), which is just as well, since you'll only wear the more expensive trinkets (or the best imitations thereof). Go for diamonds, emeralds, rubies or sapphires. Wear rings and earrings *or* a necklace and bracelet, but never all four.

It goes without saying that belts, bags and footwear will always be of the best quality. Go for neutral shades to match or co-ordinate with your fur(s), letting your hat or gloves provide the colour. Shoes will have high heels, worn with trousers and dresses alike. If you can afford them, choose shoes and boots with details like appliqués in matching, toning or gilded leather. For summer, select peep-toe shoes to expose a flash of red painted toenails. With this exclusive footwear, wear only the sheerest stockings in the palest shades – grey or beige.

FACE AND HAIR

Grow or attach a mane. Your hair should be long and glamorous or at least shoulder length and immaculate. Keep it in place Garbo-style with trailing scarves. Or use only the most beautiful hair accessories, like diamanté-studded clips and combs. (See *Ideas*.)

For make-up instructions, see THE LADY, but aim for a more sun-tanned complexion. Add glamour with brighter or deeper lipstick and false eyelashes (ideally one by one). To complete the look, your finger- and toe-nails must always be perfectly painted. For a professional manicure, you will need the following supplies: absorbent cotton wool, nail brush, dish of warm soapy water, cotton swabs, emery boards, cuticle clippers, soft towel, hand lotion, orange stick, and cuticle cream.

1. Remove all old nail polish with an oil-based polish remover.
2. Using an emery board, shape each nail into a long oval, working with smooth strokes and filing from each side.
3. If a nail is too long or damaged, use the nail clipper to cut it straight across, then round off the sides with an emery board.
4. Massage each nail with rich hand cream.
5. Soak nails in warm, soapy water for five minutes, scrubbing with a nail brush if necessary and using lemon juice to bleach stains.
6. With a cotton swab, apply cuticle cream to each finger. Then, using an orange stick wrapped in cotton wool, push back each cuticle very gently.
7. Rinse and apply hand lotion.
8. If the tips of the nails need whitening, run a white nail pencil underneath the rim.
9. Apply base coat polish to prevent the pigments from discolouring the nails and to give the colour a smooth surface.
10. Apply two coats of polish, giving each coat at least five minutes to dry. In terms of colour, dark shades give hands a delicate look, while the lighter, sunnier shades flatter a suntan.
11. To remove smudges of polish, dip a cotton swab in polish remover.

IDEAS

● Use individually sold rhinestones or diamantés to decorate inexpensive accessories such as plastic hair combs, frames of sunglasses, the back of stockings along the seamline, scarves. Apply a dot of glue with a cotton swab and position rhinestones one by one.

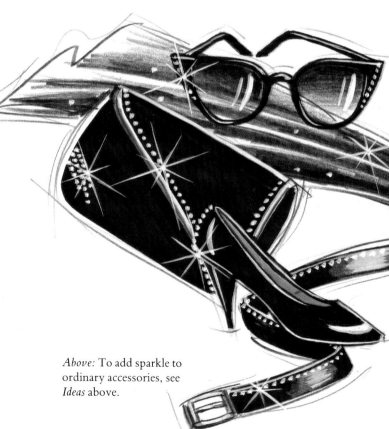

Above: To add sparkle to ordinary accessories, see *Ideas* above.

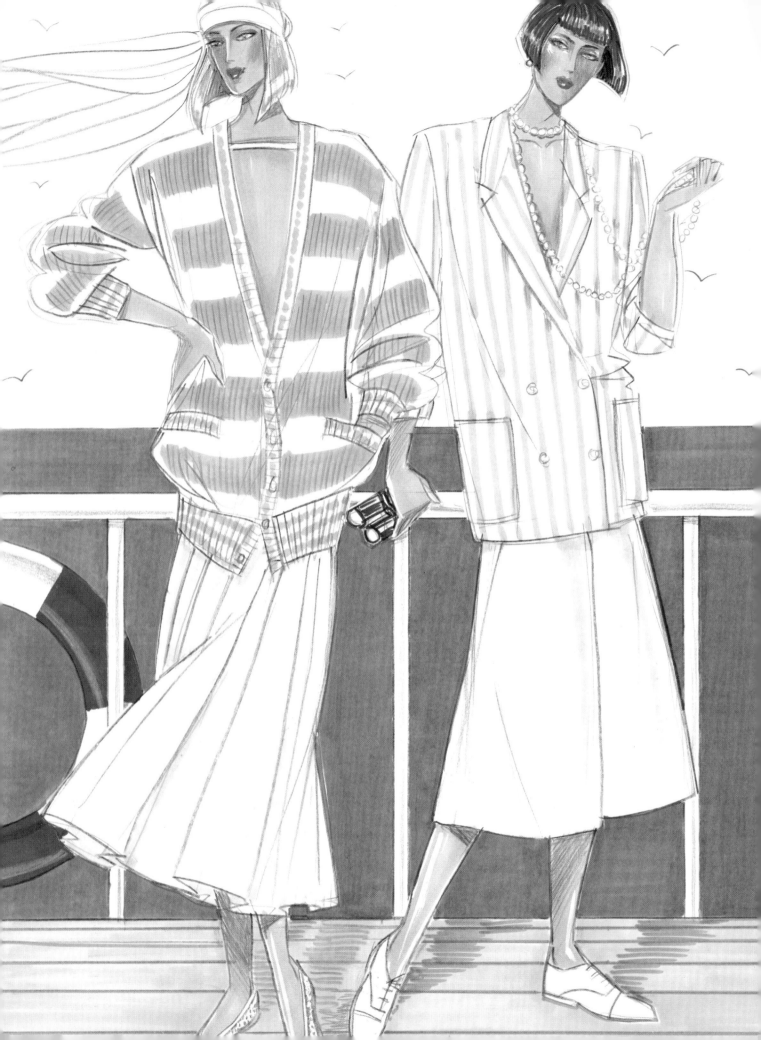

THE OCEAN VOYAGER

BACKGROUND

Have breakfast in your cabin, stroll on windy decks, bask in equatorial sunshine around sheltered swimming pools, breathe in fresh sea air while playing shuffleboard, lunch in oriental tea rooms, dine in chandeliered dining halls, dance the night away in palm-crowded ballrooms. This was the life of THE OCEAN VOYAGER. Only fifty years ago world travel was accomplished primarily by ocean liner. These palaces of the waves catered for a wealthy clientèle who expected their high standards of service on land to be equalled on the open sea. They were not disappointed.

One ship's inventory on the Holland America Line boasted 20,000 silver dishes and beverage pots, 400,000 pieces of linen and three kitchens. These were the halcyon days before the Great Depression of the Thirties which brought about an abrupt end to such luxury living.

THE LOOK

To dress like one of these privileged travellers is easy. The components are classics, easily obtainable and the result is a refined, yet casual look. THE OCEAN VOYAGER is essentially a Twenties look (see THE FLAPPER for a dressier version) and as such has clean geometric lines and proportions, reflecting the influence of Art Deco. Begin with a long V-neck cardigan. It should be hip-length and fasten with a row of pearly buttons down the front. It should be in any fine knit such as cotton, lambswool, cashmere or good quality man-made fibres, and ideally in white, cream, or a pastel shade. Navy or royal blue are appropriately nautical, too, though the resulting ensemble has a less soft and delicate look.

Wear the cardigan over your one-piece bathing suit as you stroll from pool to shuffleboard, but mostly team it with a matching calf-length, pleated skirt. The pleats

Below: **The Ocean Voyager** collects slightly less seaworthy accessories than her sister **The Sailor.** Crepe and rubber soles stay, but have slight heels, bags may be roomy and striped, but are executed in pastel shades, and she'll borrow a few refining touches from **The Flapper** – pearls and long flowing scarves add the finishing touches to this elegant seaboard look.

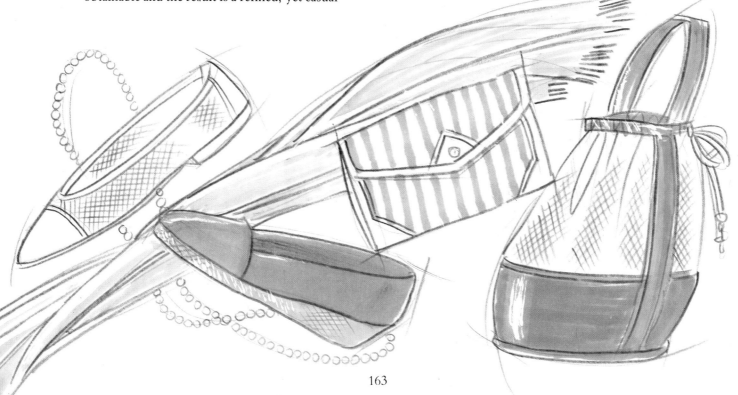

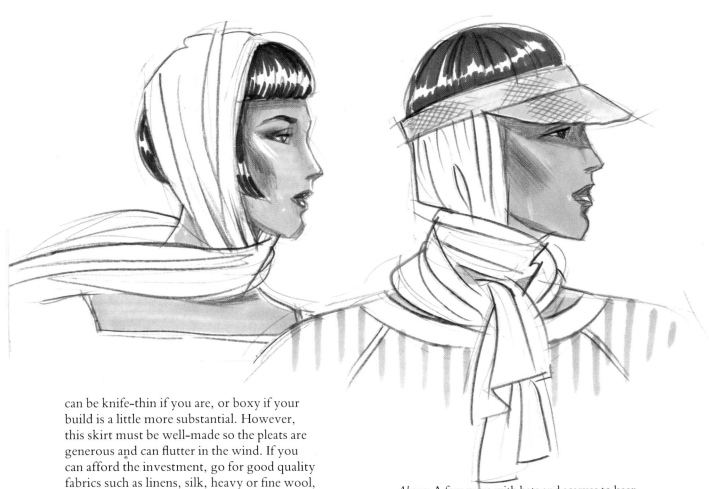

can be knife-thin if you are, or boxy if your build is a little more substantial. However, this skirt must be well-made so the pleats are generous and can flutter in the wind. If you can afford the investment, go for good quality fabrics such as linens, silk, heavy or fine wool, barathea, gabardine, or mixtures of these – they will last forever, or at least as long as you do. THE OCEAN VOYAGER is a fashion perennial and looks attractive on young and old alike.

For a more nautical version, team your navy cardigan with a contrasting skirt – red or cream. Blouses and shirts are white (or pastel shades for the softer version) and should have small neat collars, short sleeves, tailor's buttons and even fine tucks down the front.

Collapse on to a rattan *chaise longue* with a good book, wearing the same cardigan with straight-legged matching slacks. Again, quality is paramount and colours must follow one of the two schemes. Culottes also look right with the cardigan, again in white, cream or pastel shades, but in terms of length can be just below the knee, like the skirt or a few inches above the ankle depending on the length of the cardigan and the proportions of THE OCEAN VOYAGER in question.

For night time on board, see THE FLAPPER, or wear the ultimate in understatement – satiny evening pyjamas with contrasting piping and pearly buttons.

ACCESSORIES

Enliven the supreme simplicity of THE OCEAN VOYAGER's ensemble with imaginative use of

Above: A few ways with hats and scarves to keep you looking chic in the worst gale: from left, a very long scarf wrapped around the head and neck; a bare head topped with a brimless visor; a long scarf or a big square wrapped over the head, with the ends tied around the neck and knotted at one side; and the same shape scarf worn under a hat, with the ends blowing free.

accessories. Begin by wrapping your head in scarves in one of the following ways: wrap a large square, folded on the diagonal, around your head, completely covering it as in THE MOVIE STAR; tie the same shape at the nape of your neck under a small brimmed hat, or even on top of hats to hold them down in those sea squalls. Alternatively, wear long thin silk mufflers, or squares folded on the bias as headbands, in the mode of the bright young things of the Twenties. A cloche – a crowned hat with a small brim which sometimes drops over one eye – in natural or pale straw is perfect for summer. Once hat or scarf is in place, add sunglasses with pale lenses and frames. A hat with a visor will look great with the trousered version.

Wear the same long thin scarf around your neck in place of, or in addition to pearls (see jewellery below). Ideally in off-white silk or a co-ordinating pastel shade, drape it over the back of your neck, both ends hanging loose in

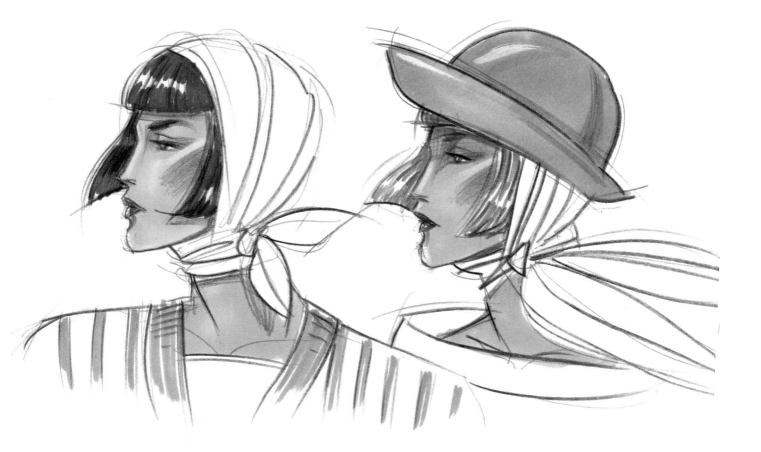

front, or throw one end over your shoulder for a carefree touch.

The accessories you wear with this elegant and refined look will tend to overlap with THE LADY and THE FLAPPER, so the investment in, say, a long silk scarf, a string of pearls, or a cloche will have many other uses, as they are fashion classics in their own right.

For footwear, wear white, taupe or pastel low-heeled shoes with skirt and sweater and tanned legs or the sheerest, off-white stockings. Twenties-style almond-toed shoes with a strap over the instep and a button fastening are ideal, as are two-toned shoes with perforated toe and heel, sometimes called 'spectator pumps'. With the more informal trousered version, wear rope-soled espadrilles. Espadrilles come in dozens of colours, are relatively inexpensive and work well with other casual clothes in THE SAILOR, THE CLASSICIST and THE SPORTSWOMAN.

For a bag, carry a co-ordinating clutch purse with the skirt, maybe with an Art Deco clip fastening; with the trousers a string or leather drawstring style is best.

Pearls or at least pale round beads are *de rigueur*. They can be very, very long, double- or single-stranded, mid-length or choker tight. Don't forget them, you won't feel right without. Other pieces of jewellery will be pearly too – bracelets, drop earrings, even rings. Moonstones, opals and coral are variations on the same theme of understated feminine chic.

FACE AND HAIR

A slight golden tan is an ideal beginning to this very refined look; in place of that begin with an application of a very sheer foundation dusted with a matching powder. Apply ivory shadow over the entire eyelid, accented with a little dark blue blended into the crease with a small dab of pink shadow on the inner corner of the lower lid. Use a navy kohl pencil just under the eyelashes and a navy mascara on the lashes. Blush with a pinky shade, gloss lips with a pink or rose lipstick.

Hair can be bobbed as in THE FLAPPER or any loose style that looks nice blowing in the wind and is not too fussy.

IDEAS

● See the illustrations at the top of the page for ways with scarves and hats.

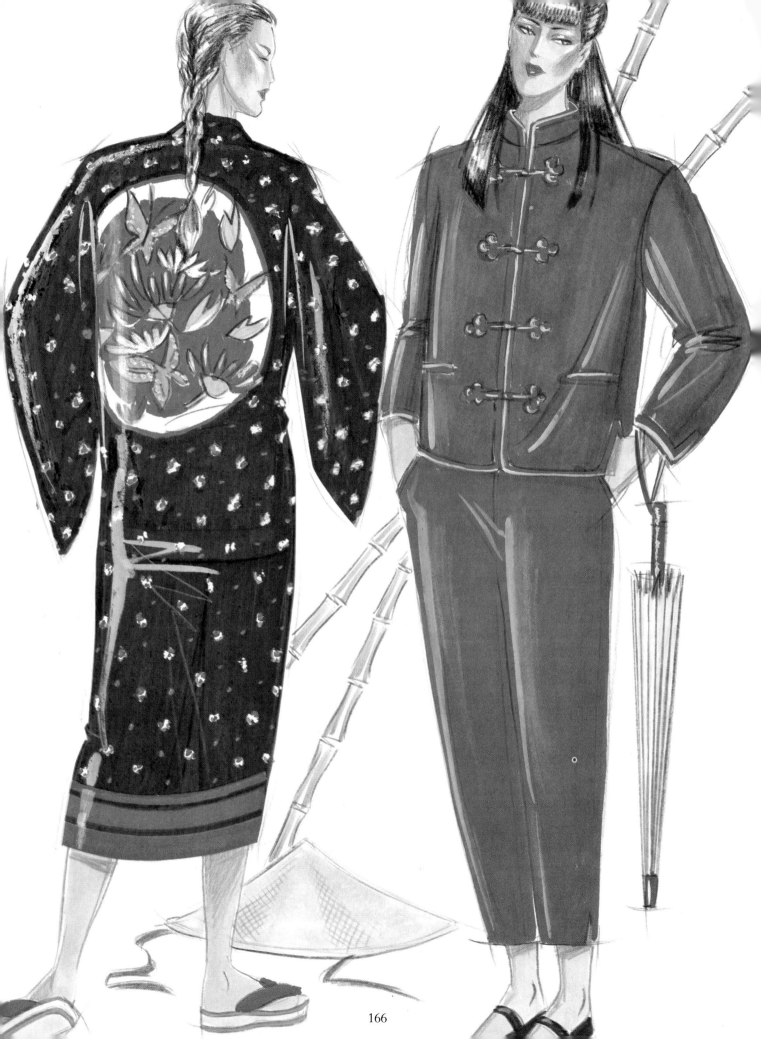

THE ORIENTAL

BACKGROUND

The expansion of trade with China in the late seventeenth century gave rise to a fashion for Chinese silks, printed or embroidered with designs of bamboo, chrysanthemums and dragons, and a growing demand by the emerging merchant classes in Europe for spices, rugs and semi-precious materials. Near the end of the eighteenth century, furniture designers like Thomas Chippendale were influenced by Oriental cabinet-makers to imitate the clean lines and lacquered or gilded panels of their furniture. In the nineteenth century, the emergence of Japan as an international power meant that the expanding middle classes could enjoy boatloads of Japanese imports including prints, fans, fabrics, pottery, furniture and clothing – a taste which provided the inspiration behind such pillars of British taste as Liberty and Co. Ltd.

The latter years of the twentieth century are proving no exception to this tendency: Japan is enjoying another exporter's heyday as the West struggles to compete with her highly efficient workforce in the fields of telecommunications, micro-chip technology and even fashion. This, coupled with the relaxation of trade restrictions with mainland China, means that we are able to choose from mounds of basketry, bamboo furniture, inexpensive clothing and embroidered handcrafts.

Various fashion historians have suggested that styles are imitated when a nation begins to emerge as a power or threat – witness the spread of blue jeans when the authority of America went unquestioned during the Fifties and Sixties. This theory would, of course, go a long way towards explaining our fascination with Oriental goods – worried as we are economically by Japan and politically by China's one billion population. However, leaving the sociology of the look behind, we are forced to merge these two countries as many of the garments for THE ORIENTAL are common to both.

Below: There's a wealth of inexpensive accessories to choose from when you're adding the finishing touches to **The Oriental.** Keep off the rain or sun with oiled-paper umbrellas, utterly plain or prettily stencilled; walk along in raffia-soled sandals or choose strapped pumps in cotton or silk with an embroidered front panel; carry your worldly goods in woven straw or shiny silk purses.

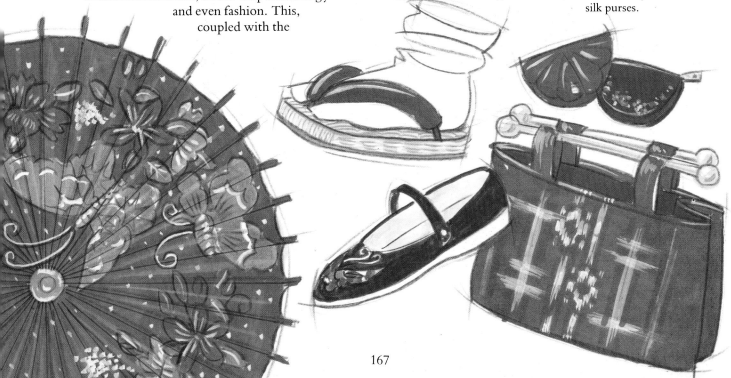

167

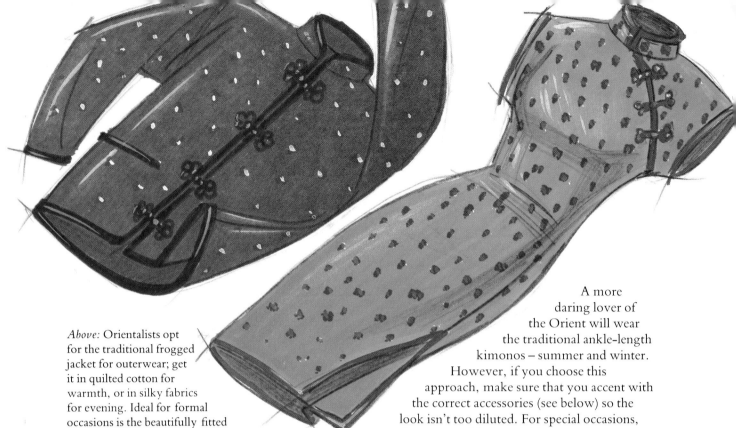

Above: Orientalists opt for the traditional frogged jacket for outerwear; get it in quilted cotton for warmth, or in silky fabrics for evening. Ideal for formal occasions is the beautifully fitted mandarin-collared cheongsam (right) in delicately printed silk or satin.

THE LOOK

Like all ethnic looks, THE ORIENTAL is amazingly versatile. You can choose heavily-ornamented garments in silks and brocades to shimmer the night away like a golden Buddha, or you can wear some of the most functional, informal clothing in the world, adopted by millions of Chinese peasants during the Cultural Revolution when Mao Tse-tung attempted to equalize China's distribution of wealth.

Begin with the kimono – a loose-sleeved, wrap-over, ankle-length garment of silk or cotton secured by a wide sash. By day, wear it waist length with tapered-leg or wide-bottomed, cut-off, pyjama-style trousers. Underneath wear a cotton T-shirt or nothing at all. Plain colours suitable for the kimono should be clear and bright, such as saffron yellow, lacquer red, midnight blue, jade green or coral. Patterns should feature traditional Oriental motifs like dragons, butterflies, grasses, birds, mountain landscapes and the compact geometrics. Buy your kimono from purveyors of Oriental goods, from secondhand clothing venues, from a martial arts supply shop (thick creamy cotton ones for judo are ideal both summer and winter), or make your own from a simple pattern – after all, there are no zips, buttons or pockets to complicate the job.

A more daring lover of the Orient will wear the traditional ankle-length kimonos – summer and winter. However, if you choose this approach, make sure that you accent with the correct accessories (see below) so the look isn't too diluted. For special occasions, the ornate ankle-length kimono takes some beating for stunning effect. For example, a brightly-embroidered silky one will take you out on summer evenings worn with nothing but tanned legs and sandals, and in winter with tapered trouser legs, traditionally black or colour co-ordinated with the kimono. Kimonos are unequalled for Occidental evening wear; they are pure and simple, easy to wear, flatter all figure types and will always look elegant and dramatic.

For slightly provocative evening wear, choose the cheongsam: a straight-skirted dress with fitted bodice, mandarin stand-up collar and a slit up one side of the skirt, usually found in an exotic silky fabric (as illustrated). It is usually fastened on the diagonal across one shoulder by frogs – a row of tiny silk-covered hooks.

More prosaic peasant's gear is even simpler to wear and easier to acquire since it has many imitators among fashion manufacturers of non-Oriental origins. For this informal version of THE ORIENTAL, wear the same tapered or cut-off trousers as above, whether they are in sheerest cotton for summer, wool for winter, or shantung silk for evening. On top, add the essential mandarin-collared blouse; it can be short-waisted to hip-length and in any fabric from slinkiest silk to wool.

For outerwear, choose the commune worker's delight – a quilted jacket, also with the distinctive mandarin collar. You'll find these in the traditional dark indigo blue (which fades beautifully with washing); in brightly printed cottons covered with butterflies and flowers; in corduroy, wool, felt, shiniest satin, padded silk, velveteen and heaviest brocade. Often piped at the edges and usually fastened with frogs or toggle buttons, they are warm and practical because of the quilting. They can also be immensely versatile.

ACCESSORIES
Kimonos, whether short or long, and hip-length mandarin blouses should be belted with an *obi* – a broad cummerbund tied in a large flat bow at the back. There are very precise, traditional Japanese techniques for tying the *obi*, but if you wrap a length of fabric or a scarf folded on the bias around your waist several times and tuck the ends in you won't be far wrong. Finish the effect with another layer – a band of twisted fabric centred over the *obi* will look right.

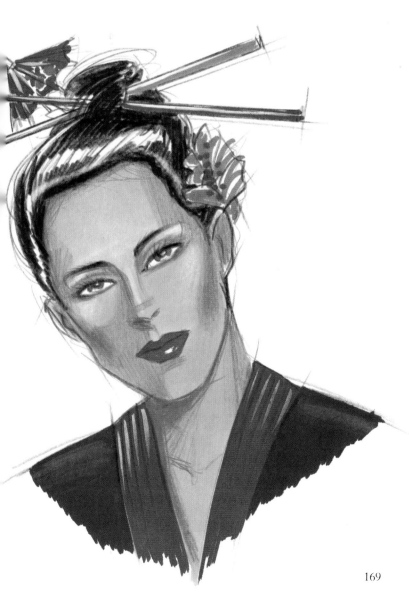

Sandals are the ideal footwear. With formal kimonos choose high-heeled styles. For daily wear, get flip-flop *zori* sandals.

Jewellery is very minimal because of the plethora of printed patterning and embroidery which are so much a part of THE ORIENTAL look. If you feel naked without adornment, choose semi-precious stones such as jade, coral, opals and pearls for earrings, carved pendant necklaces, fine strings of beads and rings – typical motifs such as dragons, Buddhas and flowers abound.

Handbags are really not a part of this look. Choose inexpensive printed paper change purses, string bags for parcels or an imported lacquered straw case. For evening, you might carry a satiny embroidered drawstring or small clutch purse. As a final touch, carry a fan or a prettily-stencilled umbrella. Or wear a coolie hat.

FACE AND HAIR
Warm your face with a golden-toned foundation unless you have naturally high colour. Shadow is confined to the lower lid area to accentuate the length of the eye; apply a sandy shade to the inner corner, blending it into a chestnut brown at the outer corner, extending this into a 'V' or wing shape at the end of the eye. Bring the same colour around under the lower lashes, applying mascara to the top lashes only. Use ivory highlighter to emphasize the highness of Oriental cheeks, shadowing with a tawny blusher underneath. Use a lipstick to co-ordinate with your clothes, keeping to the apricot–orange–red spectrum, and employing a lipstick brush to achieve a perfect outline.

Hair should be worn cut in a straight bob or in a single plait for informal occasions. With your finest kimono, wrap hair into a chignon, decorating it as suggested below in *Ideas*.

IDEAS
● Decorate your chignon by inserting long hair-pins, lacquered chopsticks, or an appropriate cocktail swizzle stick. Alternatively, add a cluster of fake or real flowers – make them chrysanthemums, natural grasses, or gladioli.

Left: For finishing touches to this look, scoop up your hair and decorate with lacquered chopsticks.

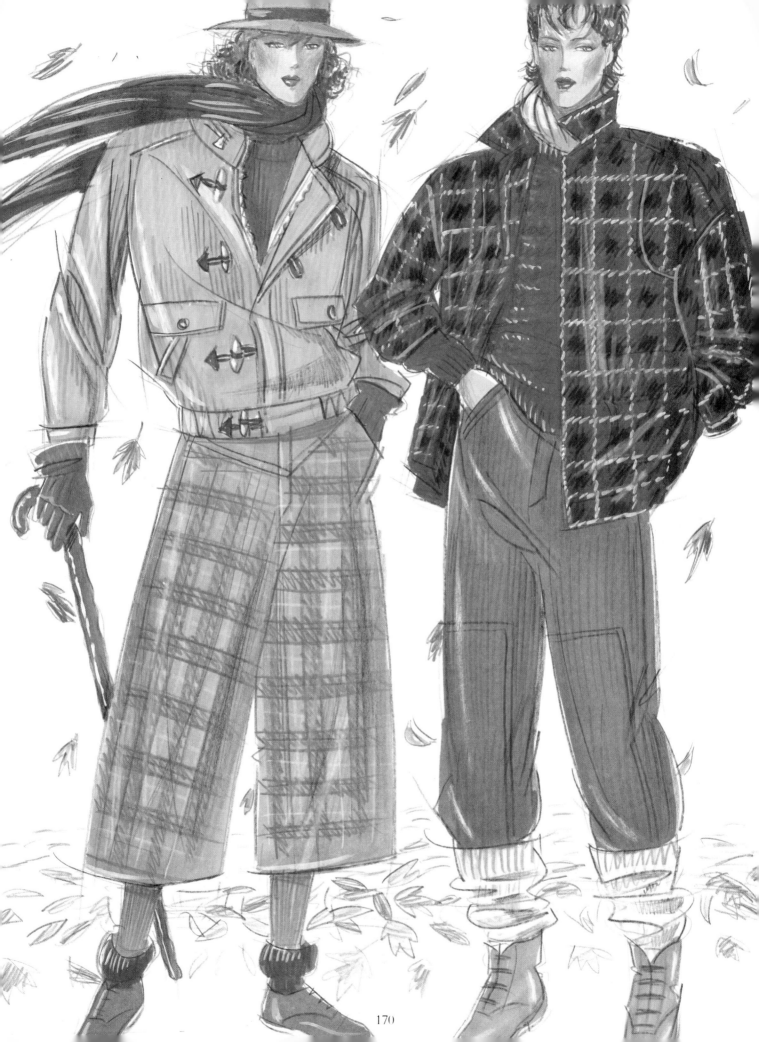

THE OUTDOOR GIRL

BACKGROUND

Tramp through the autumn woods, kick up the falling leaves, collect blackberries and rose hips for jams and jellies, and revel in the golden, burning shades of autumn. While the LANDOWNER and THE HORSEWOMAN are off a-shootin' and a-huntin', THE OUTDOOR GIRL prefers to take country life at an easier pace, allowing herself time to observe Nature at its best.

THE LOOK

THE OUTDOOR GIRL delights in all the seasons, but spring and autumn are her most favourite. Gathering elderberries and crab apples or holly, mistletoe and ivy, crossing streams, scrambling up muddy banks and pushing her way through tangled undergrowth and overhanging branches – these are the pursuits she revels in. To protect herself from such obstacles she needs substantial clothing and practical footwear.

Freed from the harsh sophistication of her cosmopolitan sisters she chooses soft, loose-fitting clothes which reflect the colours of her surroundings: loden and mossy greens of leaves and bushes, rusts and earthy browns of the woodland floor, glowing russets of the autumn trees and the rich reds of berries, sycamore and maple foliage; occasionally she'll add a soft mid-blue of bluebell or forget-me-not.

Fabrics, too, are nature's own. For your woodland look select cloths of different weights: woven wools, gentle corduroys, flannels and Viyella, knits of textured yarn, thick tweeds and well-worn, supple leather.

Fairly loose-fitting trousers in a warm, thick subtle plaid or corduroy, provide the best protection from scratching twigs and prickly

Below: **The Outdoor Girl**'s shoes and boots are for walking, her plaid scarves and socks are for warmth, but she still looks stylish!

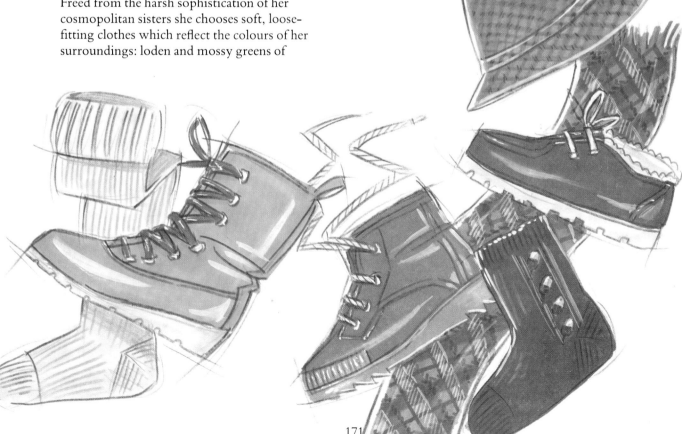

brambles. If you prefer to wear a skirt, exchange the trousers for loosely gathered culottes or a dirndl shape in one of the above Flannel or Viyella shirts in small checks, soft plaids or plain colours are as warm and comforting as they sound. Textured sweaters in bobbly yarns of woodland colours go on top. The Shetlands and lambswools of THE HORSEWOMAN and THE LANDOWNER are quite suitable, or borrow from THE FAIR ISLANDER. For an appropriately rustic look, make the sweater the central feature of your outfit. Look for pullovers with cosy collars, double cuffs and wide-ribbed bottoms. (Knitters could produce pictorial sweaters of a favourite nature subject or incorporate knitted motifs of woodland berries, fruits or flowers into a plain garment.)

On crisp frosty mornings and chilly misty evenings, warm outerwear is essential. If you choose plain trousers or a skirt, add your country cousin's lumberjacket in a muted plaid, buttoned up and bound with a sturdy leather belt. With plaid trousers, try a corduroy or tweedy blouson or a jacket cut on looser lines than the hacking coat or the Norfolk jacket; outside pockets need to be big enough to take a hoard of pine cones for the fire. Alternatively, a knitted jacket or thick cardigan (see THE SCOTSWOMAN's Aran) might be the answer; again belt it round the waist or wear open.

The final optional layer is a vast woven shawl or blanket square in varuna or heavier wool mix such as wool and cashmere, if you can afford it. Drape it round your shoulders and wrap it over your head. A serape or large and flowing poncho from THE LATIN, a large leather jerkin with an optional fleecy lining or a down-filled waistcoat are warm practical alternatives.

ACCESSORIES
Crossing endless woodland streams necessitates sturdy waterproof footwear so wellingtons are essential. But more aesthetic and still fairly sensible are crepe- or rubber-soled boots and shoes with practical and comfortable flat or low heels. The uppers should be of robust leather, tough suede or

strong canvas, in woody greens and earthy browns. Choose flat suede 'goblin' boots, with turn-over cuff, or sturdy lace-up calf or ankle boots fastened with laces wound round rows of metal studs; sheepskin-lined boots, or tough hard-wearing walking shoes fit the bill too.

Socks must be of the warmest kind; flecked and textured woollen yarns in double or treble ply will give extra insulation when worn over ribbed wool tights. Thermal socks are essential inside rubber boots. Tuck trousers into socks and lace your boots on top; or wear knee socks over tights in ankle boots with tweedy skirts or culottes.

Plaid scarves, mufflers and wool gloves will cover other exposed extremities; tie a muffler round your neck or head or fold a loosely-woven wool square with self-fringe (see THE FAIR ISLANDER) diagonally in half and wear

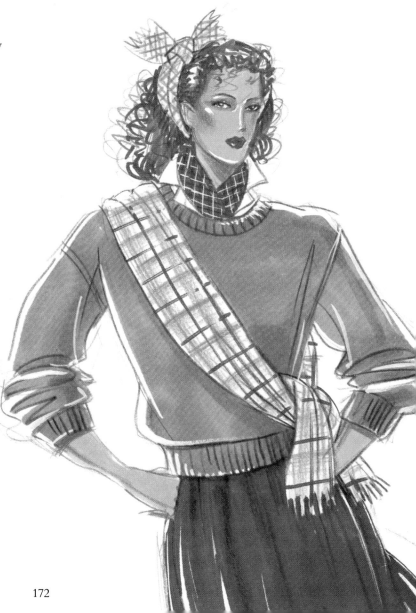

Right: Scarves do more than wrap necks – try them as headbands and worn on the diagonal.

172

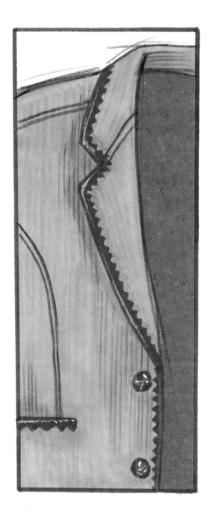

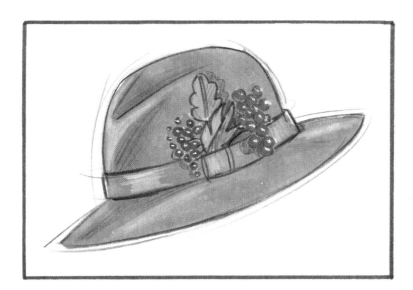

Above and left: Make your clothes last a little longer by binding worn edges in leather and by replacing buttons; make your hats prettier by decorating them with woodland finds. (See *Ideas* below.)

over your head, in neck of your turned-up jacket collar or arranged loosely over the shoulders of coats and jackets.

Favourite cravats and ribbons also have a place in THE OUTDOOR GIRL's wardrobe; a paisley or plaid cravat in fine wool will tuck neatly into the neck of a Viyella shirt. A slouchy, soft hat in felt (farmer-style) and a large leather satchel bag, or even better, a willow woven basket (for carrying field mushrooms, blackberries and wild garlic), are your final items of equipment.

FACE AND HAIR

THE OUTDOOR GIRL's face reflects her dedication to nature: camomile, nettle or rosemary are infused in boiling water, then cooled for hair rinses; egg white or yolk used to treat oily and dry skin respectively. However, the most important qualities to this look are a face glowing with healthy vitality and hair which is supremely shiny and well cut, no matter what the style.

Make-up is thus really secondary and used very sparingly. Eyes might be shadowed with russet or soft sludgy green, with a lick of brown mascara and a semi-gloss rust or berry colour for lips. Cheeks will flush naturally after a brisk walk or after a dust of russet or rosy blusher.

IDEAS

● Collect woodland bits and pieces on a nature ramble, walk in the woods or from your own back garden: seed sacks and pods, small sprays of dried flowers and twigs with hips or other berries. Spray with clear varnish for protection and use to trim felt hats or in jacket buttonholes. Glue or wind stems on to pin fasteners to make rustic brooches.

● Extend the lives of worn-out cuffs, pocket edges or cardigan fronts by adding leather bindings. Replace plastic or similarly unimaginative buttons with traditional criss-crossed leather ones.

● Use soft-coloured yarns to embroider rustic designs onto wool sweaters, gloves and even socks. Choose motifs such as fruit, berries, leaves or flower buds. Try a single one above the breast or a regulated all-over pattern along an edge.

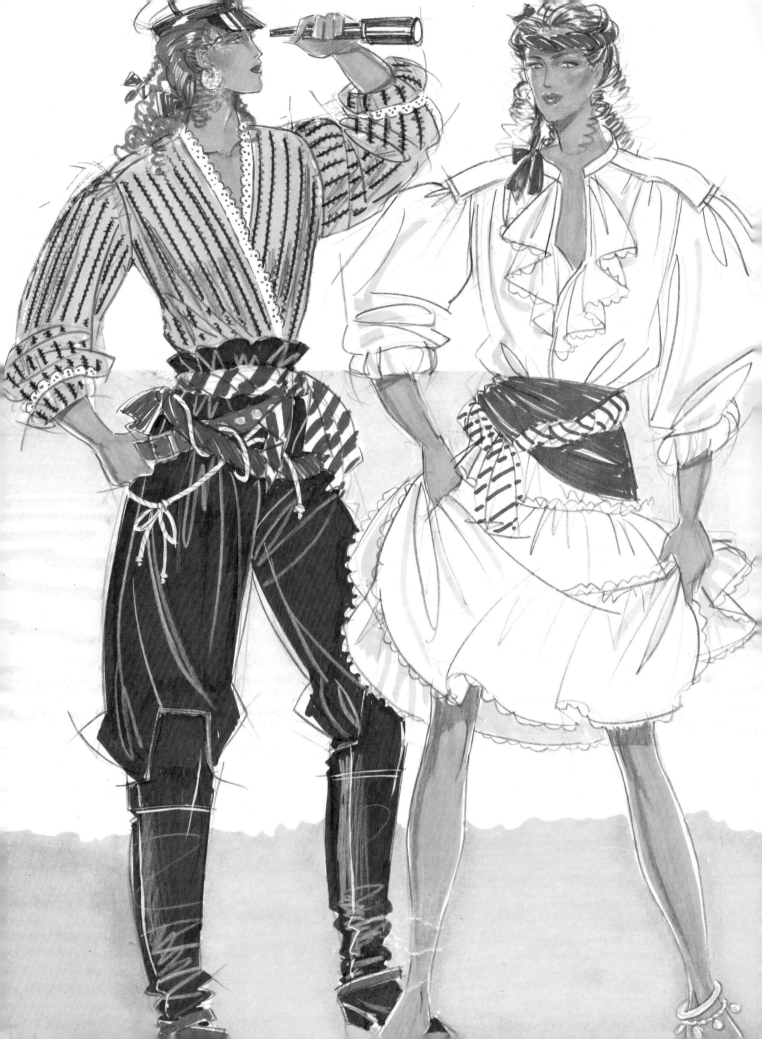

THE PIRATE

BACKGROUND

Yo, ho ho and a bottle of rum! Remember Captain Hook in *Peter Pan*? Or Long John Silver in *Treasure Island*? Their names evoke a whole breed of sinister characters, peg-legged eye-patched, armed with a pistol or a sword and a parrot on the shoulder. As it happens, both these anti-heroes from children's fiction were based on a very real problem: for three hundred years between the sixteenth and nineteenth centuries, roving bands of buccaneers prowled the north African coast and the Caribbean islands robbing the fleets of the great maritime nations. Fierce sea battles were fought, treasures lost, captives taken; pirates were the plague of the sea. Their eclectic appearance was derived from the wide range of goods they captured. If you're attracted by the romance of the Spanish Main,

steal a loose-sleeved white shirt from THE GYPSY, swipe undergarments from THE SHEPHERDESS, and baggy trousers from THE ARABIAN, secrete a feather from THE YOUNG ROMANTIC, and lift a waistcoat from THE DANDY, imitate the rag curls of THE IMMIGRANT and rob THE GENTLEMAN of his gold watch.

THE LOOK

Pirates, though often ferocious men, could be foppish too, liking the effect of a ruffle or two, or a jewel or three, or wearing luxurious silks and velvets (looted no doubt). And because of the abundance of frills, this is a perfect look for women – and it can be worn every day or dressed to the hilt for parties and special occasions. It is a fairly complicated yet messy look, taking some effort to achieve, so for the hurried and impatient among you, steer clear. You would, after all, have had hours to experiment with the clothing you'd stolen and days to admire yourself in your broken looking glass.

Below: **The Pirate** is barefoot or wears tall shiny black boots; she uses rope to wrap rags for belts and headbands, to cinch trouser tops, keep trouser bottoms out of the salty sea and to lash on her binoculars and stolen 'jewels'.

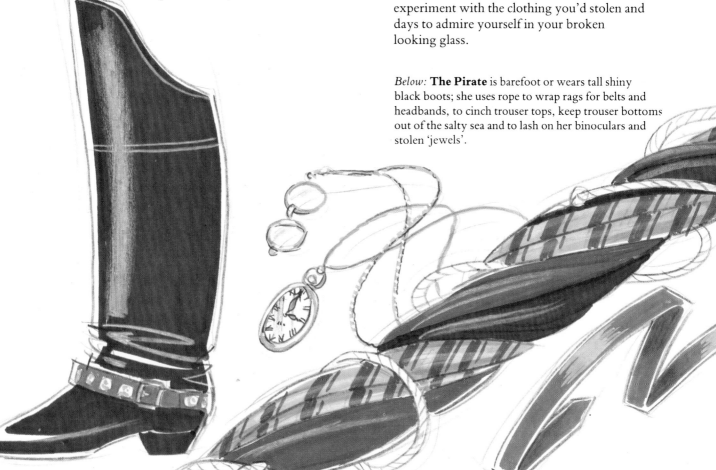

Right: For outerwear, nothing beats a long, fitted deeply-cuffed jacket, complete with big brass buttons. Wear it with trousers or short skirts – it looks even better if you're wearing a watch fob around your neck and a parrot on your shoulder.

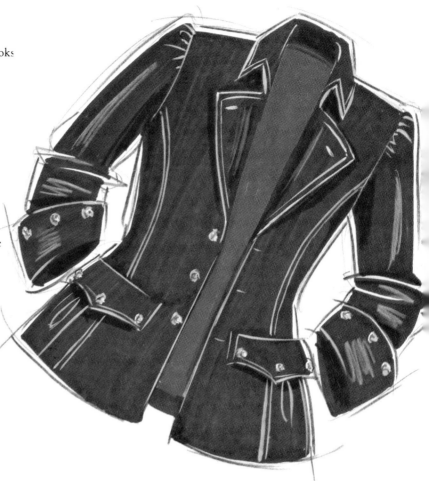

Begin then, with a loose-sleeved white blouse, either with notched collar or V-neck and with lacy ruffles galore. Wear this with dark, baggy trousers which are gathered at the waist, wrapped or rolled at the cuffs, or try a too-big pair which are hitched up, and belted at the waist as in THE IMMIGRANT. If you'd prefer to be a lady pirate, substitute a short white cotton petticoat with a deep edging of ruffles or lace for the trousers, but in this case wear the blouse over the skirt, belting it as directed below.

Should you be sailing in the scorching heat, forget the blouse and wear a sleeveless vest or camisole instead. It can be quite plain, cellular knit, lace-edged, very tight or very big.

On top, wear a frock coat, long captain's jacket, or even a navy or black blazer. Period clothing can be hired from theatrical costumiers or found in secondhand clothing stores; otherwise, raid a man's wardrobe.

ACCESSORIES
The above outfit may be a slightly off-beat combination, but it is nothing compared with the eccentric accessorizing required to transform it into a real Pirate.

Traditionally THE PIRATE wears a hat or some form of headdress. It can be a captain's cap complete with a visor and gold braid, or you can fashion an authentic pirate's tricorn hat from a large-brimmed felt hat, as directed in *Ideas* below. Headbands made from ragged strips of fabric also look right, if worn across the forehead as the introductory illustration shows. For a simpler headdress tie a spotted kerchief casually round your head, knotting all ends at the back (see THE OCEAN VOYAGER).

Rags are an important and unusual feature of this look. Use them twisted for belts, wear them as scarves and kerchiefs, lace them to tighten baggy trouser legs, wrap them round damp hair to make rag curls, tie them in bows for adorning rag curls, and sport them across one shoulder as a kind of mock parade ribboning. (Old white cotton sheeting torn into strips is ideal).

The other ingredient used for holding up a pirate's often ill-fitting clothes is a thick black or brown leather belt, at least two inches wide with a heavy brass buckle. These wide leather belts will be worn over blouses and T-shirts whether they are tucked in or not. Cinch them tight or let rags define your waist and let the leather one hang loose so it falls off your waist, as the introductory illustration shows.

Jewellery is brassy – wear gold doubloons on leather strips; adorn your person with antique gold pieces such as fob watches, brooches and magnifying glasses and large gold earrings. Use brooches to decorate your pirate hat or to secure an ostrich feather, or in other off-beat places such as on your headband or on your fabric belt. Lengths of heavy gold and silver chain are also in keeping (see *Ideas*.)

On your feet, wear nothing if the weather and occasion permit; failing that, nautical boating shoes or better yet boots of any length from calf-high to excessive over-the-knee styles in a supple leather that any self-respecting pirate would be proud of. These luxuries of the wardrobe are amazingly versatile if you live in a cold-weather climate as they work perfectly with other looks such as THE GYPSY, THE YOUNG ROMANTIC and THE IMMIGRANT.

FACE AND HAIR

As this is a summertime boyish look, wear no foundation if you are sufficiently suntanned. Failing that, a bronzed gel will do the trick. Use bright blue pencil or navy kohl just inside the rim of the eyes, as near as possible to the lashes. Mascara top and bottom lashes in navy and let cheeks glow with a warm rusty red blusher if you're not glowing with sun or windburn already. Hair should be as wild and as full of body as possible. Add waves to short hair with setting lotion and heated rollers, to longer hair with rag curls brushed into soft waves.

IDEAS

• Make a hat any pirate would give his Jolly Roger for: roll up opposite ends of a large-brimmed hat, securing each side with a safety pin, antique brooch, stud earring or stitch. To this add a red or white ostrich feather, as the illustration shows, or stick on a skull and cross-bones motif.

• Fix a too-big T-shirt by knotting a handful of excess fabric in front and/or by tying a single knot at the shoulders of sleeveless and camisole styles.

• Make inexpensive chains by buying lengths of brass chain 14–20 inches-long and in various diameters from one-quarter to one inch from hardware supply shops.

• For a real touch of authenticity, make a tattoo on your bare upper arm with a blue felt tip pen. Make an anchor or skull and cross-bone shape, filling it with a red felt tip, and finally outline in with a fine black one if necessary.

• If you can't afford wide leather belts, consider making them from a double layer of black or brown felt and a 3–4 inches (8–10 cms) silvery buckle (from specialist sewing shops).

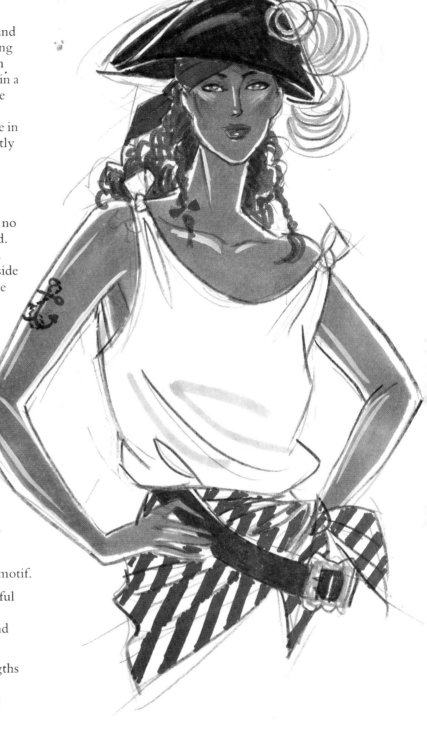

Above: Grab a man's sleeveless undershirt from your first mate, gather the excess at the top of your shoulders into a knot and you'll have a perfect hot-weather solution.

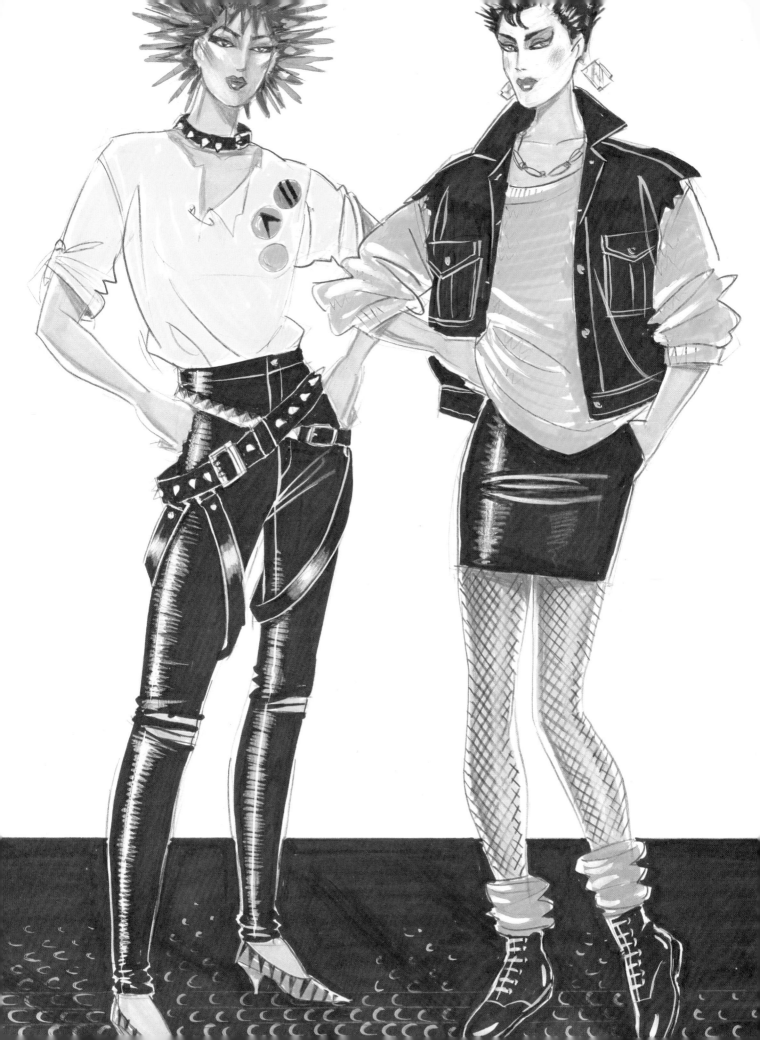

THE PUNKETTE

BACKGROUND

A theme which began as a musical alternative in the late Seventies has spawned a major revolution in the way we look. Punk rock was born on the backstreets of London, but forced its way into the mainstream with its frenetic beat, offensive (sometimes obscene) lyrics, basic harmonies and aggressive performances by kids dressed in extraordinary clothing.

Anarchy ruled supreme on the stage and in the halls where these live bands performed their deliberately raucous music – fans spat, brawled and bounced in ill-assorted, secondhand clothing, decorated by such worthless objects as safety pins and razor blades.

Only five years later, punk had been diluted, then polished, coloured and re-packaged into a huge fashion and music business. The kids who were clothed in cast-offs must be amused, maybe shocked, to see designers like Zandra Rhodes and Vivienne Westwood charging hundreds for their imitations. Punk clothing has become much more saleable – it

Below: **The Punkette** collects plastic and metal accessories, preferably in shocking neon shades and in aggressive patterns like razor stripes, lightning streaks or big cat prints.

is aggressively sexy, even sexist, with tears in all the right places, safety pins and zips gaping to reveal inches of bare flesh, metal studding much in evidence.

By now punk has been and almost gone, but even if you were not part of the movement, it has infiltrated all our wardrobes. Our skirts can be worn shorter, we are less afraid of violent garish colours (evidence THE DANCER), our hair stands up a little more with a bit of back-combing, and short hair is back on boys and girls alike. You may not have the time, inclination or bravura to dress like THE PUNKETTE every day, but if you're attracted to its wild style, keep it for parties and nights on the town.

THE LOOK

THE PUNKETTE is an uneasy mixture of clothing gleaned from the beatnik, the Fifties rocker, the Sixties mod, and a freakshow.

Unfortunately, there is no easy way to achieve this look in its entirety without going to a designer who creates bizarre clothing such as those along London's Kings Road. Alternatively hold on to your money, go for the original streetwise look, and become a

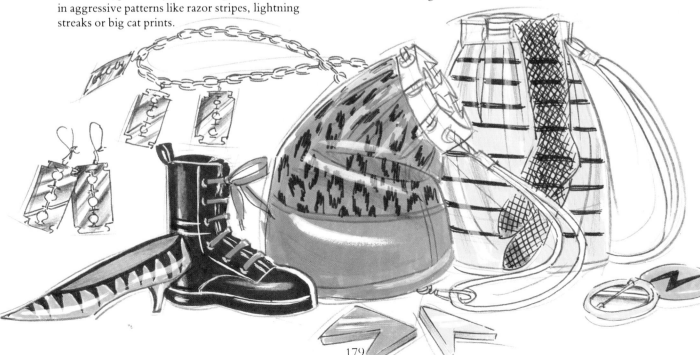

179

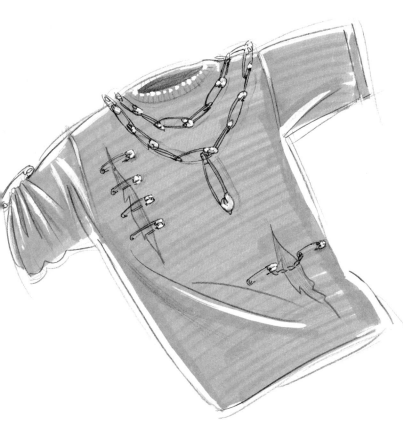

Above: Ways of dealing with a mundane T-shirt: a safety pin on left sleeve exposes your arm a little more; a tear at the left side is closed with a row of small safety pins; at the neckline, large and small pins are linked together to make a necklace, and at the bottom of the T-shirt, two safety pins close the gap using an inch length of inexpensive chain.

little aggressive with your existing clothes. Using scissors to make a small cut, start a tear in a garment, expanding it to the desired length by ripping or additional cutting. (Tearing slits works particularly well with stretchy knit fabrics.) Leave the tears gaping open, or fasten one side of the tear open with a brass or steel safety pin. If you've made the tear too long, close it up with a row of safety pins, or narrow the gap with a length or two of fine chain, either sewn in place on either side of the tear or pinned or stapled.

The same technique can be used on cotton T-shirts, and sweat-shirts whether short-sleeved for summer or high-necked for winter. Rip slits in the arms, maybe along the back too, or make radial slits along the neckline. You might also cut off one shoulder or shorten one arm, or just roll up the sleeves, securing the cuff with a safety pin.

Tight trousers in any style from pedal pushers to stretch pants, zouaves to jeans can be subjected to a similar treatment. For example, you might rip open the knee of tight pants, or add a gash or two near the ankle. Incorporate bondage straps – using lengths of leather shoelaces, strips of suede or rags to match or contrast with your trousers. Use these to wrap the legs of pants, but not in the artistic manner of THE GYPSY or THE COSSACK – make your punk lacings as uneven and as knotted as you like. Tie more strips around your thighs and knees, holding them in place with safety pins if necessary: even join trouser legs with an 18-inch (46 cms) length of fabric or chain, pinning it in place. Wear a shaggy or animal-printed sweater in raw shades. With a long enough sweater, wear it as a dress with footless black leggings and pointed flat shoes.

In terms of colour, it's black, black and more black. All-black clothes have, of course, been around for a long time; the beatniks of the Fifties wore nothing else, but they never had black eyeshadow and black fingernails and black lipstick! Once you've recovered from all the black, incorporate all the brightest of the brights too – shocking pink, electric blue, acid yellow in hideously clashing combinations. Be as vicious as you can in choosing tones that vie, patterns that jar. The whole idea is to set the teeth on edge. Go for an idiosyncratic mix of textures – zebra-striped hair with big-cat printed clothing, green streaked hair with garish versions of Scottish tartans and black leotards, white faces with mohair sweaters and plastic skirts.

For outerwear, nothing beats the black leather jacket, complete with chains and studs. Get it short-waisted or long, wear it big or tight, choose it sleeveless or long-sleeved so that you have to roll the sleeves up. Wear it with minis and trousers alike. Alternatively, wear any of the outerwear suggestions given in THE ROCKER or THE CAT WOMAN – even a jacket from THE SOLDIER.

ACCESSORIES

Tights, leggings, leotards, leg warmers, socks all play an important part in the wardrobe of THE PUNKETTE. You can conveniently use the ones you've torn or laddered. Wear tights and leotards as a first layer under short skirts or short shorts; wear leggings as trousers with long baggy, shaggy sweaters; wear leg warmers and thick socks on top of those. This unusual layering is very important – think nothing of wearing skirt over trousers or overalls even, or one torn pair of tights over another. After all, you're trying to look the direct opposite of well kept.

Footwear, too, knows no limits. Wear Louis-heel pointy pumps from the Fifties, lace-up, crepe-soled walking boots, sometimes called 'Bovver boots', soft and floppy calf-length boots, even ragged tennis shoes. Again, go for unlikely combinations, like leg-warmers worn on top of boots, black tights with tennis shoes and shorts in warmer weather, walking boots with socks and short skirts anytime.

Jewellery should be equally bizarre – it can be as crude, kitschy or hideous as you like. Wear badges with suggestive messages, or the cocaine-cutter's friend, the plated razor blade on a chain. Alternatively, make your own cheap pieces as directed in *Ideas* below. Safety pins appear on your person as well as on your

Below: A Punky face, complete with inexpensive earrings, gelled hair and appropriately heavy makeup – see *Face* and *Hair*.

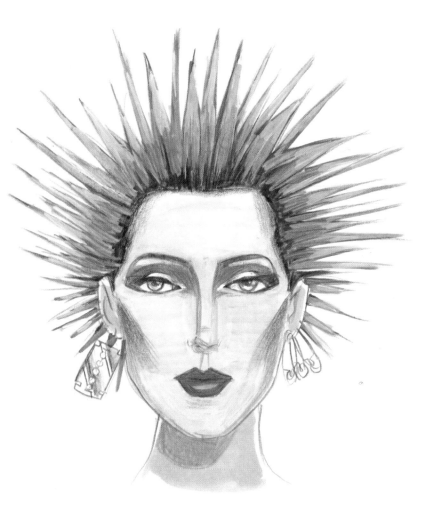

clothes – wear them through pierced-earring holes in ear lobes, or linked together to make bracelets, necklace and anklet chains.

Handbags can be any style so long as they're cheap – those from the Fifties and Sixties rate highly. Better yet are plastic duffel bags, string bags, or zany plastic hold-alls.

FACE AND HAIR
Start off with a very pale, even white foundation, dusted with an ivory or white powder. Use a brown pencil to extend the eyebrow downwards towards the cheek, stopping at the edge of the eye. Then take a black pencil to draw a thick line next to the top and bottom lashes, bringing this line out to meet the extended eyebrow. Using very dark grey, navy or even black shadow, colour the inner and outer corner of the eyelid, working it along the nose on the inside, and to the brown line on the outside. For a very hard look, use the shadow from the crease line up to the eyebrow, creating a virtually solid block of dark colour.

Colour cheeks with a bright pink daub of blusher, or leave them untouched. Define lips, creating a new extreme shape if you like with an outline of dark brown or black kohl pencil. Fill in lips with dark claret or even black.

Backcomb the entire head, then pin into sections. Apply setting gel to each section and pull hair into points all over the head and leave to dry; the overall effect should resemble a starburst. Ideally have a proper 'punk' cut. Spray in gaudy colours to remove it one step further from nature.

IDEAS
• Make-up schemes can be changed to suit the clothes you choose; in that case, you might change the above instructions and use fuchsia pink or bright blue in addition to the darker colours on the eye. If so, paint fingernails pink or blue as well.

• Hair can be similarly varied – you might want to spike only the central part of the head, or just around the face. Or maybe just leave the whole head backcombed and fixed with a heavy application of hair lacquer.

• Make inexpensive jewellery from lengths of fine chain sold at do-it-yourself stores and safety pins. Chain for necklaces and jewellery and clothing can be joined with a safety pin.

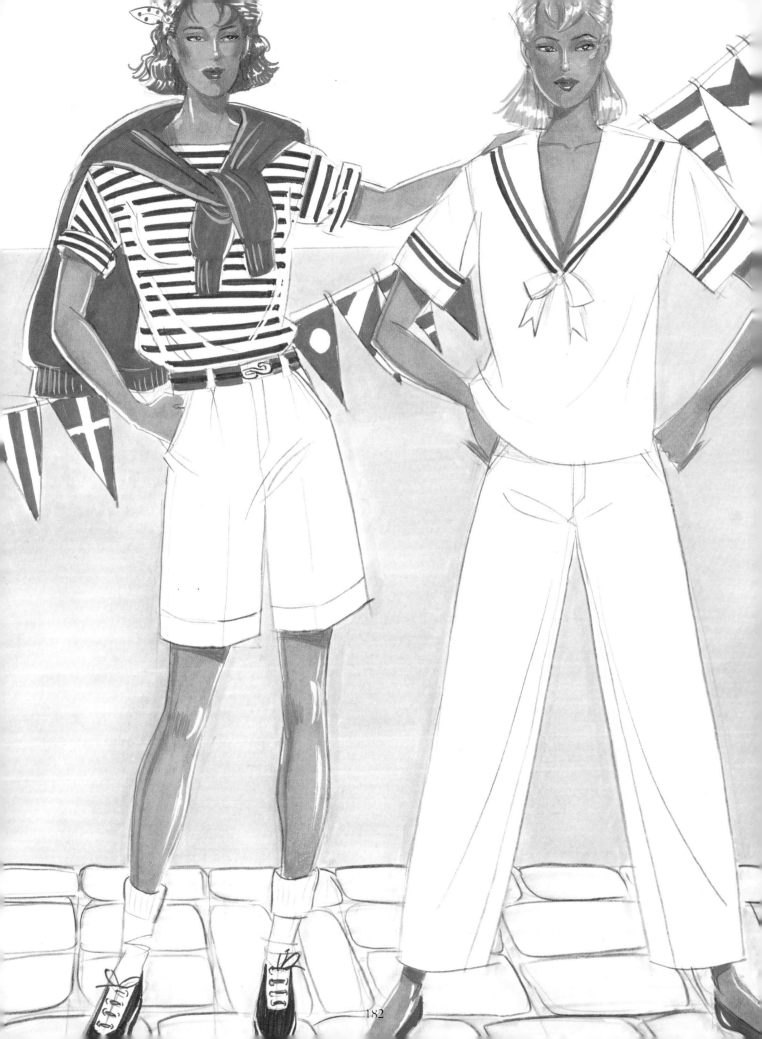

THE SAILOR

BACKGROUND

Splice the mainbrace, hard to starboard, weigh anchor and don't miss the boat! Your cottons are crisp, your linens immaculate and your theme is the Navy's blue, white and red.

Yachting has been a popular sport for much longer than one might imagine. Britain and the USA were vying for the trophy of the America's Cup yacht race in the mid 1850s. In more recent decades yachting has become a major international sport. Nowadays, throughout the world, wherever there is a harbour or port, you'll also find THE SAILOR.

Her favourite habitat may be the sun-kissed harbours of the jet set: the Mediterranean ports of St Tropez and Cannes, or the marinas of the Caribbean, Florida or Maine. Or she may frequent the local port and just love mucking about on boats. Summer is your season and this look is the perfect style for week-ends or holidays at any river or seaside resort; it can be dressed up or down according to whether you moor at sophisticated St Tropez or the most remote isle.

THE LOOK

The matelot style is best for messing-about-on-the-boat days. You will be on the right tack with white, navy or deep sky-blue shorts, culottes, pedal pushers, sailor's trousers or jeans – all in cotton. Then choose interchangeable tops: short or long-sleeved boat-necked cotton T-shirts in sailor stripes or plain colours and the ubiquitous cellular knit polo sports shirt, of the Lacoste type. Plain T-shirts can have nautical designs on the front, the name of the yacht, an anchor or a coil of rope, perhaps. For chilly evenings a sweatshirt or a sweater is essential; tie it over your shoulders or round your waist when not wearing it. A Breton sweater, with buttons along one shoulder, in navy and white or navy and red stripes is highly in keeping as are Guernsey pullovers in similar, but plain, colours. Alternatively, wear a solid navy, scarlet or white wool cardigan over a stripey T-shirt.

Below: Steer to the red, white and blue and you won't be far off course – shoes can be canvas or leather but must have rubber or crepe soles; hats should have brims to keep sun and spray out of your eyes; and bags should be roomy for all the gear you stow on board.

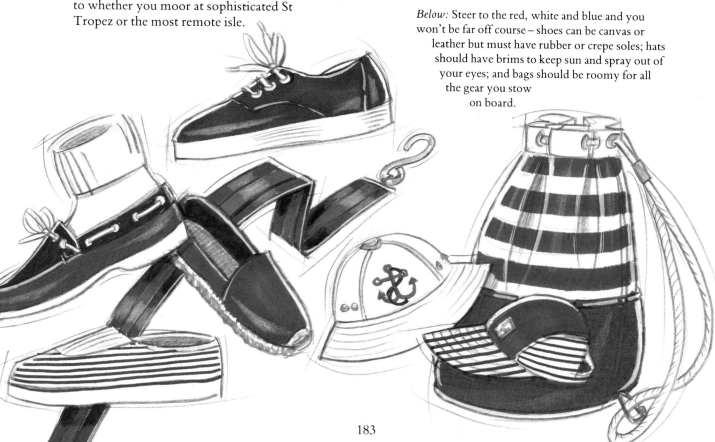

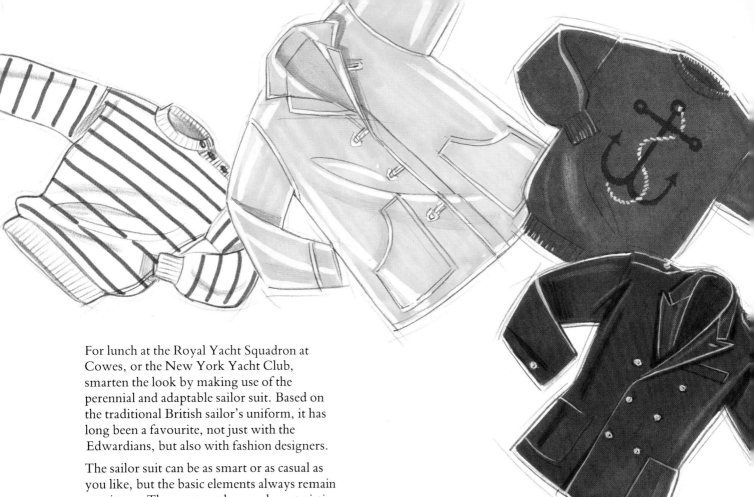

For lunch at the Royal Yacht Squadron at Cowes, or the New York Yacht Club, smarten the look by making use of the perennial and adaptable sailor suit. Based on the traditional British sailor's uniform, it has long been a favourite, not just with the Edwardians, but also with fashion designers.

The sailor suit can be as smart or as casual as you like, but the basic elements always remain consistent. The top must have a characteristic square-cut sailor collar, hanging down to your shoulder blades at the back and tapering to a V-neck at the front. The suit top can be in navy, white or red and the collar, decorated round the edges with rows of braid or ribbon, in the same or a contrasting colour. Long shorts, culottes or a skirt are all possible alternatives for the bottom half of the suit, and, of course, it comes in dress form too. (This is basically a summer style but when made of navy wool it is suitable for winter too.) A classic look, it is hardly ever out of fashion but if you cannot find it in the usual places, look out for surplus stores which often deal in naval (as well as army) surplus equipment. Here you will also find the authentic sailor's trousers, complete with wide-buttoned front flap and real bell-bottoms.

Emulate the Admiral and take the wind out of everybody's sails on ultra-smart occasions by wearing a double-breasted navy blazer, with two regimented rows of brass buttons; its cuffs can be embellished with gold stripes to indicate your rank! Wear it with white or off-white flannels or a crisp linen skirt in navy, red or white. Try a white silk shirt or a stripey crew-neck sweater in a silky yarn under the jacket. Alternate colour schemes

Above: For outerwear, **The Sailor** chooses a classic yellow sou'wester to add a bit of brightness to inclement conditions or the true-blue navy blazer for more formal occasions. Sweaters can have a nautical motif, or be one of the traditional "salty" styles such as the striped Breton.

and fabrics: gabardine blazer with linen or flannel trousers, for example, or linen jacket with cotton ducks.

And finally, should the heavens open, rush below deck and grab from the hold a tough nylon or oilskin coverall; in yellow or navy, hoods, sou'westers, coveralls and boating wellies will be essential. You will find these 'oilies' in traditional ship's chandlers alongside a host of other sailing accessories.

ACCESSORIES
Follow the sailor's example on footwear: traditional sailing shoes are of navy blue canvas with broad white rubber soles. However, espadrilles are also very much in keeping or you could wear any type of flat cotton or canvas pump.

A yachting cap is a practical accessory by day; it keeps hair less wild in the wind, shades eyes from the glare, and protects the head from strong sun. Choose a cotton or canvas cap with a traditional peak; trim it with nautical insignia, rope band or braided anchor (see *Ideas*). In navy with gold peak trim or with a full white crown and navy peak, it will enhance the blazer look and, for the height of correctness, white gloves.

Belts can be cording, leather or elastic creations; choose stripey ones in dazzling nautical colours. Sailcloth, canvas or oilskin kitbags with drawstring closings are the practical answer to carrying around your gear. Or use a canvas satchel in nautical colours – and don't forget the sunglasses.

FACE AND HAIR
Yachting folk thrive on fresh and bracing salty air; and sailing inevitably produces a healthy, tanned complexion – the combination of the salt, the water and the wind ensure this. Away from the sea, help nature on her way by the application of a tinted moisturizer with a sprinkling of fake freckles (see THE LITTLE BOY). Shadow eyes in cream, with maybe a hint of blue on the lid and in the crease, finishing eyes with navy mascara. Protect lips with a slightly tinted gloss. The time to bring out the paint box is when you take to the admiral's blazer; if scarlet is part of your chosen colour scheme, select a matching red for a strong mouth and allow the eyes to feature more prominently, with a line of navy very close to the lower lashes.

Healthy, clean and natural are again the three provisos for hair; you might go for a few blonde or lightish highlights for a sun-streaked effect.

IDEAS
● Kerchiefs are useful yachtswoman accessories, especially if they are spotted or striped. Use the same one in lots of different ways: as a belt; round the neck with a knot in front, more loosely to give the impression of a sailor collar, or with the knot at the back; tied as a headband with knot on top or underneath, or folded in a triangle and tied under the hair at the back.

● Trim a white or navy collar with bands of ribbon in contrasting colours to give the appearance of a sailor collar; use remnants to trim breast pockets and cuff edges.

● Transform a plain navy jacket into a blazer by the addition of brass buttons and gold braid trim. Look for buttons in junk shops and braid from upholstery suppliers. Add an appliqué badge to the breast pocket.

● Use soft ropes or cords to make your own appropriate belts; experiment with single or double lengths knotted at the front, or try a series of smaller loops linked together with metal boating hooks; or braid several strands together into a flat belt.

Below: To cinch **The Sailor**'s waist, choose white or coloured nylon rope, tied in a double knot; alternatively, use the nautical splice to attach the rope to a yachting clasp.

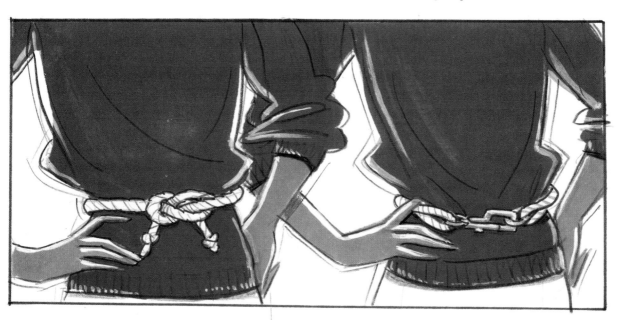

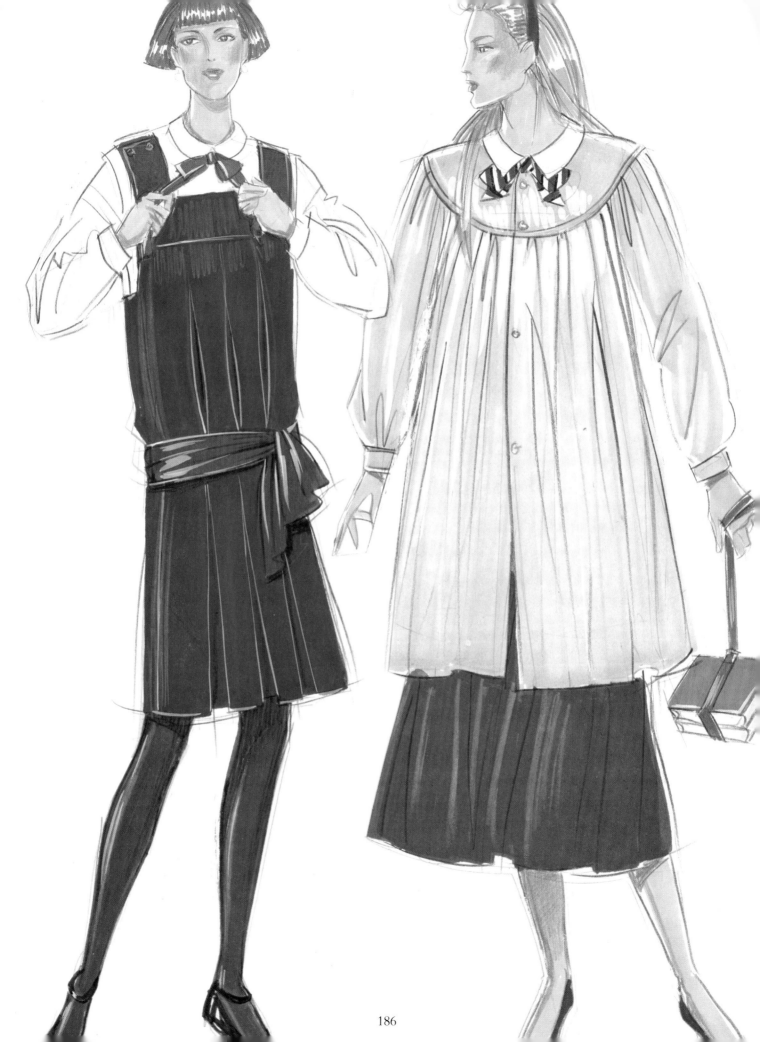

THE SCHOOLGIRL

BACKGROUND

Don't fidget at your desk! Stop running in the halls! No giggling during class! Be in bed by nine o'clock! Do you remember what it was like to be a schoolgirl? Whether you went to a private school or not, whether you had knock knees or were a natural athlete, whether you were bookish or lazy and whether you had an idyllic spell or those awful years of adolescent awkwardness, THE SCHOOLGIRL's approach to dressing is a delightfully simple solution now that you're finally grown up. This is not the anything-as-long-as-it's-jeans gear now permitted in most American schools; it's not the dowdy and shapeless clothing worn by the English 'gals' of St Trinians; nor is it the extremely prim and proper version worn in France.

Instead, our SCHOOLGIRL is an amalgam of the best from a girl's school wardrobe, gleaned from international sources and re-assembled into a new look. It comes from the classrooms and corridors around the world – smocks from France, Peter Pan collars from England, white stockings from America, and endless navy and white from uniforms around the world.

Below: Like **The Little Boy**, **The Schoolgirl**'s accessories can be found quite cheaply – school satchel, hair ribbons, striped neckties and white anklets don't cost much.

THE LOOK

THE SCHOOLGIRL is ideally suited to those with a taste for plain colours and simply clothing. There's little frill, not much strict tailoring and hardly any pattern. It requires little effort and is quickly gathered together. In short, it's the perfect look for women of all ages who like simplicity and chic. Although essentially an old-fashioned way of dressing, because of the functional nature of the clothing and the hard-wearing fabrics they're made of, it is ideal for lovers of the prim and proper with its starched white shirts, no-nonsense colour scheme and sensible low-heeled shoes. All you have to do is add the pert impishness characteristic of the brightest schoolgirls everywhere.

Begin with a starched white blouse (or palest pink, blue or yellow if you prefer). It should have a round collar which may be any size from a demure little Peter Pan shape to a larger, deeper Puritan collar. It should button down the front and must be worn with a necktie or soft bow (see *Accessories*).

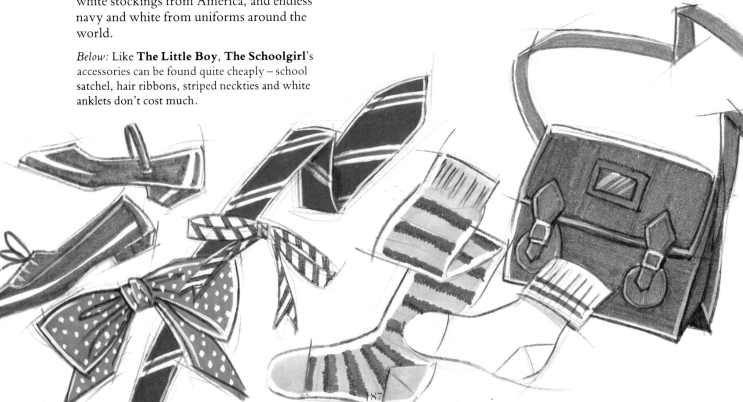

Wear it with a plain pleated skirt and matching cardigan (like THE CLASSICIST) or better yet with a gymslip or pleated-front sleeveless dress worn by English schoolgirls in the Thirties and Forties. Becoming more fashionable today with designers in luxury fabrics, the gymslip is most readily available from school outfitters where you'll be able to buy one or two very inexpensively in traditional colours such as navy blue, bottle green, burgundy, grey, brown or black.

In addition to, or instead of, the gymslip, THE SCHOOLGIRL can wear a smock. Not the famous shepherd's garment, but the fullfronted dress of the nineteenth-century French *collégienne*. Falling from a yoke across the front and back, or hanging in pleats or soft gathers from the shoulders, this smock can finish just above the knee or just below. Like the gymslip, it comes in traditional colours and tough fabrics like gabardine, corduroy and poplin. However, you'll also find smocks in very fine wools and cottons, even corduroy or velvet. These refined versions of the prosaic cotton painter's smock are ideal for special occasions and should you choose to wear the smock for evening, let a ruffled or lacy collar peek out of the top. If you are a more provocative and mischievous schoolgirl, wear your smock or gymslip above the knee.

When walking to school or waiting for the schoolbus, wear any traditionally-styled overcoat – see THE BUSINESSWOMAN, THE CLASSICIST, THE LADY, THE LITTLE BOY for suggestions or go to school outfitters for the classic trench or balmacaan style. Choose a colour to match your gymslip, or go for a contrast: maybe a bright red as a foil to the understated navy or grey of your dress.

ACCESSORIES
It is important to wear appropriate neckwear with the round-collared blouse or you will

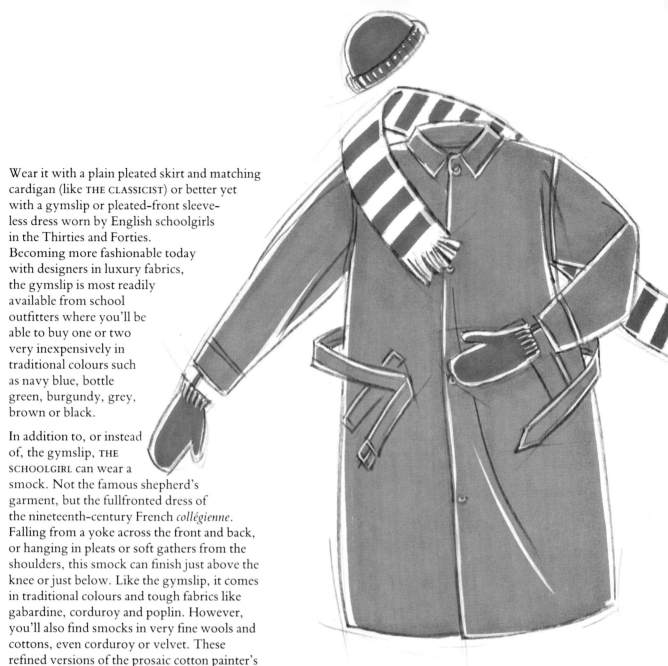

Above: An uncluttered coat in one of the traditional colours teamed with striped scarf, beanie and woollen mittens keep the cold away from **The Schoolgirl.**

look terribly dull – try a striped or spotted necktie, knotted as directed in THE GENTLEMAN worn under the collar of the blouse with just the knot and a few inches of the tie showing. For more flamboyance tie a brightly coloured ribbon in a neat bow at the neck, or for a touch of the artist, use a scarf folded on the diagonal to make a big floppy bow. Classic bright red accessories work well with greys, blues and green, while more daring girls might like paisley or dotted silks, tartan, flowered and striped ribbons – why not change your neckwear each time you dress as THE SCHOOLGIRL?

Legs should be covered in tights to match or enliven the gymslip or smock – sheer or thick depending on the occasion. Thick knitted ones might be ribbed, have cable designs on the outside leg, or even Tweedle-Dum and Tweedle-Dee horizontal stripes. For dressing up, wear opaque tights white or cream – they look especially cute with black patent ankle-strapped shoes. To cut a dash wear red ribbed tights. Unorthodox little brats might wear white ankle socks over tights; nice little girls wear them with tanned legs in summer.

Wear a fringed sash of wool or silk around your middle, tied low on the hips with the gymslip or smock, blousing the top over it. If you're wearing a more dressy smock define your waist with a patent belt; innocents should wear their smock unbelted.

Footwear will be functional except when Daddy takes you out, in which case you'll wear your patent shoes. Otherwise, choose sturdy loafers, slip-on pumps, lace-ups, even brogues, in tan, black or navy leather.

Traditionally, schoolkids used long brown leather straps to bind books and papers together, but these are really a little impractical and dated. Your best handbag for wearing with your best frock might be a fine leather or patent one, but for every day you'll carry a canvas or leather school satchel (see THE LITTLE BOY). You can pay the earth for these from designer shops or get one for very little from school outfitters. Cheaper yet are the plastic alternatives in bright colours which might add a needed bit of zap to your clothing. Choose shoulder straps for all your bags – they'll free your hands for throwing snowballs and skipping with your rope.

Heads will be kept warm wrapped with a long, striped woollen scarf in winter or topped by a colourful felt beanie or beret in a traditional shade or a brighter one to match your bag or tights. In summer, wear a Panama straw hat or boater.

FACE AND HAIR
Hair can be cut pageboy-style complete with deep fringe (bangs) and a central parting. Or it can be held off your face and out of your eyes with a covered headband or ribbon. Alternatively, secure it in one or two

Right: Revitalize old headbands as suggested in *Ideas*.

ponytails like THE INNOCENT; plait it like THE COWGIRL; for Sunday best, dress it in ringlets like THE IMMIGRANT's rag curls. However, keep it simple if not straight – nothing wild or extreme for THE SCHOOLGIRL.

Make-up? Forget it. At the absolute maximum you might mascara eyelashes, slick lips slightly with tinted gloss, and line near lashes with the finest of pencils, but that's it. When you get just a little older, emulate THE INNOCENT.

IDEAS
● When knotting ribbons, ties and scarves at the neck of your blouse, consider the double bow – it looks delightfully full.

● If Mummy and Daddy won't allow you to wear make-up, cheat a little – use Vaseline to slick lips and make your eyebrows and lashes behave, and of course, it's the perfect polish for your patent shoes.

● When your old headbands get a little tired looking, wrap them with new velveteen or grosgrain ribbons, as the illustration shows.

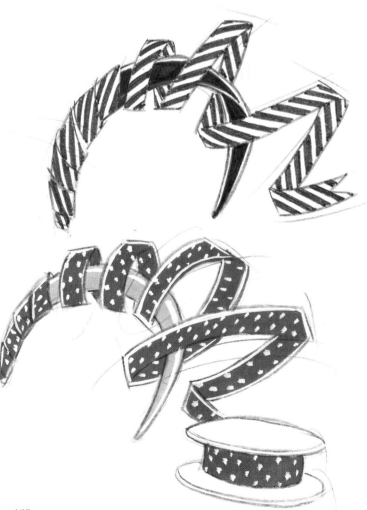

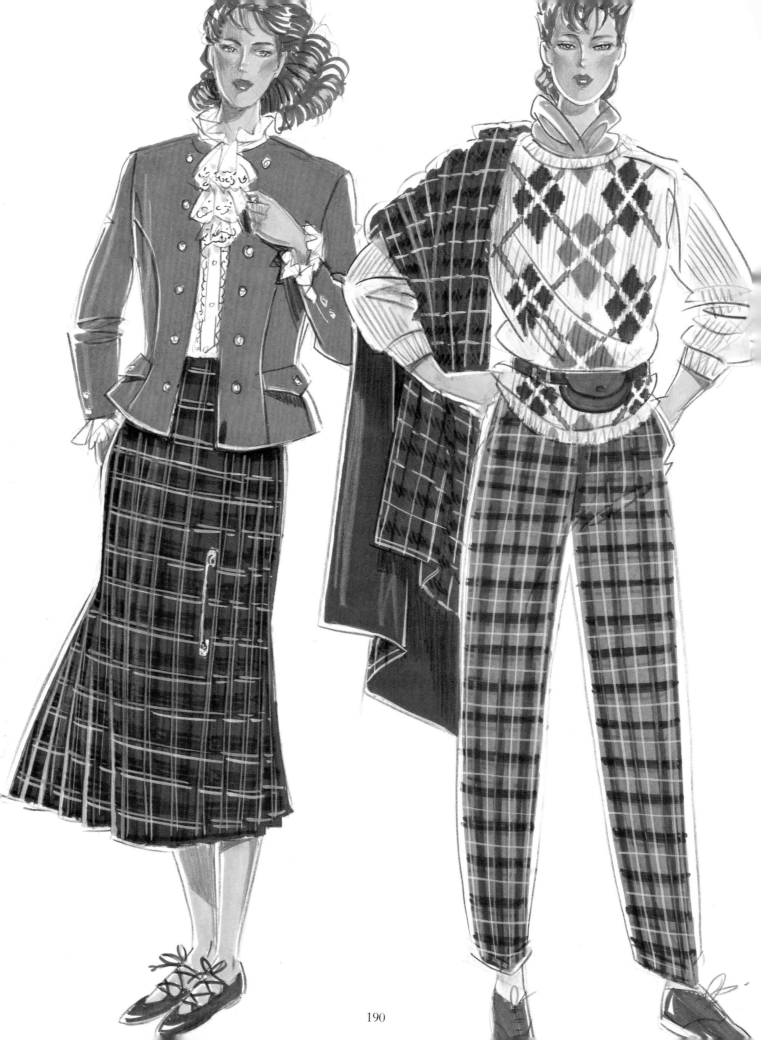

THE SCOTSWOMAN

BACKGROUND

The SCOTSWOMAN has spread her fashion influence far and wide. Tartan is the fabric most immediately associated with her wardrobe and the kilt her favourite item of clothing. The Scottish Highlanders have been wearing kilts and long, broad lengths of plaid draped over their shoulders for warmth and protection, since the fifteenth century. Each clan evolved (and still retains) its own distinctive tartan; the reds and greens of the Royal Stuart, the black, blue and bottle green of the Black Watch are perhaps the best known. This national dress was banned after the failure of Bonnie Prince Charlie's 1745 rebellion and the use of tartan illegal until 1782. It is worn today by many Scots and has become one of the most popular British looks, finding great favour also in Europe and America.

THE LOOK

The kilt is the key to this most comfortable and wearable of looks; although a traditional garment, it can be quite versatile, particularly as it is available in a mass of plaids and tartans of different hues and in a variety of lengths. For everyday winter wear, choose a knee-length kilt, complete with kilt pin, as the basis of your outfit. Keep the tartan subtle. With your kilt you will want a plain cotton or wool shirt, a Shetland sweater and a soft and comfortable tweed jacket in Harris or another traditional Scottish tweed. Loden jackets, thick creamy Aran sweaters or cardigans with leather buttons also provide much needed warmth for this cold weather version of THE

Below: Aye, my lassie get yourself some ghillies and fringed brogues, then some plaids and tams and sporrans (little purses) so you can enjoy your Highland fling as **The Scotswoman.**

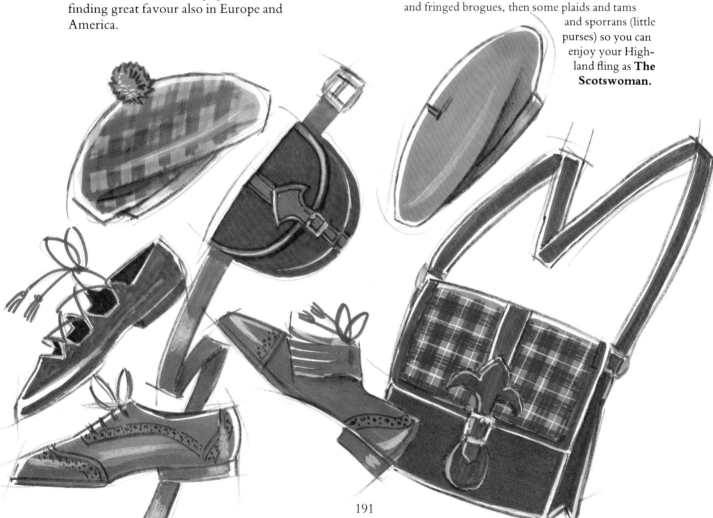

SCOTWOMAN. A word of warning, though: every imaginable garment, from trousers and waistcoats to hats and jackets, are available in tartan fabric; limit yourself to one tartan item, or at most two, in your outfit.

To dance your way through Hogmanay Highland flings, at which the Dashing White Sergeant, the Hamilton House and the Eightsome Reel are danced, more formal Highland dress is appropriate. The ubiquitous kilt appears once more, this time in an ankle- or calf-length version, preferably in a 'dress' tartan of brighter, richer colours. Add to it a fine white blouse, preferably with a beautifully frilled white lacy jabot; a floppy bow is a good alternative. A bottle green or black velvet fitting jacket completes the look. (This can also be worn with a knee-length kilt for smarter daytime occasions.)

Vary this evening style with fuller gathered or pleated tartan skirts and fitted peplum jackets (see THE GIBSON GIRL for details) in matching fabric or plain velvet.

ACCESSORIES
The correct footwear is essential for stomping across the moors and mountains, the landscape where this look originated. Without

it your feet will not survive those long walks in the company of curly-horned sheep and Aberdeen Angus cattle. Front-lacing shoes such as ghillies are archetypal and come in hard-wearing strong leathers; for less rigorous occasions prettier examples in softer leather can also be found. All kinds of brogues with lace-up fronts, punched patterns, cut leather fringes or tassels are the answer for really rough conditions, and, if worn correctly with Argyll knee socks or thick ribbed tights, look great. For evening, all that Scottish reeling requires a pair of classic black patent shoes with silver buckles or more delicate ghillies with pretty laces, ballet shoes or pumps.

Sporrans, leather belts, pouches and tough bags in country styles are THE SCOTWOMAN's natural accessories, together with co-ordinating plaid or tartan scarves. Long, or square and folded diagonally, these can be tied round the head as well as the neck to keep out the cold mists which rise from the bonny banks of Loch Lomond. Aran or Shetland gloves or mittens and an Aran or discreet plaid tam o'shanter will keep extremities protected.

A final big sweep of the traditional clansman's blanket wrap (a vast scarf) in a plain wool or striking tartan, swung over the shoulders and

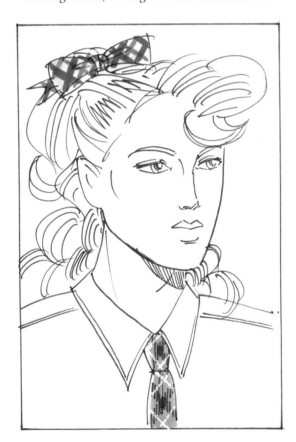

pinned in place with a clan pin or big brooch, will provide added warmth.

Adornments are bold and Celtic in inspiration: rough sludgy-green coloured stones (from the Isle of Iona) set in silver, and amethysts that can occasionally be found in the boulders on the Scottish coasts. Silver, rather than gold, is traditional. Look out in junk shops for old silver clan pins, bearing the motto and motif of the clan, or entwined silver filigree work in Celtic scroll and foliage patterns (excellent reproductions of early Celtic jewellery can be obtained in some museum shops).

FACE AND HAIR

THE SCOTSWOMAN shows her ancestry in her looks: a mixture of the Celtic traditions of the Western Isles and descent from Lady Macbeth perhaps. If you've wild and wavy auburn tresses, a translucent skin and crystal-clear blue eyes, you are a natural for this look. If not, don't worry; tone down your natural face colour with a pale foundation, but you will still need some cheekbone colouring to prevent the brighter tartans in your wardrobe taking over. Eyes should be clear and strong, but shadowed in subtle shades of grey, dusky mauve or browns.

Hair is as wavy and wind-blown as you like, but make sure it's shining and ultra healthy. If it's long and straight tie it back like Bonny Prince Charlie in a loose, low ponytail held with a black velvet bow.

IDEAS
● Add a white jabot to a white blouse; make your own layers of frills or search the old clothes shops and antique markets for an old lace collar. Attach it permanently with a few stitches or make it detachable with press studs. Lace ruffles or floppy frills can also be sewn to shirt cuffs and should show at the wrists of the velvet jacket.

● Tie tartan ribbons in different ways: round the neck in a floppy bow; as a neater bow tie, or like a man's full length tie; round the head with a knot on top; in a bow round a ponytail.

Below and opposite: Four ways of adding a bit of plaid using a tartan ribbon to put the finishing touches to **The Scotswoman:** tie a headband around the neck in a big floppy bow or in a discreet tie under blouse collars; as a necktie (see **The Gentleman** for the knotting instructions) and to top a ponytail.

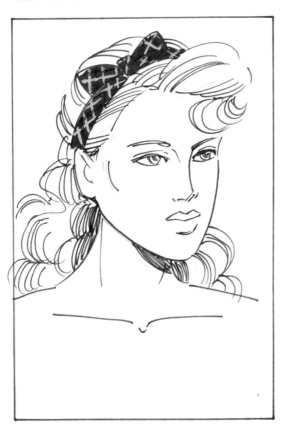

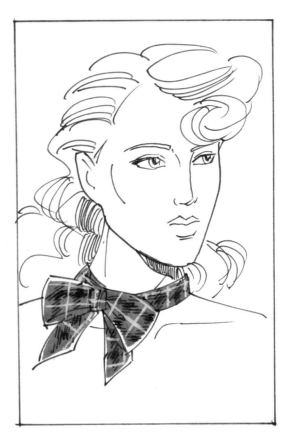

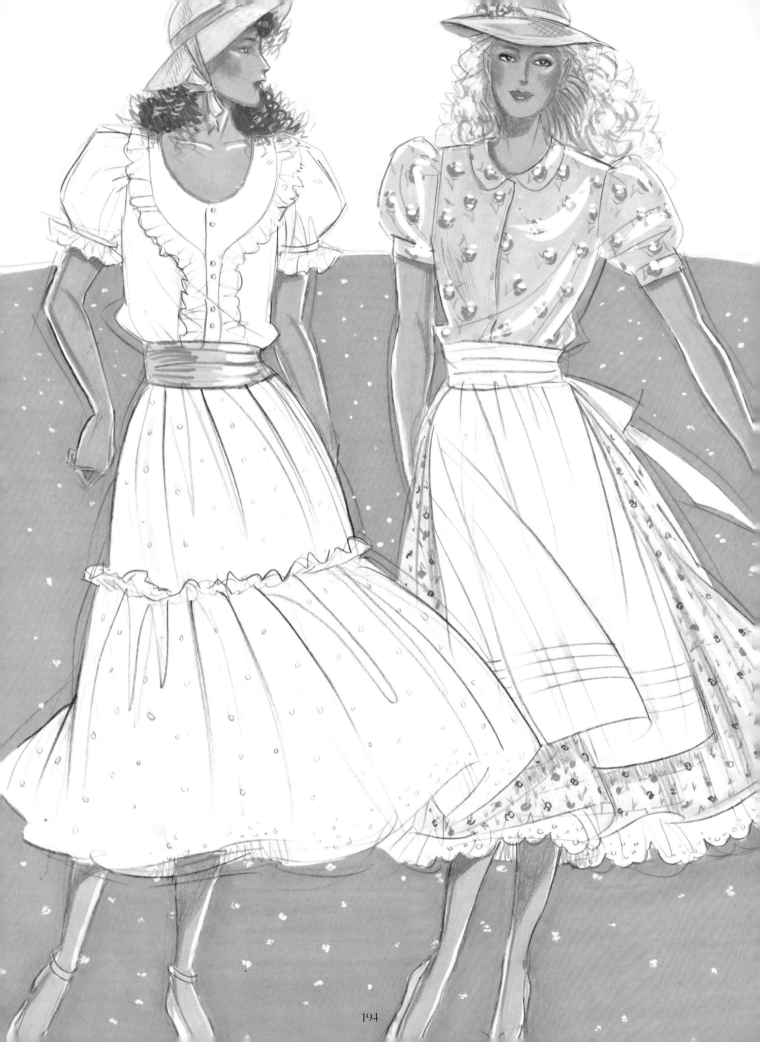

THE SHEPHERDESS

BACKGROUND

Remember Little Bo Peep who lost her sheep and fresh-faced Heidi from the Swiss Alps? For most of us, shepherdesses belong to our childhood storybooks where little girls are pretty and good and everything has a happy ending. However, these fairy-tale shepherdesses were outdone by the most famous 'real' shepherdess of them all, Marie Antoinette, Queen of France just prior to the Revolution in 1789. Bored with court life at Versailles, she would don her Bo-Peep bonnet, dainty dress and polished shepherd's crook and vanish for the afternoon to her pretty reproduction cottage in a carefully mown pasture scattered with fluffy, well-washed sheep. Here (still safely within the grounds of the palace) she played out her fantasy of the simple life.

THE LOOK

To look pretty as a picture can be a little complicated because of the layers, but the results are well worth the trouble. It has one small drawback: petticoats and whites must be dazzlingly clean and well-starched. This is not the look for those who loathe ironing or the committed traveller!

Being with an immaculately laundered white petticoat. This should have scallops, lace, or broderie anglaise, embroidery or ruffles round the hemline (or a combination of these). On top, wear a white camisole or lacy undershirt similarly trimmed. If the weather is hot, stop there, maybe adding a simple sash. Pantaloons or camiknickers make an unusual but appropriate addition under your petticoat – look for them in lingerie departments or in antique clothes shops. For street wear, continue with another petticoat and/or a white or demurely flowered overskirt letting an inch or so of the under-petticoat peep out. Skirts and petticoats should be full and gathered, knee-length or longer, tiered or not and preferably in cotton. If you have a suitable skirt which is above the knee, wear it on top of the final layer, as a sort of apron. (Obviously, with all these layers, this is a look

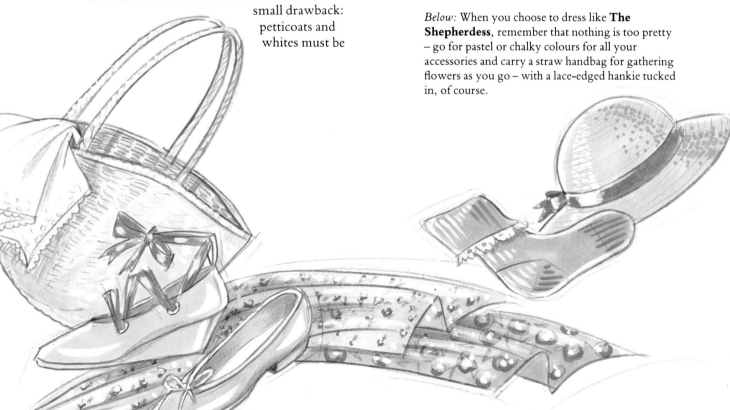

Below: When you choose to dress like **The Shepherdess**, remember that nothing is too pretty – go for pastel or chalky colours for all your accessories and carry a straw handbag for gathering flowers as you go – with a lace-edged hankie tucked in, of course.

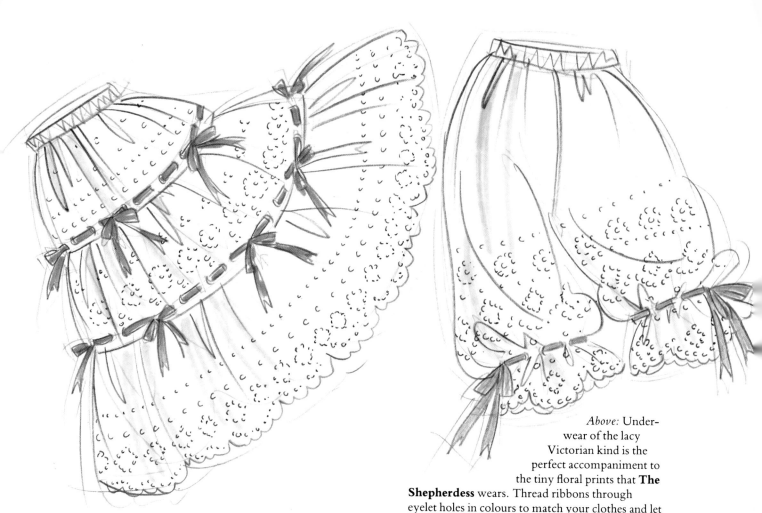

Above: Under-wear of the lacy Victorian kind is the perfect accompaniment to the tiny floral prints that **The Shepherdess** wears. Thread ribbons through eyelet holes in colours to match your clothes and let ruffles peek out of hemlines for the ultimately sweet summery look.

for those with a small waist; although all the gathers cleverly disguise generous hips and thighs.)

Over the camisole, wear a white blouse, preferably with puffed sleeves and characteristic embroidery, lace or similar frilly effects. It can be any style, buttoned or not, collared or otherwise and in any lightweight fabric from cotton to silk. (If you have a spare plain white blouse without frills, see *Ideas* below for instructions on applying lace.) Alternatively, you can wear a pastel or flower-sprigged blouse. Bear in mind that this is not the look for bright colours: THE SHEPHERDESS should be all in white or in a medley of pastel shades. Above all, the effect should be sweet and gentle.

If the weather is chilly, add a shawl in a print to match or co-ordinate with your skirt(s) or a short-waisted pastel cardigan (see THE INNOCENT). Ideally, however, reserve this look for those balmy days when woollies are not required.

ACCESSORIES
Certainly the most essential accessory for THE

SHEPHERDESS is her straw hat. It should be natural straw and with a widish brim. The hat can be worn unadorned or festooned with flowers (fake or otherwise) and ribbons – after all, what should you do in the pasture all day but decorate your bonnet! (See *Ideas* for hints on decorating yours.) Secure the hat with a hat-pin or with a ribbon tied under your chin; for a more casual effect wear it hanging down your back.

Other accessories will be white or in pastel shades. Shoes, belts, stockings and jewellery are the only places for solid pastel tones such as pink, yellow, aqua, soft red or baby blue. For example, if you're dressed in white, you might choose pink for all your accessories; if your outfit is flowered, pick out one of the colours and use it for your accent colour.

Ribbons are immensely useful for trimming this outfit. Wear them around the brim of your hat, at your waist, to tie back your hair, to tie up your shoes (see *Ideas* below). Avoid velvet and velveteen ribbons with the summer-weight fabrics appropriate to this look, opting instead for satin, grosgrain or taffeta textures. Ribbons woven with tiny flower designs also look especially effective with all white clothing.

On your feet wear simple pumps, ballet slippers, espadrilles, any slightly dressy shoe with a low to flattish heel or even a dainty lace-up ankle boot. Team footwear with white or pastel stockings or tanned legs. Wear white cotton ankle-socks with your shoes if you have slim calves.

Jewellery will be simple or quaint, pretty or plain, but old-fashioned, not new. Try a pearl choker or small round beads in the accent colour. Add a delicate ring or bracelet, but don't overindulge.

FACE AND HAIR

Hair, and make-up too, will be sweetness and light. Depending on the shape of your face and the length of your hair, gather hair in one of the following way: take a lock from each side and join at the back of the head, make two ponytails at each side, starting just above the ear or make a single one at the back of the head; plaits will also look right, either single at the back or one at each side. With any of these styles, hair must be secured first with a coated rubber band, then the fun begins. Wrap a length of ribbon round the rubber band a few times to conceal it, then tie it in a bow, letting

the ends dangle. Use two co-ordinating ribbons if you like. Finish the job by adding a cluster of fake flowers, especially if you are not wearing a hat – small clusters of any summertime bloom will look picture-perfect.

Make-up should be sweet and simple – just like THE INNOCENT.

IDEAS

● Use broderie anglaise or any white cotton lace to trim ankle-socks, blouses, petticoat and skirt edges. Buy it already gathered and hemmed, then simply tack into place, Ungathered lengths can be used as ribboning for hair and hat ornament.

● Trim a plain straw hat with ribbons using several colours of ribbons if you're wearing prints, or the chosen accent colour otherwise. Use a single length or several layered in various thicknesses as the illustration shows. Ribbon can also be twisted and braided to interesting effect for hat and waist ornament.

● Small bundles of fake flowers can be used with or instead of ribbons on your hat. Choose simple summer flowers like daisies and small roses rather than the larger, heavier blooms. Arrange five small bunches at equal intervals around the base of the crown; sew a large bunch over the spot where the ends of the ribbons are joined; sew single flowers to the end of ribbons; or use them on the underside of a large-brimmed hat to flatter your face.

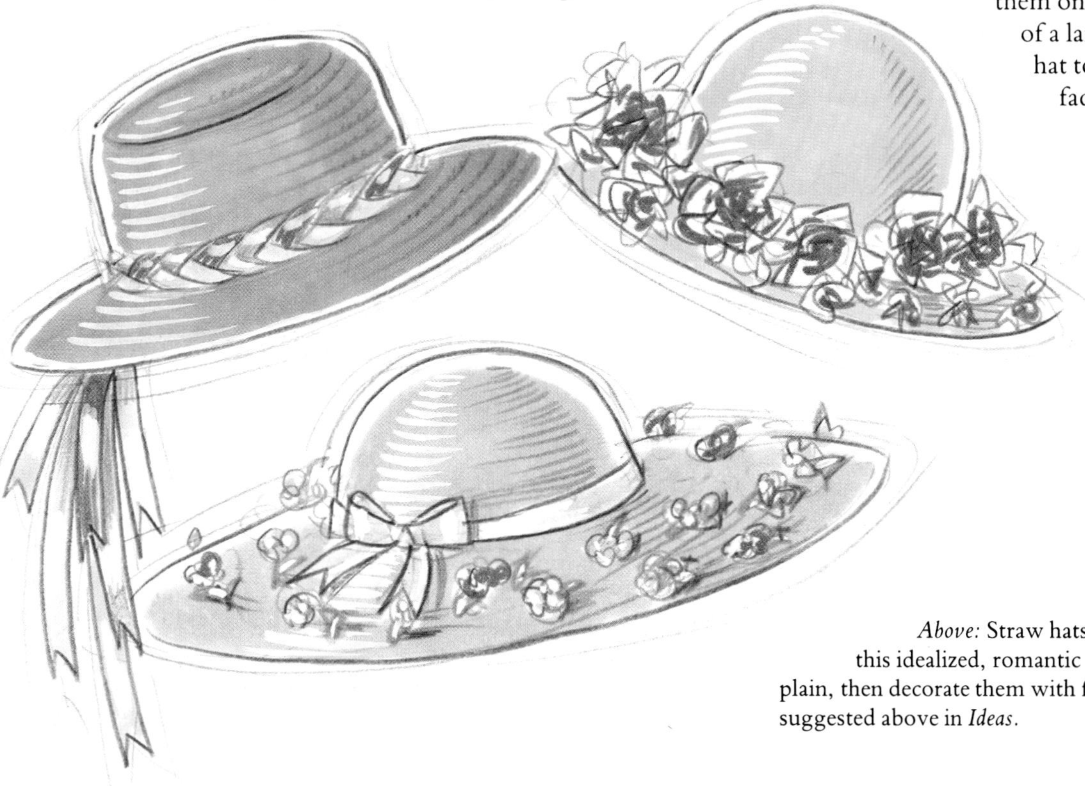

Above: Straw hats are essential for this idealized, romantic look – buy them plain, then decorate them with fake flowers as suggested above in *Ideas*.

197

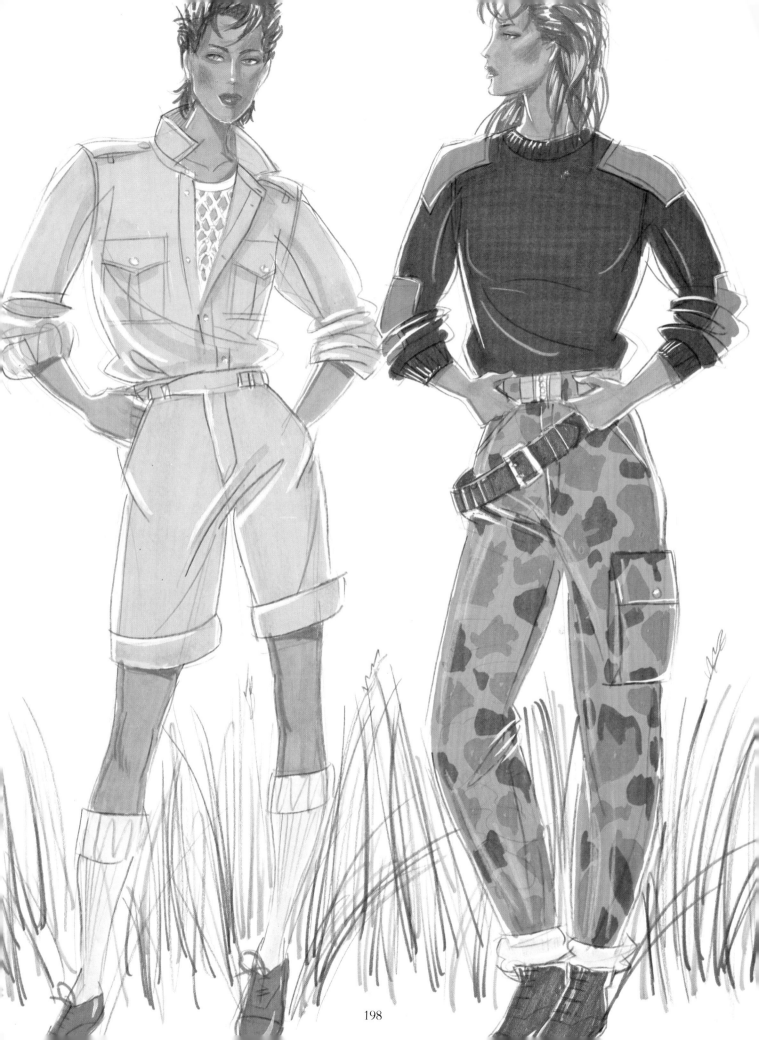

THE SOLDIER

BACKGROUND

Standing to attention, marching with the band; the rattle of military regalia and the sound of the trumpet. All echo the pomp and ceremony of the traditional soldier. But remember also those Latin-looking camouflaged revolutionaries, crawling through the steaming jungle on hands and knees. Two very distinct styles, but that's to your advantage: by day you can play the guerrilla in functional hard-wearing khaki kit, by night the dashing military man in full regimental dress.

A craze for military nostalgia brought forth hordes of young swingers dressed as generals, captains and sergeant-majors, often a blurred mixture of all ranks. The cover of the Beatles' 1967 *Sergeant Pepper's Lonely Hearts Club Band* album depicted the 'Fab Four' in zany military attire, thus setting the seal of approval on frogged frock coats, resplendent with medals, brass buttons and epaulettes.

Below: **The Soldier**'s gear is as no nonsense as she is – shoes are sensible, bags are roomy, belts double as carryalls and have sturdy brass buckles, hats have brims to keep the sun and rain out of eyes.

But the new tough-outdoor-soldier look also came to the fore in the Sixties – for years the practical and durable workwear of the regular soldier had been sold in army surplus stores; but it was not until the wave of military nostalgia came in that this accessible look found appeal. Suddenly camouflage, khaki, sand and olive green-hued multi-pocketed fatigues, patched ribbed sweaters, leather greatcoats and water-proofed trench coats appeared on every street corner. This was the garb of the trenches of the Second World War, of Korea and Vietnam; of Che Guevara and his guerrillas – even *Sergeant Bilko* and *Mash*!

The basic, and the most authentic, components are usually readily available in army surplus stores, thrift shops or street markets for minimal prices. Some items, like the grey-green trench coat, have become so popular that they are now standard equipment in many a woman's wardrobe.

THE LOOK

The most useful military look, and one that can be worn at any time, in any season and on almost every type of figure, is the hard-wearing practical style of the urban guerrilla. Choose an outfit which combines several of the traditional colours, or alternatively stick to one: khakis, sandy tones, olives and grey-greens are perfect; greys, navy and beiges also work well. Your kit must include a pair of baggy fatigue trousers, in either a plain colour or a camouflage fabric,

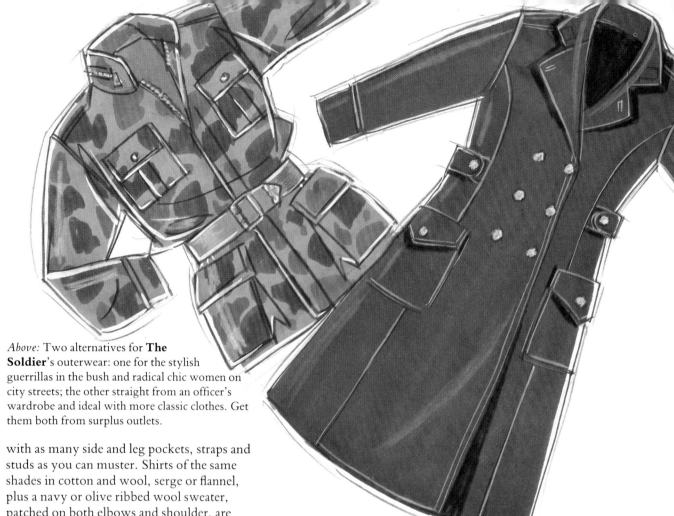

Above: Two alternatives for **The Soldier**'s outerwear: one for the stylish guerrillas in the bush and radical chic women on city streets; the other straight from an officer's wardrobe and ideal with more classic clothes. Get them both from surplus outlets.

with as many side and leg pockets, straps and studs as you can muster. Shirts of the same shades in cotton and wool, serge or flannel, plus a navy or olive ribbed wool sweater, patched on both elbows and shoulder, are essential equipment.

For a lightweight jacket choose from two styles: the sand-coloured, (sometimes in navy blue), tight-fitting, single-breasted, gold-buttoned parade jacket with matching or brown leather belt, or the large, cotton khaki or camouflage print jacket with button-down patch pockets, large epaulettes, sturdy zip fasteners and metal studs. For further protection, swirling capes, heavy wool greatcoats (or leather if you can find one) and trenchcoats, with inverted back pleat and tight belt , will withstand the worst weather conditions.

Keep the same lines for summer but lighten the fabrics: a khaki or sandy cotton shirt, with rolled up sleeves, simple epaulettes and breast pockets, should be tightly belted into similarly coloured, front-pleated military shorts, cuffs turned back too if you like – and matching jungle helmet, if you dare! Exchange the shirt for cellular cotton T-shirts for the warmest weather. Cotton culottes and tailored skirts, perhaps with a single central pleat, give a more formal feminine appearance.

There is nothing more stunning than a lady

dressed to the hilt in full ceremonial regalia for outrageous evenings or fancy dress events. We are not suggesting you brandish a sword on such occasions, but you can have fun with, sashes, braids, medals, helmets, and gauntlets, all in striking bright colours. Snap to attention in tight dark trousers or breeches worn under a scarlet, royal blue, white or black regimental tunic with a stand-up collar. A satin blazer can always have its collar turned up and pinned in place to a military tunic, and tuck trousers into boots for the Iron Duke effect. (See *Ideas* below.)

ACCESSORIES

For the sparkling ceremonial look, add a satin sash or thick ribboning in a bright, contrasting colour wound tightly around the waist and draped over one shoulder, and tied under the other. Sew on gold braid edgings to collar and cuffs, gilt regimental buttons, 'clothes-brush' epaulettes, your distinguished service medals, a peaked cap trimmed with braid and badge and the shiniest shoes or knee length boots ensuring you live up to your forebears' reputations.

To go with the heavy-duty camouflage or khaki kit you will need very practical army accessories. Most characteristic are the belts, shoulder straps and pouches in brown leather or olive webbing. A wide belt with integral zipped pocket or leather cartridge pouch is a must and very useful for carrying small change. If you like, add a diagonal leather shoulder strap clipped to the belt at front and back for authenticity.

Lace-up khaki canvas or leather ankle boots, worn with thick socks, tall low-heeled leather boots, with trousers tucked inside, or leather lace-ups, polished to such a shine that you can see your face in them, will enable you to cover the roughest terrain or alternatively pass muster on the parade ground. Protect lower legs in summer with knee-socks which match your shorts or culottes.

Gauntlet gloves tucked into an epaulette, peaked cap or beret (complete with regimental or revolutionary badge) and a strong canvas satchel or leather cartridge bag are the finishing touches. No trinkets on the soldier – a fighter can't be fussing with such trifles. Today's military man finds a solid digital watch most useful so indulge your taste for micro chip technology and get the chunkiest

Below: An ordinary jacket can be transformed for party or parade ground with a few yards of gold braid and near-invisible stitches, as shown on the right of this red jacket.

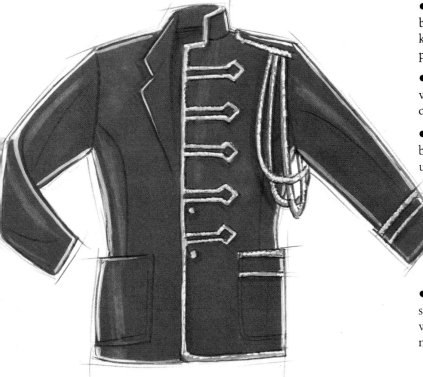

most complex one you can find. In the evening, allow a little fantasy to enliven military correctness: maybe just a pair of simple gold earrings and a simple ring or two.

FACE AND HAIR
Start with a slightly tanned foundation unless you have the real thing. Shadow the eyes with a brassy shade on the upper lid, a khaki shade on the lower, blending a little rust into the inner corner. Apply dark brown kohl pencil along the lashes on the lower rim, extending the line into the inner and outer corners a little, blending it into the khaki shadow to emphasize the eye. Apply a bronzed blusher to the cheekbones, finishing with an outline on the lips with a rust pencil, filling in with a rust or apricot lipstick depending on your colouring, with maybe a glimmer of gold lipstick on top. Apply make-up in the same way for full regimental dress, but use pink, navy and grey shadows, rosy blusher, navy kohl pencil and red lipstick.

Daytime hair can be neat and efficient in true army fashion: no hair touching the collar, please, which means plaits, chignon or bun, or just tucked tidily under a cap. But this rule does not apply to mercenaries or guerrillas; jungle warfare allows you to have your hair as wild as you want. For evening, let it be outrageously full and flowing or slick it right back to give a really ice-cold Prussian look.

IDEAS
• Dangle useful objects on your leather army belt with dog clips: watch, penknife, whistle, keys; and use a leather belt pouch as your purse.

• Patch worn sweaters on the shoulders as well as on the elbows with khaki fabric for a correct military effect.

• Look for original solid brass regimental buttons and badges in junk shops; polish them up and add to your chosen garment.

• Use coins as substitute medals and hang from striped ribbons to prove you are a real die-hard campaigner. Or find the real thing in antique markets and restore to their original condition, with replacement ribbons.

• Add braids and tassels to cuffs, collars, shoulders, jacket edges and fronts of evening wear. Upholstery braids are perfect – the more extravagant the better.

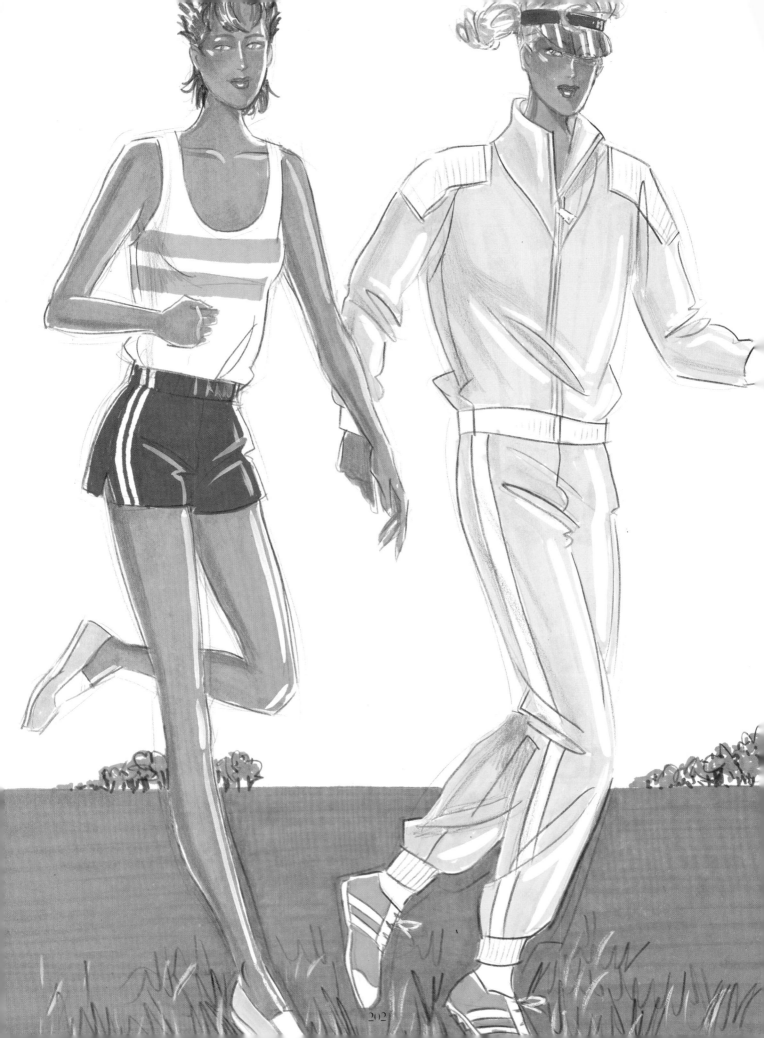

THE SPORTSWOMAN

BACKGROUND

THE SPORTSWOMAN has been with us since the Twenties. When skirts got shorter and hair was bobbed, young ladies were suddenly on the move. With their new political and social freedoms and the loose, casual fashions that epitomized them, women took up outdoor activities with enthusiasm, and soon the more ladylike sports such as tennis, walking, croquet and swimming were requisites of fashionable society. Whereas the Victorian young lady was expected to be able to play the piano and sing a pretty duet at social gatherings, no bright young thing could hold her own in the Twenties or Thirties if she was unable to wield a tennis racket gracefully. 'Anyone for tennis?', coined by Noel Coward, just about sums up that carefree period.

In the Eighties, sport has re-emerged as *the* trendy leisure activity, but these days it's taken much more seriously. Now women are getting into sport with the determination previously thought to be a male prerogative. New ideals of beauty are being formed – the feminine woman is one who runs, even marathons, who works out in a gym till the sweat pours, who plays her tennis hard and to win, who even lifts weights and trains on Nautilus machines. The sexy woman is strong, muscled, fit and healthy; and she looks good and happy on it.

Predictably, fashion manufacturers have responded enthusiastically – now sporting-inspired clothing appears in totally non-sporting circumstances. Additionally, movies like Hugh Hudson's *Chariots of Fire* (1980) beautifully captured the joys of running. Only thirty years before, film audiences enjoyed more balletic and sensual athletic efforts, courtesy of Olympic swimming star, Esther Williams, in films such as *Million Dollar Mermaid* (1952) and *Dangerous When Wet* (1953).

Sociologists explain the fitness phenomenon by suggesting that we have much more leisure time to fill, and are turning to the simple pleasures of physical activity in an increasingly complex world. Additionally, people will increasingly seek satisfaction from their own individual efforts and accomplishments. Sport, unlike most of our jobs, is something the individual can control.

Below: Go for zappy colour combinations when dressing as **The Sportswoman.** Stripey details look great and suggest speed, while brighter colours cheer you on when you're feeling less than energetic.

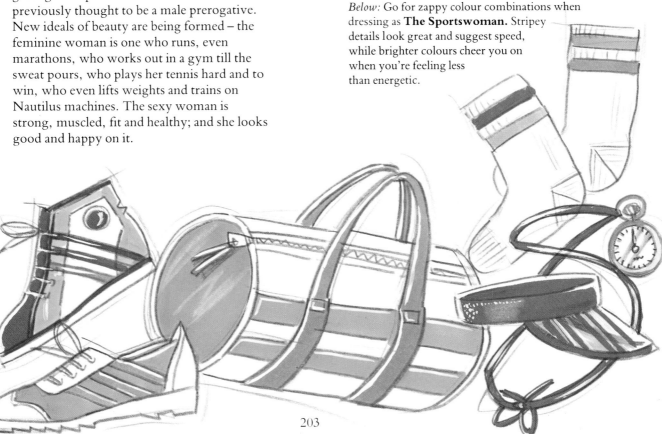

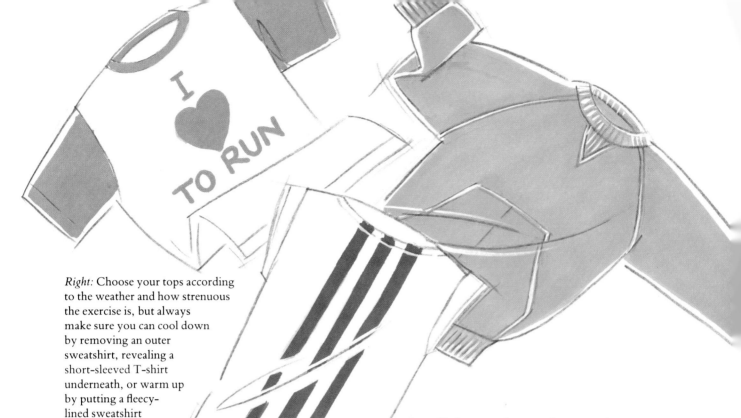

Right: Choose your tops according to the weather and how strenuous the exercise is, but always make sure you can cool down by removing an outer sweatshirt, revealing a short-sleeved T-shirt underneath, or warm up by putting a fleecy-lined sweatshirt back on.

THE LOOK

THE SPORTSWOMAN is always the picture of health, and since there is no short cut to achieving that wonderful glow, you might as well achieve it honestly. There is no mystery as to why one feels better after exertion. Practised regularly, your chosen sport will make you feel better, give you that healthy glow and will affect every area of your life – from work to love – for the better.

As with THE DANCER, the clothing of THE SPORTSWOMAN has become common wardrobe currency, and for most sports and most everyday activities, nothing can beat the tracksuit. Its soft fabrics, generous cut, and fitted cuffs, legs and waist allow great comfort and freedom of movement. Its practical fabrics mean an end to ironing, its characteristic fleecy lining keeps you warm in cool weather, and cool in warm weather, and it comes in every colour imaginable. For choice, opt for pure cotton separates, sometimes called 'sweats' for obvious reasons and because they are updates of the perennial sweatshirt. Avoid the newer man-made fabrics and more fitted styles: although man-made fibres keep their shape better, they also harbour perspiration odours and produce little fibrous balls which soon make them look old.

In really hot weather or when pursuing rigorous sports, choose cotton or satin running shorts; the former are generally cheaper and more practical, the latter have a sleek stripe down the outside leg and a light-catching sheen. Like 'sweats', these too come in clear bright shades, soft pastel and traditional colours like navy and can be worn with the tops of tracksuits, sweatshirts, T-shirts or singlets. You can also wear leotards or bathing suits under your shorts to great effect.

The T-shirt is the other staple garment of THE SPORTSWOMAN. Large, out-size or closely fitting, it is available in a multitude of different colours, with stripes or slogans, with collar or round-neck, with or without pockets and buttons. Have a selection in different styles to match your jogging-suits, shorts – and, of course, your moods. Sporting snobs will have the choicest T-shirts which sport the name of a running club, gym or dance studio. Classicists will prefer the Aertex Lacoste-style tops in the wide range of colours now available. Again, make sure all T-shirts are pure cotton for comfort.

For outerwear with both sweats and shorts, choose fleecy-lined sweatshirts in the traditional long-sleeved, round-necked style, or zip-fronted and hooded, appliquéd with sporting symbols and messages, decorated with manufacturer's insignia or not, as you choose. Alternatively, nylon or cotton parkas and large sweaters also look and feel great.

ACCESSORIES

Running shoes and tennis shoes are available in a wide range of different colours today, so that you can team them up with your chosen colour scheme. Shades from palest pinks have now overtaken the traditional white gym shoe and are available in most sports outfitters. Your socks will be fleecy inside the sole, unusually ribbed, thick and soft, probably in a cotton and acrylic combination. Look for them in white, topped with colourful stripes, in clear colours and in any length from ankle short to calf-length. For extra warmth on cool days, add leg warmers over tracksuit bottoms. To hide your legs or just to keep them a little warmer, wear coloured tights under running shorts, opting for a shade which complements your clothing.

Keep your hair out of your face so your eye's on the ball, with the help of a headband. Wear it over the forehead and ears or across the forehead to the back of the head like the great tennis stars. Though they look wonderfully stylish, headbands have a serious function in preventing perspiration from dripping into eyes, just as wrist bands help prevent sweaty hands. Wear both, choosing absorbent fabrics such as towelling; start with bright white, then collect colours and stripes.

Should you be running around in the glaring sun, nothing beats a visor (sunglasses are useless as they easily bounce off). Whether attached to headband or hat, in translucent coloured plastic or in a starched, stitched and stiffened fabric, visors are unbeatable. Similarly, brimmed hats or caps serve the same function in THE SPORTSWOMAN's life and add the perfect finishing touch to her outfit. Consider baseball caps, golf caps, ski visors and soft knitted caps for cold weather.

With your sporty clothes, carry a sports bag. Make it canvas or nylon, in whatever colour matches your scheme, as big as you like, tote, drawstring or duffle style; it will carry all your junk clobber in appropriate style. Wear waist-wrapping purses found in ski shops and worn by skiers and runners to hold change, keys and lip salve. At your neck wear nothing more than a gold or silver chain; better still, a shiny whistle or stopwatch on a nylon cord,

Right: Whether you wear a silvery referee's whistle or toy versions in bright plastic, they are the perfect 'jewellery' for **The Sportswoman.**

and at your wrist, the essential shock-resistant, digital and waterproof wristwatch – a very economical investment today.

FACE AND HAIR

If you've only just begun to get your healthy glow, apply a tinted moisturizer until the real thing arrives but remember your face will perspire with exercise. Blush cheeks with a creamy apricot or pink shade, darken lashes with a waterproof mascara, gloss lips with a slightly tinted gel or clear gloss.

Hair can be worn free but should be secured with a headband as above. If it's short give it a bit of body with hair setting gel each time you wash it; if it's long, tie it back in a ponytail or plaits or keep it off your face.

IDEAS

● If you're on a budget but coveting the gorgeous pastel sports clothes now available, instead purchase the cheapest white gear – sweatshirts, shorts, even socks and shoes, and dye it, using colour-fast dye. Purchase two co-ordinating and complementary shades, and dye a complete set of gear in each shade. Then mix and match to your heart's content.

● Create a cheap and natty necklace by tying colourful toy plastic whistles on a bright bit of string or nylon cording.

● If you have an authentic whistle or stopwatch, you might change the cording which holds it by using various colours of nylon cording and dog clips.

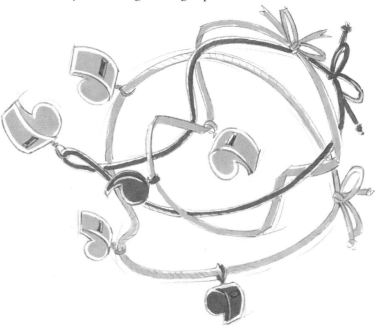

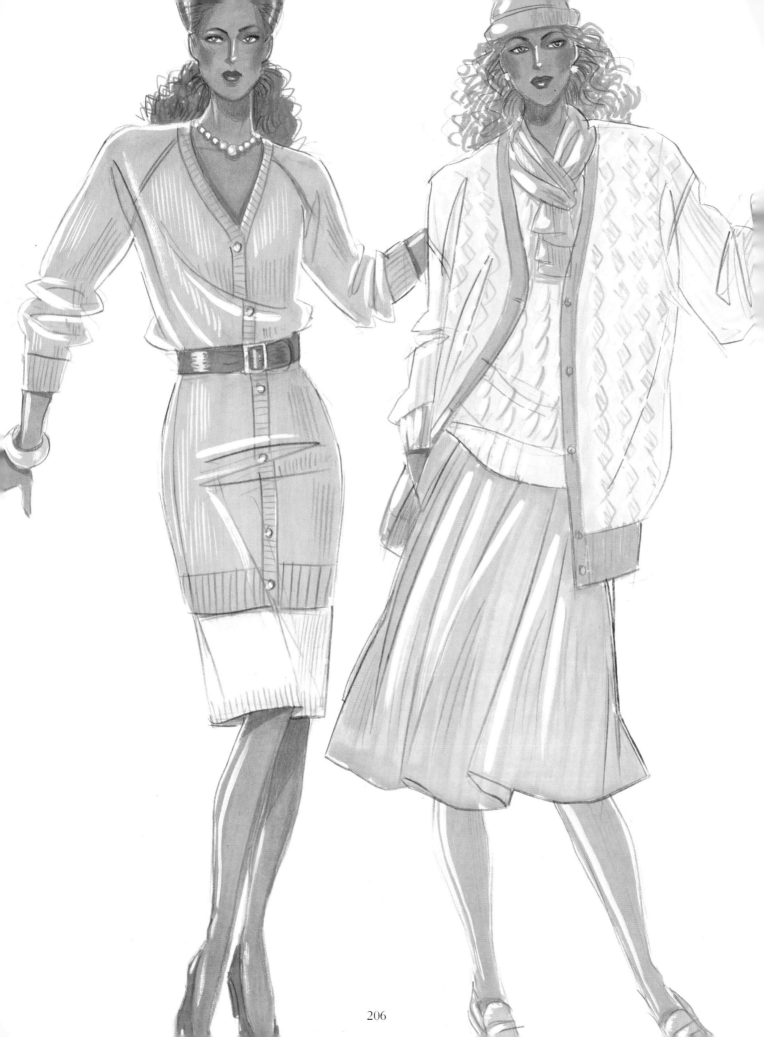

THE SWEATER GIRL

BACKGROUND

Sweaters entered the ranks of fashion in the early years of this century along with sporting activities for young ladies; as sports such as tennis, walking and swimming became desirable leisure pursuits for the emancipated young woman of the day so sporty clothing became a whole new and exciting area for the fashion industry to explore (see THE SPORTSWOMAN). The cardigan came before the sweater and was popularized by such tennis stars as Suzanne Langlen, fifteen-year-old champion of France in the early Twenties.

But it was the Forties and Fifties that saw the establishment of THE SWEATER GIRL in popular imagination. (The title was originally applied to the buxom Jane Russell in Howard Hughes' film, *The Outlaw* (1943).) innovations in knitwear were made throughout the Fifties and Sixties with the invention of new equipment, more sophisticated knitting machines, new synthetic yarns, and innovative weaving techniques and designs. But perhaps the greatest single influence on knitwear in the past two decades has been the fantastically intricate and adventurous colorations and interweavings achieved by the Italian designer Missoni.

Below: For **The Sweater Girl**, it's knits galore – hats, gloves, scarves and legwear can all be knit, in anything from the most sensuous cashmere to the coolest cotton.

THE LOOK

If you want to look cool and chic, opt for the long knitted cardigan or tunic and skirt, in pale or chalky shades, of the Twenties, as outlined in THE OCEAN VOYAGER. If you prefer more fitted and tailored styling, go for the puff-sleeved, self-textured or Fair Isle patterned sweaters and waistcoats of the Thirties and Forties (see THE FAIR ISLANDER).

However, if you want to imitate THE SWEATER GIRL of the Fifties, the considerations are altogether different. In this case, get yourself a finely-knitted matching cardigan worn over a short-sleeved pullover, sometimes referred to as a 'twin set'. Make sure the cardigan has pearlized buttons down the front, and wear the duo with a very flared or very straight calf-length skirt. The original sweater girls wore their sweater like a second skin, then poured themselves into toreador pants or tight skirts.

You might start your relationship with knits with a matching sweater and skirt. The sweater can be cardigan or pullover of any style; the skirt will have an elastic waistband, ribbed or otherwise. However, the effect of such predictable separates will depend on the way you accessorize. For example, if you add a pearl necklace, a thin leather belt on top of

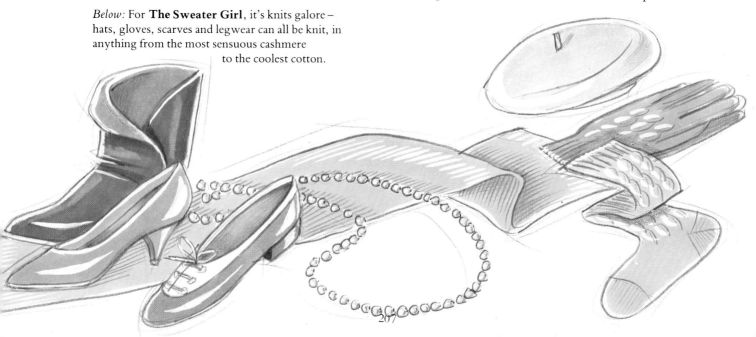

207

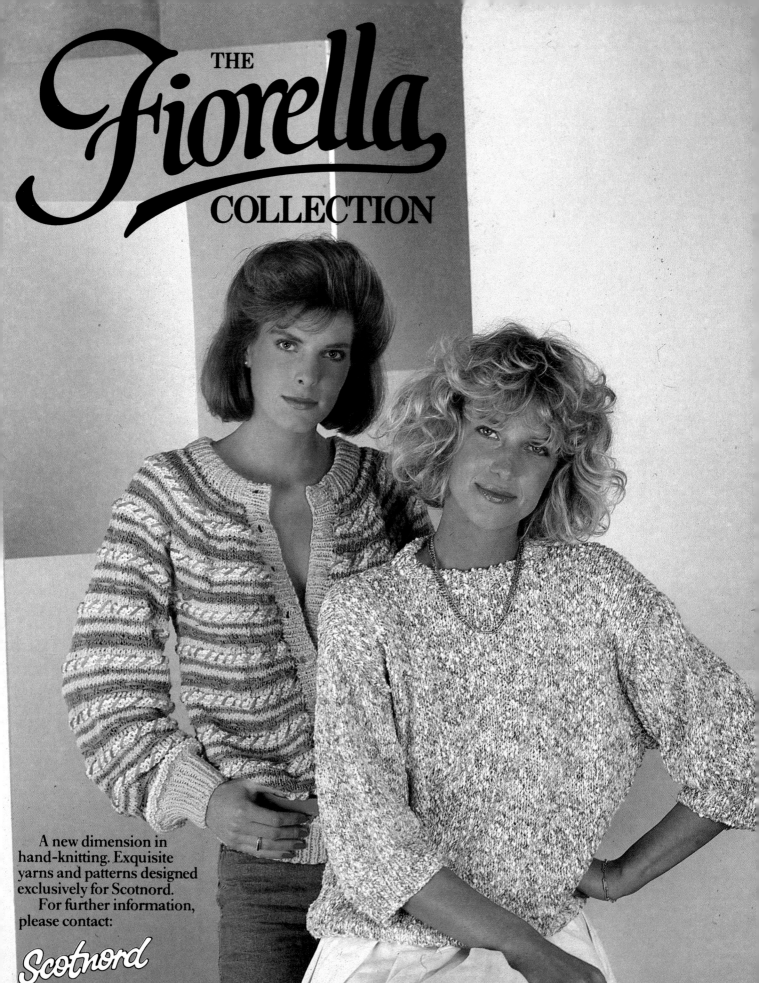

THE *Fiorella* COLLECTION

A new dimension in hand-knitting. Exquisite yarns and patterns designed exclusively for Scotnord.

For further information, please contact:

Scotnord

Broich Terrace, Crieff,
Perthshire, PH7 3BW.
Tel: 0764 3801/4.

Alafoss Lopi. Naturally the best.

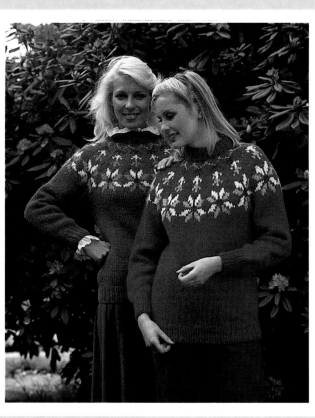

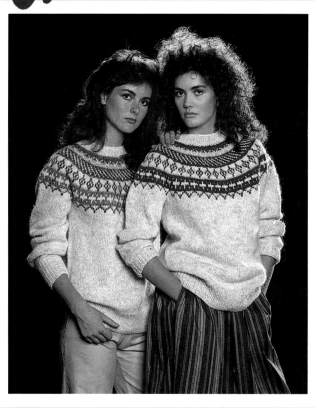

✳ The best selling Lopi available.

✳ The best range of patterns – over 67 to choose from.

✳ The best colour selection – over 40 shades.

✳ Don't settle for less, buy the best. Alafoss Lopi naturally.

Scotnord

Alafoss

PURE NEW WOOL

Broich Terrace,
Crieff, Perthshire PH7 3BW.
Scotland.

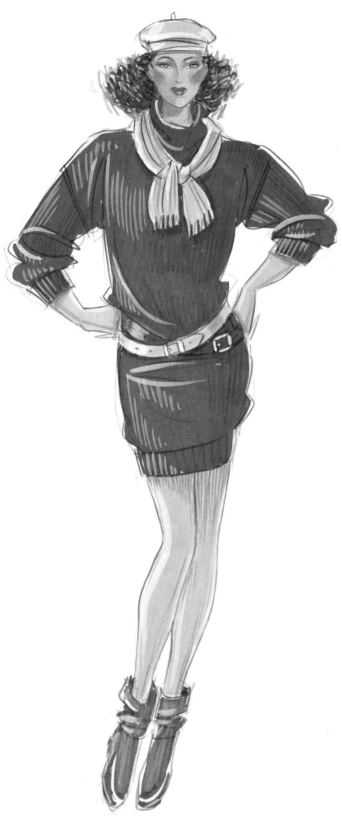

variety of styles; only the very thin should wear very full knitted skirts because of the bulk and no-one should wear them very tight, unless with tongue-in-cheek. Additionally, try to prevent fitted styles from 'seating' or stretching in the hip region – this looks very unflattering and tends to make the skirt hang unevenly. There's no solution to this problem other than dry cleaning by a professional firm.

When gazing at your selection of sweaters and knitted skirts do not be afraid to mix and match textures and colours. Work backwards from one stunning cardigan, coat or jacket if you like and make it as intricately-coloured as possible so that your other clothes can pick up any of the shades and colours incorporated. For example, it might be a blousy, slubby-textured mix of mohair and nylon in olive, rust and gold; you'll be able to wear it with any of those colours as well as with tans and browns, maybe even with yellow or apricot. Waistcoats and slip-ons can be anything from fine lambswool to chunky undyed Shetland. Don't be afraid to layer.

Complete THE SWEATER GIRL look by acquiring accessories like scarves, hats and gloves in the same colourway but in different patterns and textures. For example, if your sweater has stripes in red, blue and purple, look for thinner or thicker stripes, spots or florals in exactly the same colours for accessories. Or do what Dorothée Bis did in the late Seventies, creating a knitwear revolution by mixing unusual plain colours in the same outfit – imagine a red skirt and big triangular scarf teamed with a bright yellow tunic and leggings. Again, this expensive designer look is easily imitated by careful selection. You can also be a SWEATER GIRL in knitted trousers and co-ordinating cardigan, even in a mini-length sweater and contrasting or matching woolly tights.

Left: **Sweater Girls** fond of shorter skirts could choose a mini-length sweater dress, worn with contrasting tights, scarf and tam o'shanter.

Opposite: You can transform even the most ordinary sweater with a touch of personalization. Here, embroidered ready-made appliqués in the form of initials and flowers add style to knits; a cardigan becomes a waistcoat with the removal of arms (and the edges turned under and hemmed).

the sweater, toning tights and highish heels, the outfit could take you to dinner or the theatre. On the other hand, if you add a chunky knit cardigan, woolly tights, walking shoes plus co-ordinating hat, gloves and scarf, it's perfect for walking in the woods or round the shops.

Knitted skirts, like other skirts, come in a

ACCESSORIES

To evoke THE SWEATER GIRL of the Fifties requires a strand or two of pearls at your throat or a brooch on your shoulder. Then choose a widish leather belt to accentuate your waist; on your feet slip on highish-heeled courtshoes maybe in patent leather, but certainly with pointed toes worn with pale stockings. For the healthy 'outdoorsy' version wear heavy brogues with thick rolled-down socks over tights. Co-ordinate the colours in your jersey with socks or wool tights for extra warmth and style.

SWEATER GIRLS of the moment will opt for less precarious footwear – choose any low-heeled style from pump to knee-length boot. Indeed boots look great with any of the chunkier knits. Tights, socks or stockings will range from slightly textured, lacy or ribbed styles with finer knits, to highly patterned or very thick ones with heavier knitwear in a multitude of exciting colours.

Jewellery will be minimal or very ethnically-inspired, especially with looser, bigger knits; otherwise choose very classic pieces such as chains, lockets, glass beads. Earrings can be daring or discreet.

Follow similar guidelines when selecting your handbag. Finer knits require clutch or small-handled styles, medium knits look right with shoulder bags, while very textured, mohair or bouclé sweaters seem to ask for equally gutsy bags. Of course, for a real outdoors look, nothing beats the matching hat, gloves and scarf set for style. For hardwearing accessories, go for wool; for luxury try angora or cashmere, wonderfully soft against the skin.

FACE AND HAIR

If you're trying to evoke the original Fifties look, wear your hair fairly tightly curled or waved, secured with a ribbon tied in a side bow or held in place by a plastic or velveteen headband. Follow the make-up instructions below, accenting lips with a very red lipstick and matching nail-varnish to complete the effect.

More modern SWEATER GIRLS will wear their mane fuller and more softly curled; their make-up subtler. Start with a light foundation, followed by a dusting of matching powder. Shadow eyes with a soft grey or taupe colour, depending on the tonality of the sweaters in question. Blend shadow on lid into a pearly shade applied under the brows. Outline the eye close to the lashes with a fine grey or brown pencil. Tint cheeks with a soft pink or coral shade applied on the cheekbones, finishing with a matching lipstick and nail polish.

IDEAS

● When shortening knitted skirts, don't turn up the hem in the usual way. Instead cut the required inches from the top, at the waistband, turn over the new top, insert a length of elastic as long as your waist and restitch the casing waistband.

● Don't hesitate to re-style sweaters when you tire of them – see illustration. Stretched waistbands can be re-gathered with elastic.

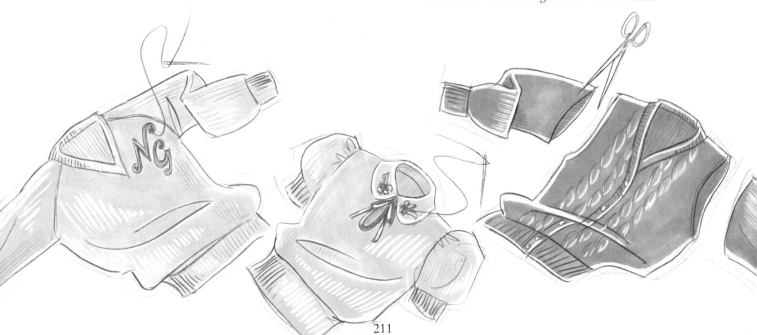

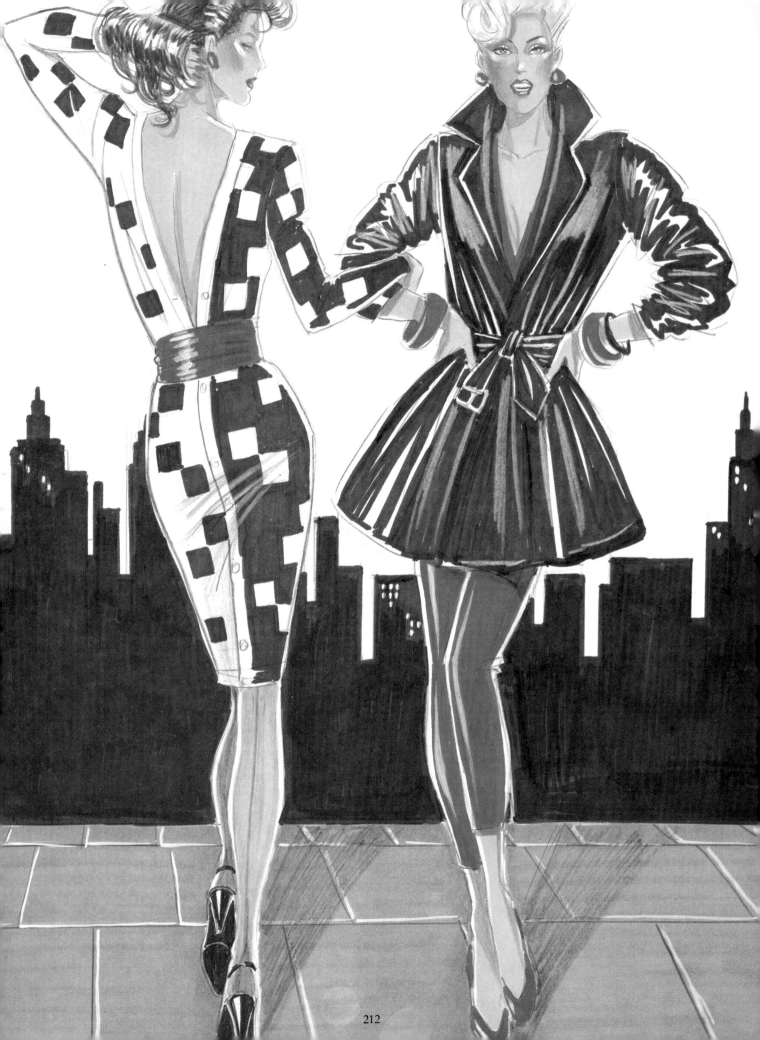

THE VAMP

BACKGROUND

THE VAMP has been with us for a long time but she became firmly established in popular imagination during the days of the silent movie. She was one of two female stereotypes who could be conveyed successfully without the use of words. Her counterpart was the pale, innocent victim, always clad in purest white. Vamps on the other hand were sexy, sultry and decidedly sinful; their aim was to get their man, and they didn't care how they did it. Names like Theda Bara and Hedy Lamarr – with their hooded eyes, heavy make-up and blood-red lips on which plays just the smallest trace of a wicked smile – still evoke the image of THE VAMP today.

The advent of the 'Talkies' in the late Twenties made such extreme characterization seem ridiculous; subtleties could now be conveyed with dialogue, so THE VAMP, while remaining a favourite of the silver screen, became rather more sophisticated (Jean Harlow). In recent years, THE VAMP has all but disappeared from the cast. However, the look remains and at its best can be the ultimate in seductive dressing – subtlety is not the domain of THE VAMP.

THE LOOK

In the serious business of seduction THE VAMP employs every weapon – from slinky, bottom-hugging clothes to plunging cleavages – without scruple. She pours herself into tight-fitting skirts, dresses, trousers (such as toreador pants) and tops, and compounds the effect with the clingiest, shiniest fabrics around. So if vamping appeals to you, choose materials like nylon cire for trousers and belted coats, satins for blouses, dresses and evening wear – indeed any natural or man-made textile which has a sheen to it.

Balance the figure-hugging bottom half of your outfit with a wide upper half, produced by wearing off-the-shoulder dresses, sweaters; blouses and T-shirts with plunging necklines. Jackets should have the wide boxy look and padded shoulders of the Forties and Fifties.

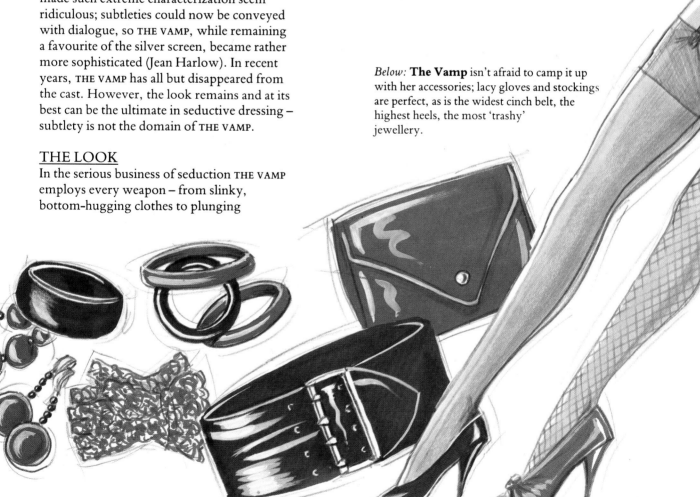

Below: **The Vamp** isn't afraid to camp it up with her accessories; lacy gloves and stockings are perfect, as is the widest cinch belt, the highest heels, the most 'trashy' jewellery.

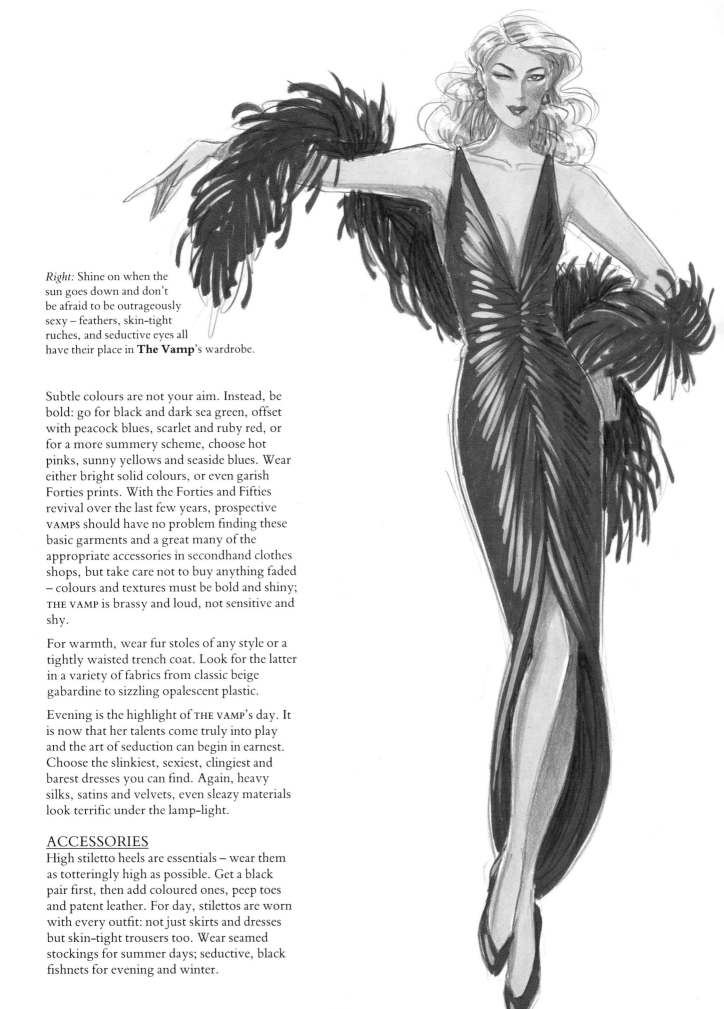

Right: Shine on when the sun goes down and don't be afraid to be outrageously sexy – feathers, skin-tight ruches, and seductive eyes all have their place in **The Vamp**'s wardrobe.

Subtle colours are not your aim. Instead, be bold: go for black and dark sea green, offset with peacock blues, scarlet and ruby red, or for a more summery scheme, choose hot pinks, sunny yellows and seaside blues. Wear either bright solid colours, or even garish Forties prints. With the Forties and Fifties revival over the last few years, prospective VAMPS should have no problem finding these basic garments and a great many of the appropriate accessories in secondhand clothes shops, but take care not to buy anything faded – colours and textures must be bold and shiny; THE VAMP is brassy and loud, not sensitive and shy.

For warmth, wear fur stoles of any style or a tightly waisted trench coat. Look for the latter in a variety of fabrics from classic beige gabardine to sizzling opalescent plastic.

Evening is the highlight of THE VAMP's day. It is now that her talents come truly into play and the art of seduction can begin in earnest. Choose the slinkiest, sexiest, clingiest and barest dresses you can find. Again, heavy silks, satins and velvets, even sleazy materials look terrific under the lamp-light.

ACCESSORIES
High stiletto heels are essentials – wear them as totteringly high as possible. Get a black pair first, then add coloured ones, peep toes and patent leather. For day, stilettos are worn with every outfit: not just skirts and dresses but skin-tight trousers too. Wear seamed stockings for summer days; seductive, black fishnets for evening and winter.

Jewellery is big, glittery and blatantly fake. Earrings should be large round clip-ons in bright primaries or large glinting pear-drop shapes in glinting gem shades. Wear thick bangles, preferably in plastic or metal, and strings of large round beads from choker length to long strands that wind round your neck several times.

Belts are outsized too. Try wide cinch-waist ones in glossy kid, patent leather or plastic, in strong shades. Pull them tight to define your waist. Bags come in the same colours and should be clutch styles.

To balance the tottering heels, try a pillbox or cloche hat plus black-net veil for winter or special occasions. The black-net veil is one of THE VAMP's most seductive ploys and she'll wear it even for daytime. Alternatively, wear the cloche or wide-brimmed hat slightly askew or provocatively over one eye.

Gloves co-ordinate with belts and bags and the same rules apply. But they may also be fingerless, in which case THE VAMP's nails should be painted a strong shade of red – anything from vermilion to deep carmine. (See THE MOVIE STAR.)

Below: The right underwear is essential when 'vamping'. Strapless bras work with décolleté sweaters and halters, camiknickers are ideal under microskirts, and suspender belts essential with all dresses and skirts.

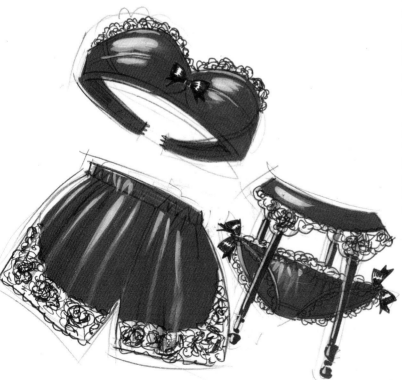

This is one look where underwear plays an important role. Vamps love to romp in satiny lingerie – pastel shades for slips and camisoles will do, but black or even red with black lace trim are more successfully vulgar. Wired bras and suspender belts, long since thrown out by her more liberated sisters, are still an essential part of THE VAMP's wardrobe.

FACE AND HEAD

Hair can be full and blowsy, crimped and lusciously permed, or sleek and severe depending on which style suits you best.

Make-up is on the heavy side. Begin with a pale foundation, followed by a dusting of matching powder. To achieve the distinctive smouldering eyes, use a silvery or gold eye-shadow on the inner corner of the lid, followed by a navy, grey or khaki shade applied from the centre of the lid to the outer corner. Use the same shade in the crease, blending it with the light metallic shade. Finish the eyes with an opalescent whitish shadow under the eyebrow itself. Pencil in darkish eyebrows if you haven't got them, accentuating the natural arch as much as possible. Finally, draw a thickish line in dark brown or black along the inside rim of the bottom eye.

THE VAMP's lips *must* be red and glossy. To achieve this, outline the natural lipline with a tan pencil, making sharp points at the bow. Fill in with the reddest lipstick you can find, using a lipbrush to control application. Complete the lush look with a dash of lip gloss and a beauty spot applied with a sharpened dark brown pencil at either the ouside corner of one eye or just above the corner of the lip.

IDEAS

● Add black lace or net to a black hat. Fold a square yard along the diagonal, wrap it around the crown of the hat, fastening with a knot, hat-pin or hair-clip, and let a length up to the point of the triangle fall over your face on one side.

● Use another two yards of black netting to make an instant evening stole. Fold the net along its length so it is doubled over or twisted a few more times, then wrap it around your bare shoulders to offset the creamy skin and plunging décolleté of your outfit.

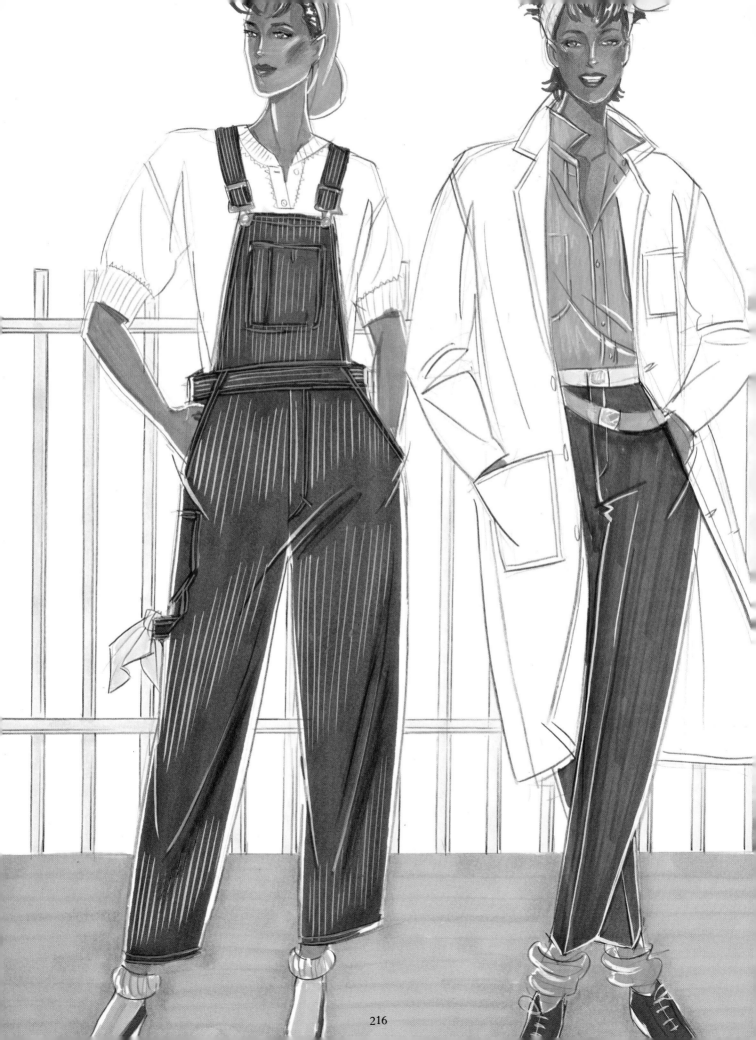

THE WORKER

BACKGROUND

On September 3, 1939, England and France declared war on Germany. Shortages of fabric and labour forced the British Board of Trade to conceive in 1942 the now famous 'utility clothing'. These clothes were to be simple, practical, inexpensive and good-looking; they also had to be made of reasonable quality material, to be resistant in the hard times. Flared skirts, fur trimmings, tucks and pleats were discarded; suits could only have two pockets and four buttons whilst embroidery, lace, turn-back cuffs and velvet collars were strictly forbidden.

At the same time, women were recruited to make bandages and to work in munitions factories. It comes as no surprise to learn that they adopted traditional workman's clothing.

THE LOOK

Those first functionalists created a practical and sensible way of dressing for work and a classic look which is still with us today. To analyse the appeal of this kind of clothing, look no further than Corbusier's famous statement that form follows function. In terms of fashion, this means that if you wield a hammer, your clothing must have a pocket or strap for it.

Not only is THE WORKER the ideal way of dressing for work, especially if your job involves getting dirty, but it can also look sufficiently chic for Saturday shopping yet down-beat enough for washing the car and working in the garden. What determines the tone of this look is the way it is accessorized and the colour scheme involved. Original functional clothing will generally be in white, navy, hospital green, garage mechanic blue, military khaki or the brighter safety-minded shades such as neon orange and electric blue. However, work gear has lots of designer imitations and you'll find these clothes in pastel cottons and in fine fabrics too.

Begin with the one-piece overall – you'll find this an indispensable garment for mornings when you're short of time and imagination. Wear it fairly fitted with matching socks, low-heeled shoes and a slightly arty piece of jewellery. For colder occasions, wear a thick wool sweater over a shirt underneath, with co-ordinating

Below: Only the roughest, toughest and brightest accessories will do for **The Worker**. Lunch pails and tackle boxes make great carryalls, men's handkerchiefs become bandanas, webbing belts are worn singly or in twos, sturdy shoes are crepe-soled for staying power.

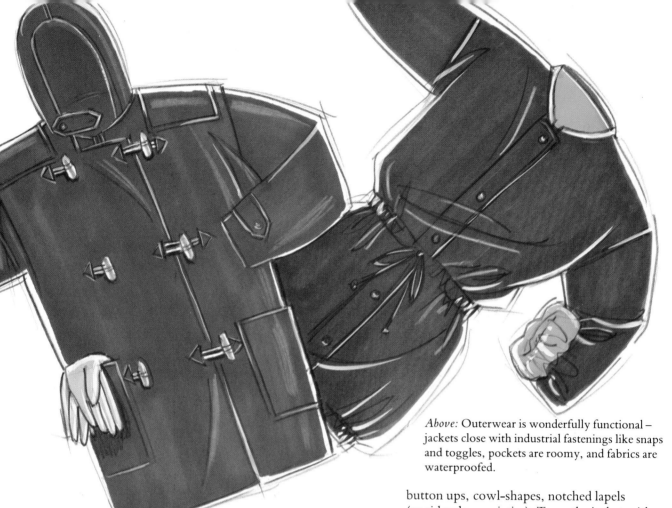

Above: Outerwear is wonderfully functional – jackets close with industrial fastenings like snaps and toggles, pockets are roomy, and fabrics are waterproofed.

leg warmers up to the knee and lace-up boots on your feet. Or wear it to the theatre or dinner in satin, silk, or a similar luxury fabric.

Bib-front overalls or dungarees are a popular derivative of the one-piece suit and again depend on the same criteria for their looks. Pastel dungarees look great with a simple white T-shirt in summer, worn with matching running shoes, while a railway worker's faded blue-and-white striped bib-front denim looks better applied to heavier tasks. Remember that you're not after a perfect fit – roominess facilitates movement. Too-long legs and sleeves can be rolled up, loose waists can be belted.

If you like this railway worker's fabric, also get a loose, copper-buttoned, patch-pocketed jacket – these look marvellous with faded denims, and lots of bright red or white accessories. Look also for a favourite of the Seventies – a very faded blue cotton shirt with overstitching and patch pockets.

From the science world borrow the classic white lab technician's coats and jackets. Made from tough white cotton twill, they have a variety of collar styles to choose from –

button ups, cowl-shapes, notched lapels (avoid nylon varieties). Team the jacket with crisp white surgeon's pants, or even a chef's straight-legged, blue-and-white-checked trousers or other tailored (non-utility) trousers, and straight skirts.

As an alternative to the all-white scheme, there's the soft green of the surgeon's outfit. Again look for tailored jackets and straight-legged trousers, but they must be accessorized imaginatively to avoid looking too much like a surgeon.

Instead of the classic round-neck cotton T-shirts, consider a workman's string vest. In maillot or sleeved styles, it can even be worn over T-shirts.

For outerwear, there is a myriad of possibilities: a duffel coat usually with a hood, fastening with toggles can be found in classic colours like navy and camel and loden green or a drawstring-bottomed coat, sometimes referred to as a gas worker's coat, are both highly suitable and easily available from utility stores.

Explore camping gear also – look for huge circles of olive plastic in the form of capes and waterproof canvas jackets. They, too, are designed for function and suit this look, as are surplus military garments.

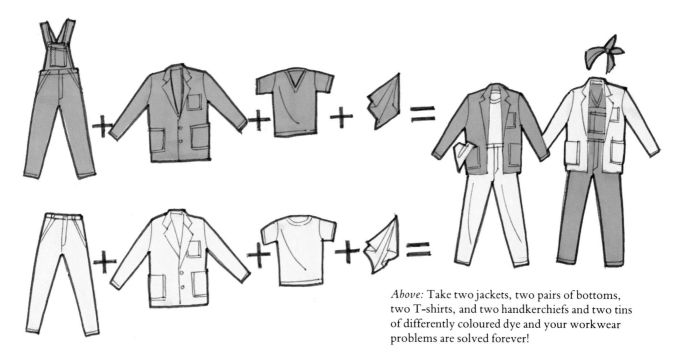

Above: Take two jackets, two pairs of bottoms, two T-shirts, and two handkerchiefs and two tins of differently coloured dye and your workwear problems are solved forever!

ACCESSORIES

Begin with boots. Ideally lace-up styles with soft crepe or leather soles, they can be cut low or ankle boots or even calf-length. With bright clothes these might even be plastic slip-on styles. Wear trousers over the boot or tucked inside with the rolled edge of a colourful sock between boot and pant leg. Wartime workers favoured sturdy lace-up brogues, worn with thick cream-coloured socks; the more daring amongst you might try a coloured sock with chunky high heels instead.

Waists need to be accentuated, either to take in a too-big coverall or simply to add a dash of colour or detail. Let the spirit of the fabric determine the belt. With brights wear zany colours or black; with fine wools try soft suedes and leathers; with military styles use surplus accessories as covered in THE SOLDIER or THE AVIATRIX. Elasticized cinch belts, in every colour imaginable, with metallic bucklings are inexpensive and look effective; similarly, any webbing fabric style will also work.

Jewellery can be as classic or as zany as you like: you might like to sport a collection of related brooches, connected by a colour scheme or theme, or to wear lots of chains, or gear such as whistles and watches from THE SPORTSWOMAN, or even several scarves.

The size of your carryall knows no limits, and has little stylistic restriction – it can be as functional as a nylon or canvas duffel bag, or as refined as a suede or leather pouch or envelope. Shoulder bags worn diagonally work well: wear a small one for change across one shoulder and a larger one for papers and cosmetics across another.

FACE AND HAIR

Apply a very sheer foundation all over the face. Shadow eyes in a sludgy green or brown on the lower lid, using a pale yellow shade under the brow bone. Use kohl in a brown or khaki shade under the lower lashes and accent cheeks with a natural peach blusher applied to the cheekbone. Gloss lips with a shrimp or coral colour.

Keep hair as simple as possible: wear it sleek and short or slick back sides with setting gel; pull it back into a plait or a ponytail; or tie a thick scarf around it (see *Ideas*). Alternatively, keep it out of your work by covering it with a hairnet, for a real touch of period authenticity.

IDEAS

• Buy two white coveralls, two white jackets and pants, two white T-shirts, maybe two large white handkerchiefs. Dye one of each in a colour to off-set the whites – maybe pale blue, bright turquoise, hot pink.

• Tie up your hair to keep it out of your work – a scarf folded on the diagonal and tied in a bow on top will look right, as will a scarf worn snood-style over the hair, knotted at the side or nape.

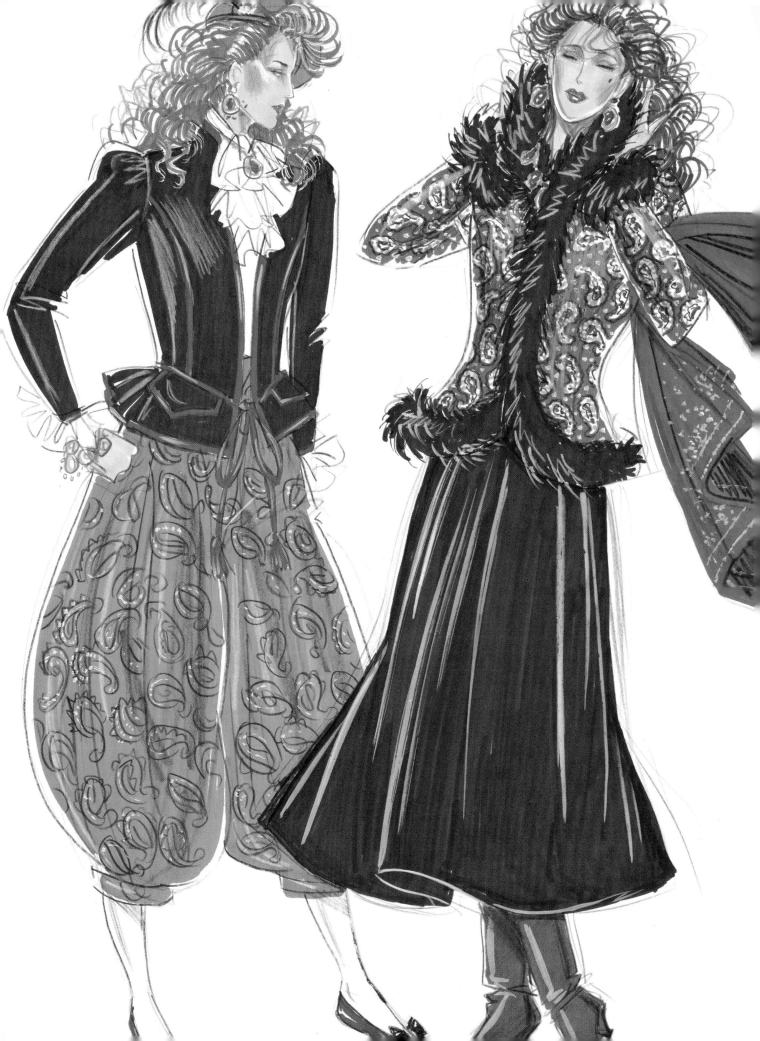

THE YOUNG ROMANTIC

BACKGROUND

Romance is with us again. Partly as a reaction to the sometimes ugly excesses of punk, partly sparked off by the heady romance of the Royal Wedding, partly as natural escapism from the hardships of the economic recession, people are again indulging their fantasies and their yearnings for nostalgia, for love, for beauty and above all for romance.

But romance today comes in different guises. Whether your tastes are *avant-garde* or more mainstream, the ingredients of Romantic dressing tend to be the same. The result depends on what and how much you combine. It is a look that flatters young and old alike; furthermore with its foundations firmly in the great periods of history it is a look whose style and appeal is perennial.

THE YOUNG ROMANTIC of today creates her image from an amalgam of fashion styles chosen from periods with romantic associations. We remember the Royalists of seventeenth-century England as much for their opulent dress as for their political convictions. In the early nineteenth century, the age of Turner and Wordsworth, Shelley and Keats, artists were obsessed with the grandeur of Nature, and the passionate, irrational aspects of human existence. Women were soft and dreamy in Empire-line dresses falling from just below the bust in long, unstarched folds of pale voile and silk. Later in the nineteenth century, the Pre-Raphaelite Brotherhood of William Morris and the Rossettis turned back to the Middle Ages for inspiration, reviving medieval ideas of the craftsmen's guilds and revering legendary tales of King Arthur and courtly love.

THE LOOK

So indulge your imagination and draw your clothes from wherever you can: your mother's wardrobe, granny's attic, antique shops, secondhand clothing stalls, flea markets, costume hire shops, designer sales – and use your ingenuity in combining them for a romantic look that expresses *you*.

Indulge in rich, opulent and mysterious textures and colours: brocades, laces, velvets, satins, silks, even furs and leathers. Cotton is too tame for this look but creamy linen can look good in a pleated and ruffled shirt.

Below: No accessory is too opulent for **The Young Romantic** – fake metal jewellery is encrusted with fake stones; hats are feathered, footwear is as flamboyant as you like.

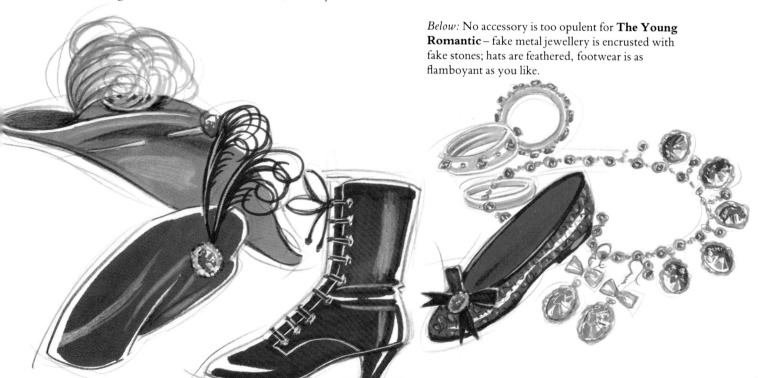

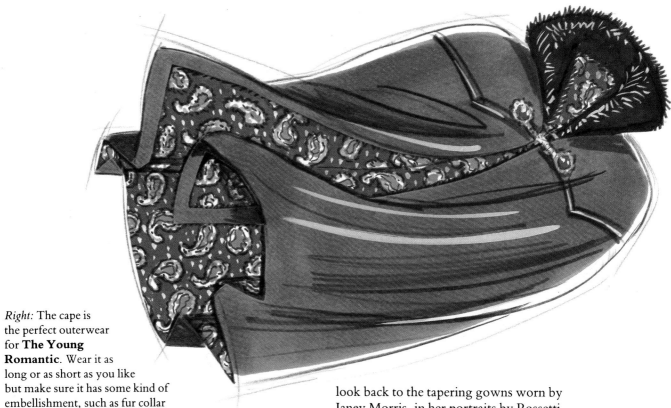

Right: The cape is the perfect outerwear for **The Young Romantic**. Wear it as long or as short as you like but make sure it has some kind of embellishment, such as fur collar or edging, a jewelled clasp or your favorite brooch at the shoulder.

Colours are sensuous and adventurous. Choose chocolate browns set off by lemon yellows, ruby reds against sapphire and peacock blues, forest and viridian greens highlighted by the deepest black, golds and pewters edged with buttery creams and strawberry pinks, deep plums with cerise and purple...

Begin this gambol through luxury with a fabulous jacket, coat or cape in any fine fabric, maybe shot with metallic accents, embroidered or beaded or trimmed with fur. This jacket might be a fitted peplum style like THE GIBSON GIRL wears, or a longer dinner or smoking style from THE DANDY, but almost any style in a luxurious fabric will do.

If you prefer dresses, go for full Victorian or Edwardian styles, or the longer line of the Empire or medieval gown. It may have straight, full or leg-o'-mutton sleeves, tucks and ruches, and should be in voluptuous fabrics like heavy satins or any of the velvets – panne, crushed, antique, flocked or printed, in a rich shade. It can be any length from above knee to ankle length.

Take your image from the wonderfully fantastical dresses designed by the Emanuels, huge crackling creations of stiff organza, silk and voile in tantalizing hues and with extravagant necklines and detailing; or look back to the tapering gowns worn by Janey Morris, in her portraits by Rossetti.

For day or evening wear opt for separates under your coat, cape or jacket but take care to balance the proportions correctly. Trousers should be relatively discreet, either tight or with waist tucks; breeches and knickerbockers are ideal but should be in a luxury fabric not the corduroy or wool of THE LANDOWNER. Skirts are full and softly gathered all round or with front tucks – and should ideally be mid-calf or longer. Or, if you like, wear tight trousers and very blousy shirts, belted as directed below. With skirts or trousers, there's only one really appropriate top – a white or cream blouse, resplendent in lace or ruffles in starched linen, gauzy voile, silk or satin. Remember, no fabric is too indulgent, no solution too extreme, no combination too unusual for THE YOUNG ROMANTIC, and opulence is the essence of every garment. For a final layer, a cape is best of all, and can be worn over most jackets – its generous folds sweeping around you to add the glamour and mystery required.

Waistcoats too have a place, wear them big or wear them fitted, just make sure they are glittery, embroidered or somehow a cut above everyday apparel.

Although this is primarily a special or party look, it works well for both winter and summer. In warmer months, substitute linen, lighter silks and satins, paler brocades, cotton velveteens for the heavier, darker fabrics of winter.

ACCESSORIES

Continue to think of periods past and times of luxury when you choose your accessories. Wear heavily encrusted earrings, even a few at a time if you have pierced ears: mix chain bracelets with bangles provided they're jewelled; choose at least three necklaces from your jewellery chest, maybe mixing colours, shapes and sizes; or wear pearls, or a rope of pearls with a length of jet or big glass beads. Consider combinations you never would for any other look – today's YOUNG ROMANTIC is always adorned – even outrageously so.

Encircle your waist with any length of embroidered or jewelled belt or with satiny or glittery curtain cording or braiding. Tie it round and round, maybe using two kinds at once. Alternatively, thick satiny or velvet ribboning will also do and might also tie up your luxuriant locks too. For a more purposeful and gallant look choose wide leather belts with filigree buckles.

Slippers, lace-up or knee-high boots will be in velvet, brocade, or the finest leather or suede, maybe with embroidered or stitched details such as pleating, appliqué or beading. Evening pumps might have encrusted buckles or clip-on clasps. Stockings will be creamy white, lacy black, or any of the sheerest darkest shades mentioned above. Gloves are also a nice touch – virtually any style except short white cotton ones will look right. Best are fur-trimmed leather gauntlets.

To cap it all off, wear a hat. It can be the Cavalier's favourite wide-brimmed style, complete with a huge billowing ostrich feather or three; it might be a small-crowned, curved brim affair trimmed with a jewelled band; or a large, floppy black velvet beret.

FACE AND HAIR

Accentuate your extreme sensitivity – if not your decadence – by applying a pale ivory foundation, followed by a dusting with matching powder. To shadow eyes, apply a plum or smoky blue shade over the lower eyelid, blending it into a raspberry shade applied under the brow. Extend the lower lid colour around the eye, drawing it into a smudgy line under the lower lashes. Further emphasize your eyes with a line of black pencil drawn very close to the top lashes and inside the lower ones. Fill in weak eyebrows with a pencil if necessary, and colour cheeks with a not-too-discreet swab of raspberry. Finish off the decadent effect by outlining lips with a plum pencil, filling in with a dark cherry lipstick. Whether long or short, hair should be as full as possible.

IDEAS

● Change laces in lace-up calf-length boots or evening slippers by substituting satiny ribbons or glittery cording.

● Brooches become necklaces when pinned to lengths of cording, braiding or ribboning, as the illustration shows.

● Use bits of fur or fake fur to trim edges of gloves, cuffs of jackets, tops of boots, hatbands.

● Use brooches for securing capes or shawls; for fixing feathers and ribbons to hats, to pin on shoes and over the knots of belts.

Below: Use fake fur to add a nice touch of luxury to the tops of accessories such as gloves and boots; use thin ribbons, plain or patterned, velvet or satin in place of mundane shoe laces, and with spare buckles, use thicker ribbons to make sashes.

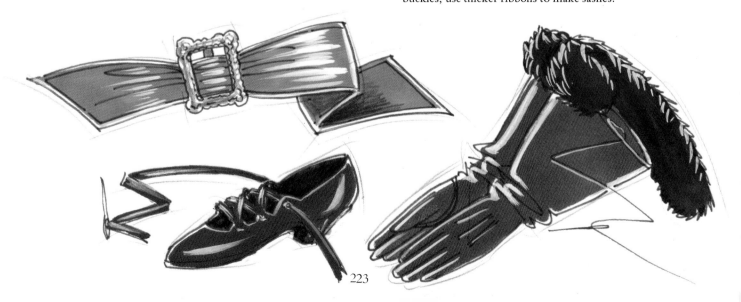

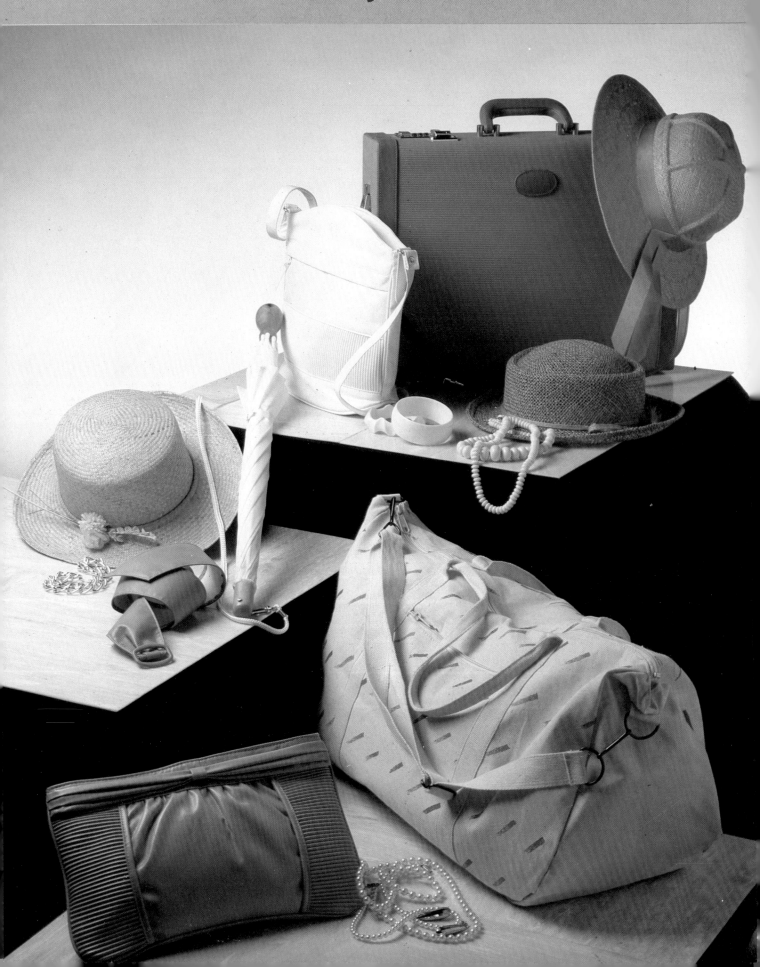